Owner's Guide to
Dog Health Care

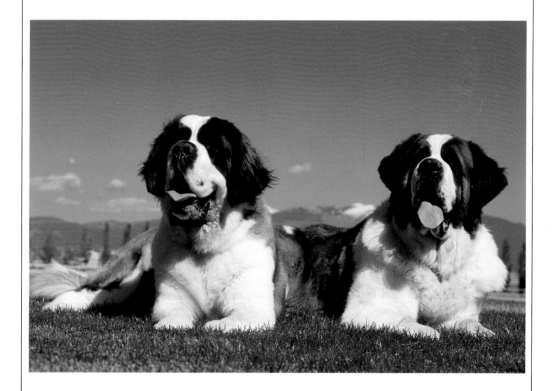

LOWELL ACKERMAN, DVM

TS-214

DEDICATION

To my wife, Susan, my daughter, Nadia, and my canine son, Alan.

Title page: Two St. Bernards owned by Patty Neumayer enjoying sunshine and optimum health. Photographed by Isabelle Francais.

Publisher's Note: *The portrayal of pet products in this book is strictly for instructive value only; the appearance of such products does not necessarily constitute an endorsement by the editor, authors, the publisher or the owners of the dogs portrayed in this book.*

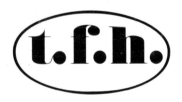

© **1995 by Lowell Ackerman, DVM**

Distributed in the UNITED STATES to the Pet Trade by T.F.H. Publications, Inc., One T.F.H. Plaza, Neptune City, NJ 07753; distributed in the UNITED STATES to the Bookstore and Library Trade by National Book Network, Inc. 4720 Boston Way, Lanham MD 20706; in CANADA to the Pet Trade by H & L Pet Supplies Inc., 27 Kingston Crescent, Kitchener, Ontario N2B 2T6; Rolf C. Hagen Ltd., 3225 Sartelon Street, Montreal 382 Quebec; in CANADA to the Book Trade by Vanwell Publishing Ltd., 1 Northrup Crescent, St. Catharines, Ontario L2M 6P5 ; in ENGLAND by T.F.H. Publications, PO Box 15, Waterlooville PO7 6BQ; in AUSTRALIA AND THE SOUTH PACIFIC by T.F.H. (Australia), Pty. Ltd., Box 149, Brookvale 2100 N.S.W., Australia; in NEW ZEALAND by Brooklands Aquarium Ltd. 5 McGiven Drive, New Plymouth, RD1 New Zealand; in Japan by T.F.H. Publications, Japan—Jiro Tsuda, 10-12-3 Ohjidai, Sakura, Chiba 285, Japan; in SOUTH AFRICA by Lopis (Pty) Ltd., P.O. Box 39127, Booysens, 2016, Johannesburg, South Africa. Published by T.F.H. Publications, Inc.
MANUFACTURED IN THE UNITED STATES OF AMERICA
BY T.F.H. PUBLICATIONS, INC.

Contents

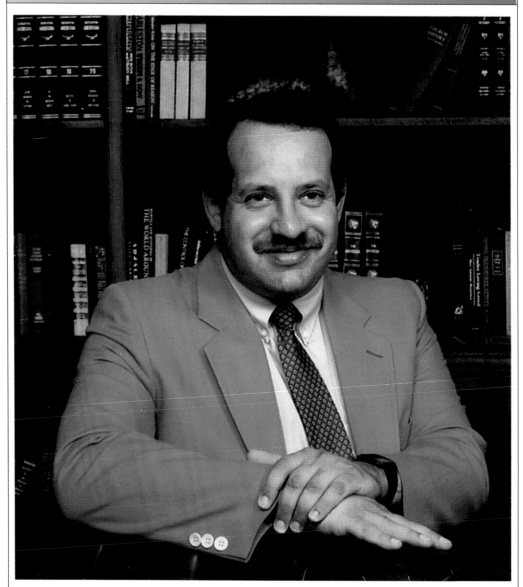

BIOGRAPHY

Dr. Lowell Ackerman practices veterinary medicine in Mesa, Arizona and Thornhill, Ontario, Canada. He is a Diplomate of the American College of Veterinary Dermatology and also has a Ph. D. in nutritional counseling. Dr. Ackerman has written several other books, including ones on canine dermatology and canine nutrition, as well as over 125 articles in various journals and magazines. He has lectured extensively on canine medicine across the United States, Canada, and Europe.

Preface

Canine medicine has come a long way since its simple beginnings. Today, veterinary specialists are performing many of the same procedures on dogs as medical doctors are on people. Pacemakers are being implanted, root canal surgeries are being performed, and CAT scans are being utilized. Specialists exist for almost every facet of veterinary medicine. There are veterinary cardiologists, dentists, dermatologists, neurologists, ophthalmologists, radiologists, surgeons, and others.

With the explosion in medical information available, with diagnostic testing becoming so sophisticated, and with so many treatment options, it is virtually impossible to be an expert in all aspects of canine medicine. So, it is not surprising that dog owners have a difficult time finding information on specific ailments, how they are diagnosed, and how they are properly treated. This book is intended to provide a synopsis of this information in a format that is entertaining as well as educational.

You will find that the terms used in this book are slightly different from those commonly used in magazines and basic books. "Clinical signs" replaces "symptoms," and "radiographs" replace "x-rays." This is because animals don't have "symptoms." Symptoms are those things that people describe about how they are feeling. You may feel feverish, but your dog either has an elevated temperature or not; there is no debate. Since dogs can't speak, they can't have symptoms, only clinical signs. Similarly, x-rays are beams of light of a specific wavelength. We can't see x-rays, but we can see the image they create on special photographic film as they pass through parts of the body. Therefore, we look at radiographs, not x-rays, of patients.

One might debate the need to be so specific in a book on canine health care, but it does impact on our understanding of medicine. Also, it is sometimes disconcerting to owners when medical decisions are not clear-cut, but nothing in medicine is carved in stone. Are vaccinations always 100% safe? No, not always. Does a low thyroid hormone test mean my dog has hypothyroidism? No, not necessarily. Is surgery the best way to manage dogs with hip dysplasia? Sometimes! In this book, we will explore these concerns and many others.

One of the biggest problems inherent in assembling a book on canine health care is that some topics cannot be covered (for space reasons) and the ones that are covered provide information that can quickly become outdated. The material in this book is the most current available but, thanks to medical progress, new information becomes available on a daily basis.

One of the most interesting (and controversial) aspects of writing a book on health care is that it is almost impossible to avoid bias. It has been estimated that only about 10% of medical procedures and therapies have been rigorously evaluated with controlled trials. This is true in human medicine as well as veterinary medicine. Which is more successful for coronary artery disease—bypass surgery or angioplasty? Only now are trials being conducted to answer this question. And yet, almost every physician has his own opinion as to which is better and which he would recommend to his patients.

We have the same quandary in veterinary medicine. Which procedure is best for treating dogs with advanced hip dysplasia? What is the best course of therapy for cardiomyopathy? Are high-protein diets good or bad for dogs? How important is the hereditary component in demodicosis? What is the best way to manage glaucoma? We don't really know the answers to these questions but almost everyone has an opinion they'd be willing to contribute. This book offers several opinions where appropriate, but certainly not all opinions.

Controversy in medicine is a good thing—it stops us from being complacent and keeps us searching for the real answers. Keep this in mind while reading this book and discussing the contents with others. There are very few certainties in medicine; most preferences are based on opinion, not fact. I hope this book keeps you asking important questions and searching for the truth in canine medicine.

Lowell Ackerman, DVM

Canine Nutrition

INTRODUCTION

Nutrition is a fascinating subject that interests most pet owners, breeders, groomers, trainers, and pet supply professionals. The only problem is that there appears to be considerable controversy between nutritional facts and an individual's interpretation of those facts. Most books available on the subject of canine nutrition have been written by individuals in some way affiliated with pet food companies. While the information included in all of these books is valuable, the different conclusions each book may draw on subjects suggest that the answers may not be as clear-cut as they may seem.

Nutrition is a fairly precise science but the conclusions we infer from the known facts are not always a logical extension of those facts. Our interpretation of the facts is what ends up being controversial and, far from being a conspiracy, this freedom of information allows individuals to draw their own conclusions, sometimes inaccurately and in a biased fashion.

Therefore, the only defense we have, as consumers and concerned dog owners, is to understand the facts and learn to draw our own conclusions based on those facts. This allows us to bypass the propaganda that we might get from individuals or companies trying to sell us their version of the facts.

DAILY REQUIREMENTS

Nutrients are substances obtained from food and then used by the body. Most of this use has to do with growth, maintenance and tissue repair. There are six different families of nutrients: proteins, carbohydrates, fats, vitamins, minerals, and water. Within these six families are over 45 individual nutrients that are needed by dogs to maintain health. Most people like to focus on protein and on vitamins and minerals. However, water is the most abundant nutrient in our dogs' bodies and the most indispensable. Dogs can survive a long time without eating, but, if they become over 12% dehydrated, they are unlikely to live very long.

Essential nutrients are those nutrients that must be provided in the diet or deficiencies will result. There are certain proteins, certain fats, certain vitamins and certain minerals that are most important, and we must endeavor to provide them in a proper balance to our dogs. This is what we refer to as "balance" in the diet.

One of the biggest misunderstandings owners have about nutrition is the assumption that the ingredients in the food determine its ultimate value. Ingredients are things like chicken, beef, soy, corn, and lamb. The confusion arises when owners look to ingredients for clues rather than nutrients. Remember, nutrients are water, proteins, carbohydrates, fats, vitamins and minerals. Specific nutrients meet a dog's nutritional needs on a daily basis. The quality of a diet is therefore determined by the appropriate blend of nutrients, not ingredients. The ingredients are important because they contribute to other aspects of the food, such as palatability (taste), digestibility, and cost.

There is much talk of daily requirements of nutrients, but there is as much variability in canine requirements as there is in that for people, probably more so. Dogs are individuals and there is no formula that will predict exactly what their nutritional needs are as a constant, throughout their lives. There is no factor that will predict optimal levels of nutrients for any animal, either. Dogs, like people, are individuals and have individual requirements which should be addressed if they are to remain healthy.

In fact, we should be wary of any published requirement that is applicable to all dogs. Remember, nutritional requirements are based on averages. There is also a significant difference between minimal daily requirements (MDR), the amount needed to prevent deficiencies, the recommended daily allowances (RDA) and the optimal daily recommendations (ODR) for each individual dog.

The National Research Council (NRC) publishes minimum requirements but this organization is not a part of the United States Government, does not conduct any of its own research, and does not enforce any claims made by pet-food companies. Most of the NRC requirements are based on preventing deficiencies in dogs kept under experimental conditions. As such, they are only loosely related to real-world circumstances. Therefore, although the NRC is a valid and useful organization, dog foods based on these minimal requirements are not necessarily the best for our dogs.

The Association of American Feed Control Officials (AAFCO) is an advisory body that provides some additional useful information about diets. It also doesn't police the industry but offers testing procedures whereby diets are fed to healthy dogs, and the health of those dogs is periodically evaluated. To be declared a complete and balanced diet for a particular life stage (e.g., maintenance, growth, reproduction), AAFCO has designed testing protocols which must be performed before the particular label claim may be made. Companies that subscribe to this protocol will say on their labels, "Substantiated by testing performed in accordance with the procedures established by the AAFCO." This certification is important because it has been found that dog foods currently on the market that provide only a chemical analysis and calculated values but no AAFCO trial may not provide adequate nutrition. Dogs fed some of these non-AAFCO-

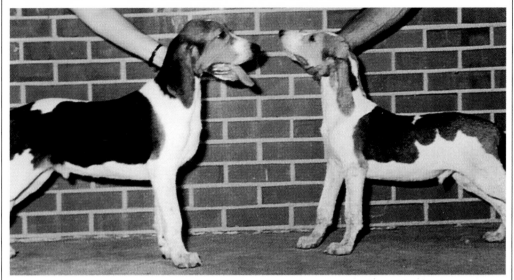

Littermates fed a national brand (left) and a regional brand (right) of dog food shown at the conclusion of a 10-week growth period. Both had identical body weights and lengths at the start of the study. Courtesy of Dr. Thomas L. Huber, Department of Physiology and Pharmacology, College of Veterinary Medicine, University of Georgia, Athens, Georgia.

trialed diets developed clinical signs suggestive of zinc and copper deficiencies.

In 1990, the AAFCO Canine Nutrition Expert (CNE) subcommittee was formed and revised the nutritional profile requirements for dog foods. Dog foods that meet the AAFCO Nutrient Profile for a designated life stage must contain concentrations of nutrients that fall within all minimum and maximum levels outlined in the report. The table is of primary benefit to those manufacturers that do not conduct dog-feeding tests to prove the nutritional value of their foods. Unfortunately, there is no requirement for chemical analysis of essential nutrients in the final product, and no bioavailability of the nutrients must be demonstrated by digestibility studies. Therefore, this information is of no value to the dog owner who wishes to evaluate the food or compare its nutritional value with other dog foods.

Even newer requirements (1992) have been designed by the Pet Food Institute and are referred to as the Nutrition Assurance Program (NAP). The Pet Food Institute is the national trade association of dog and cat food manufacturers. Under this program, only live-animal feeding tests are accepted as proof of nutritional adequacy and the trials must be performed in accordance with AAFCO protocols. The program does not examine the relationship of the diet to long-term health or to disease prevention. Products meeting this claim will list on the pet food label, "Animal feeding tests using AAFCO procedures show that (brand) provides complete and balanced nutrition for (life stages)."

In Canada, the Canadian Veterinary Medical Association (CVMA) has taken the situation one step further. They developed the Pet Food Certification Program to test a manufacturer's products and to certify those products as meeting CVMA standards. To comply, products are tested by the CVMA, feeding trials are performed, and the product is monitored to ensure that it continuously meets CVMA's high standards for composition, digestibility and palatability.

LIFE STAGE REQUIREMENTS

Dogs are very versatile when it comes to meeting their dietary needs. Nutrients that are critical for pups are less important for adult dogs. Bitches have different needs when they are pregnant or lactating than when they are spayed or not used for breeding. Finally, as our dogs age, their nutritional needs also change. Superimposed on this is the realization that other factors, such as sporting competition, the show circuit and disease, also have an impact on nutrition.

PUPPY REQUIREMENTS

Soon after pups are born, and certainly within the first 24 hours, they should begin nursing their mother. This provides them with colostrum, which is an antibody-rich milk that helps protect them from infection for their first few months of life. Pups should be allowed to nurse for at least six weeks before they are completely weaned from their mother. Supplemental feeding may be started by as early as three weeks of age.

By two months of age, pups should be fed puppy food. They are now in an important growth phase. Nutritional deficiencies and/or imbalances during this time of life are more devastating than at any other time. Also, this is not the time to overfeed pups or provide them with "performance" rations. Overfeeding large breed dogs can lead to serious skeletal defects such as osteochondrosis and hip dysplasia.

Pups should be fed "growth" diets until they are 12–18 months of age. Many large breeds of dog do not mature until 18 months of age and so benefit from a longer period on these rations. Pups will initially need to be fed two to three meals daily until they are 12–15 months old, then once to twice daily (preferably twice) when they are converted to adult food. Proper growth diets should be selected based on acceptable feeding trials designed for growing pups. If you can't tell by reading the label, ask your veterinarian for feeding advice.

Remember that pups need "balance" in their diets and avoid the temptation to supplement with protein, vitamins, or minerals. Calcium supplements have been implicated as a cause of bone and cartilage deformity, especially in large-breed puppies. Puppy diets are already heavily fortified with calcium, and supplements tend to unbalance the mineral intake. There is more than adequate proof that these supplements are responsible for many bone deformities seen in these growing dogs.

ADULT DIETS

The goal of feeding adult dogs is one of "maintenance." They have already done the growing they are going to do and are unlikely to have the digestive problems of elderly dogs. In general, dogs can do well on maintenance rations containing predominantly plant or animal-based ingredients as long as that ration has been specifically formulated to meet maintenance level requirements. This contention should be supported by studies performed by the manufacturer in accordance with AAFCO (American Association of Feed Control Officials). In Canada, these products should be certified by the Canadian Veterinary Medical Association to meet maintenance requirements.

Many manufacturers of premium dog foods market their products on the basis of ingredients. Most of the super-premium diets have a higher content of meat and meat by-products. Most of the cheaper brands of dog food have a higher content of cereal. However, it is not always easy to tell the difference by looking at the pet food label. Remember too that when selecting canned pet foods, over 75% of the contents are water. This can also be confusing when you examine the label. It may list chicken or beef

as the main ingredient but when you examine the analysis, it lists "moisture" at 78% or thereabouts.

There's nothing wrong with feeding a cereal-based diet to dogs on maintenance rations; they are the most economical. When comparing maintenance rations, it must be appreciated that these diets must meet the minimum requirements for stress-free housepets, not necessarily optimal levels. Most dogs will benefit when fed diets that contain easily digested ingredients that provide nutrients at least slightly above minimum requirements. Typically, these foods will be intermediate in price between the most expensive super-premium diets and the cheapest generic diets. Select only those diets that have been substantiated by feeding trials to meet maintenance requirements, those that contain wholesome ingredients, and those recommended by your veterinarian. Don't select based on price alone, on company advertising, or on total protein content.

GERIATRIC DIETS

Dogs are considered elderly when they have achieved 75% of their anticipated life span. Obviously, this is quite variable and differs with each breed. A Great Dane may be considered old at six years of age, while a Poodle may not be seen as elderly until ten years of age. There is so much variability between individual dogs that even these breed generalizations are only guidelines.

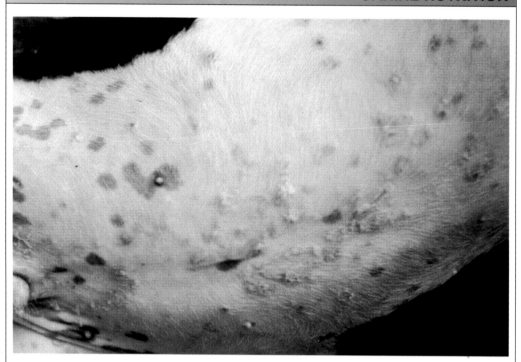

Skin problems, reminiscent of zinc imbalances, seen in dogs fed a regional generic dog food. Courtesy of Dr. Thomas L. Huber, Department of Physiology and Pharmacology, College of Veterinary Medicine, University of Georgia, Athens, Georgia.

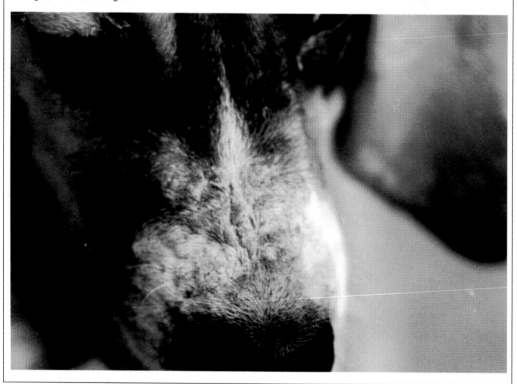

There are certain changes that occur as dogs age that alter their nutritional requirements. As pets age, their metabolism slows and this must be accounted for. If maintenance rations are fed in the same amounts while metabolism is slowing, weight gain may result. Obesity is the last thing one wants to contend with in an elderly pet, since it increases their risk of several other health-related problems. As pets age, most of their organs don't function as well as in youth. The digestive system, the liver, pancreas and gallbladder are not functioning at peak effect. The intestines have more difficulty extracting all the nutrients from the food consumed. A gradual decline in kidney function is considered a normal part of aging.

A responsible approach to geriatric nutrition is to realize that degenerative changes are a normal part of aging. Our goal is to minimize the potential damage done by taking this into account while the dog is still well. If we wait until an elderly dog is ill before we change the diet, we have a much harder job.

Most elderly dogs do better on diets that are easily digested. Since fiber is one part of the diet that is poorly absorbed by all dogs, geriatric diets are typically low in fiber. There are some medical conditions that benefit from fiber, including diabetes mellitus, colitis, and constipation, and the geriatric diets can be augmented with psyllium (e.g., Metamucil®), guar gum or pectin if a higher fiber content is required. Because the digestive system becomes less efficient as dogs age, diets that are more digestible are also more likely to provide needed vitamins, minerals, amino acids, and essential fatty acids.

It is very important to understand the dynamics of vitamin and mineral nutrition in the older dog. Because of changes in digestion and metabolism, older dogs need higher levels of vitamins A, B_1, B_6, B_{12}, and E than they did when they were younger. Most maintenance diets are much too high in sodium (salt) for the geriatric animal and the levels are restricted in the "senior" diets. These diets also take into account the changing dynamics of calcium and phosphorus metabolism and reduce slightly the phosphorus content to lessen the workload of the kidneys.

Elderly dogs need to be treated as individuals. While some benefit from the nutrition found in "senior" diets, others might do better on the highly digestible puppy and super-premium diets. These latter diets provide an excellent blend of digestibility and amino acid content but, unfortunately, many are higher in salt and phosphorus than the older pet really needs.

DIETS DURING PREGNANCY AND NURSING

Care of the pregnant or nursing bitch presents certain nutritional challenges which must be considered and met. Prior to being bred, the bitch should be in excellent dietary status to enhance her chances of conception and then maintained on an increasing nutritional plane as her body strives to meet the needs of pregnancy and then lactation (milk production). It is important to understand that the nutrient requirements may increase as much as four times over usual adult maintenance levels. Providing proper nutrition to the reproducing dam directly influences the quality of the milk she produces, the survival of the pups, and their birth weight.

Usual maintenance diets are not suitable for the pregnant or lactating bitch. They do not provide enough energy to meet her needs on a daily basis. An easily digested, high-calorie diet should be introduced before the fourth week of pregnancy, when nutritional demands begin to skyrocket. Acceptable diets usually contain more meat than do regular diets and only certain super-premium and canned dog foods actually meet these criteria. Many commercial canned cat foods also meet the criteria and are useful in toy and miniature breeds of dogs. These claims should be supported by actual feeding trials, not just lab analysis.

Underweight bitches may have difficulty meeting the nutritional needs of the pups after whelping. Overweight bitches have more trouble with delivery, have less efficient lactation and increased risk of complications for the puppies and themselves.

After whelping, the dam has an additional nutritional drain. She now has attentive pups hungering for her milk and the challenge of meeting her own needs in the process. As the pups grow so does her need to provide for their nutritional needs. This reaches a zenith when they are about three to four weeks of age, at which time she may be consuming two to four times the amount of calories she did when she wasn't pregnant. After this time the pups start to take more of an interest in solid food and demand for milk then diminishes. When the pups are fully weaned at six weeks of age, the food consumption of the dam is down to about 50% above non-pregnant levels and continues to diminish.

FEEDING THE WORKING OR COMPETING ANIMAL

The needs of the canine athlete are significantly different from those of the typical sedentary housepet. The stresses, both physical and mental, that these dogs experience increase their requirements for most nutrients. Their need for energy (calories) may be even greater than that of the pregnant and lactating bitch.

The canine athlete often requires "performance" rations that provide calories in a very energy-dense ration. These diets tend to be high in fat and readily digestible. The ideal diet for dogs competing in field events is a balanced "performance" ration that provides a significant amount of the calories in the form of complex carbohydrates such as corn, wheat, rice and potatoes. This is the same strategy used by human athletes. For those dogs that perform at exertion levels well above those of the regular canine athlete (e.g., sled dogs), most of the energy will need to be provided as fat. High-fat diets are not recommended for the average canine athlete. Inappropriately feeding these diets to regular athletes may cause digestive upset, diarrhea, and vomiting. Also, high-fat diets should never be fed to dogs with susceptibility to pancreatitis. Ask your veterinarian if you are not sure. These diets should be reserved for dogs performing exceptionally strenuous tasks.

NUTRIENTS

The six basic nutrients that are needed for health are proteins, carbohydrates, fats, vitamins, minerals, and water. Proteins, carbohydrates and fats provide energy (calories) in the diet. Water is critical because the bodies of animals are made up of 70% water. Vitamins and minerals are important in regulating many aspects of our lives.

There are many misconceptions about the relative merits and detrimental effects of proteins, carbohydrates and fats. Proteins are often regarded as "good" nutrients, fats as "bad," and most people don't quite know what to think about carbohydrates. The fact is that each of these items has its beneficial as well as detrimental aspects when considering pet nutrition. No one ingredient should be considered better for pets than another. On the other hand, most people regard vitamins and minerals favorably and sometimes don't realize that problems can occur when they are administered to pets inappropriately.

Water

Water is critical for life and provides the medium for chemical reactions, lubrication and temperature regulation within the body. The major component of blood is water, as is joint fluid, cerebrospinal fluid, digestive fluids and the fluid within the eye. In fact, 60–70% of the entire body is made up of water.

Fresh, clean water must always be available to dogs. Never restrict access to fresh water even if you feel your pet is drinking more than it needs. In this instance, contact your veterinarian and have your dog evaluated. Dehydration is serious and can occur in a very short time if a pet is losing fluids and not replacing them adequately. Dogs will not drink too much water if given free access. Water does not accumulate normally in the body and will be excreted as urine to keep the system in optimal water balance.

Make sure that the water provided to dogs is always fresh and clean and changed at least daily, if not more frequently. Ensure also that the bowl is clean and regularly disinfected. Stale water that has been sitting for days is no more attractive to dogs than it would be to us.

Proteins

Despite the fact that most advertising about dog food concentrates on the percentage of protein, you might be surprised to learn that dogs have no real protein requirement at all. What dogs (and cats and people) really need is essential amino acids, not lots of protein. Amino acids are often considered to be the building blocks of protein. They link up with one another to form both simple and complex proteins. When dogs eat protein-containing foods, the protein is broken down during the digestive process and the amino acids are absorbed from the intestines to be re-used for the body's own needs.

Protein, like fat, tends to make diets tastier, especially when animal proteins are provided. However, dogs do not need meat to survive. They can eat and digest both animal and plant proteins, though their systems are most adapted to processing animal protein.

There are ten "known" essential amino acids in the dog, and recently, it became apparent that L-carnitine may be essential for some breeds of dogs. Most animal protein contains reasonable amounts of all the essential amino acids and many non-essential ones. The richest sources of vegetable protein are legumes, including soybeans, lentils, kidney beans and black-eyed peas. Although they contain essential amino acids comparable to meat, the amino acid balance can be further improved by adding rice, corn or grains. The other advantage to these plant proteins is that they contain no cholesterol and little, if any, saturated fats. Protein quality is usually achieved by "complementation," combining protein sources to provide an optimal blend of the essential amino acids.

Poultry, meat and fish meals are often considered good-quality proteins, along with milk by-products, eggs and liver, but an ingredient list does not tell how "wholesome" the ingredients really are. When you see poultry meal on the label, you may think of a succulent chicken or turkey dinner, but is that reality or just good marketing?

Most dogs in North America consume much more protein than needed. This has resulted more from pet food marketing than from nutritional research. Dogs have requirements for essential amino acids and these can adequately be met from vegetable protein combined with moderate amounts of animal protein. Feeding excess animal protein to dogs contributes to obesity and high intake of saturated fats; it is harmful to animals with kidney, liver or heart disease. Meats with the highest fat content are lamb, beef and pork. The leanest sources of animal protein are fish, poultry and wild game.

Fats

Fats are derived from fatty acids, which are important building blocks for a whole range of important substances and are needed to maintain normal, healthy cells. Therefore, not all fats are the enemy; some are essential for our health and that of our pets.

Fats are common ingredients in dog foods because they make the food much tastier and because they are "energy dense," providing over twice as much energy (calories) as either carbohydrates or protein. Just as there is no requirement for protein in a dog's diet, there is also no real requirement for fat either. The only true requirement is for the essential fatty acids, especially linoleic acid. This can be accomplished by feeding 2% of the diet as linoleic acid, found in vegetable oil.

Most commercial dog foods are high in saturated fats and cholesterol because the pet-owning public wants their dogs to eat meat, and lots of it. It should be no surprise that where there's meat, there's fat, and the fat is very high in calories.

With fatty acids, when double bonds are added to the chemical structure, they become unsaturated. When two or more double bonds are present in a particular form of fat, it is described as a polyunsaturated fatty acid, "poly" meaning many. To illustrate, oleic acid in olive oil has one double bond (monounsaturated), linoleic acid in safflower oil has two double bonds, alpha-linolenic acid in flaxseed oil has three double bonds and eicosapentaenoic acid in fish oil has five double bonds. In general, the more double bonds, the more healthful the fatty acid. By contrast, most meats contain fats that are primarily saturated.

Essential fatty acids are important to a dog's health but most pet foods contain significantly more fat than needed and much of it is often saturated. This creates a double threat because it provides excess energy (calories) which can contribute to obesity and saturated fats and cholesterol (from meat) can result in medical problems. There is little benefit to using animal fat in a dog's diet other than as a source of calories or as a flavoring. There is no requirement in the dog's diet whatsoever for saturated fats.

Linoleic and alpha-linolenic acids get converted in the body to other fatty acids with natural anti-inflammatory properties. Unfortunately, sometimes dogs (and people) do not have enough of the enzymes to make this conversion complete. This problem can be partially remedied by supplementing directly with oils that contain eicosapentaenoic acid (fish oils) and gamma-linolenic acid (borage oil or evening primrose oil). These supplements are usually marketed for the control of allergies, arthritis, and perhaps heart problems in the dog.

Products with a relatively high percentage of linoleic acid include the oils of safflower, sunflower, soybean, sesame seed and flax. These are suitable to use as coat care supplements. However, sources of gamma-linolenic acid such as borage oil or evening primrose oil are preferred in dogs with skin problems, or with degenerative joint disease (arthritis). In the omega-3 series, important compounds include eicosapentaenoic acid (EPA) and docosahexaenoic acid (DHA). These compounds are found in high concentrations in the muscles of cold-water fish (e.g., salmon, trout, mackerel and sardines) krill, and marine mammals.

When using supplements of omega-3 and omega-6 fatty acids, caution is advised in selecting products for use. These fatty acids are quite temperamental and can be easily destroyed by exposure to heat, light and air. Therefore, it is advisable that these supplements be kept in opaque containers and that they be kept refrigerated, or at least protected from heat. Products should be tightly capped and not unnecessarily exposed to air. Unfortunately, this care may not have been taken during the production and processing stages.

Carbohydrates

Carbohydrates can be simple (sugars) or complex (starches) and are added to the diet of dogs as a source of energy (calories) and to provide bulk to the diet. But, dogs have no specific nutritional requirement for carbohydrates. There are no "essential" carbohydrates in the dog as there are essential amino acids or essential fatty acids. And yet carbohydrates are an important nutrient in dog foods.

Carbohydrates get a lot of bad press about being fattening, but this is just not true. Carbohydrates contain the same number of calories, by weight, as do proteins. The complex carbohydrates, all derived from plants, contain no cholesterol either. And, the complex carbohydrates also provide fiber or "roughage," which helps keep the digestive system running efficiently and regularly.

The simple sugars reach their highest levels in semi-moist dog foods. These diets contain large amounts of simple sugars like sucrose and syrup and comparatively less starch than dry foods. In fact, 20% or more of these diets may be made up of sugar. Because these sugars are quickly absorbed, dogs eating semi-moist diets may produce less stool but they frequently produce much more urine. Because of their high-calorie content, these diets may also promote obesity.

Starches are made up of sugar chains. Starch is the plant's way of storing energy, just as animals store energy as fat. The simpler the formation (e.g., in rice, white flour and corn starch) the easier the body can convert these to sugar and thence to fat. The more complex carbohydrates (e.g., in grains, bananas, potatoes and corn meal) are more slowly digested, less likely to convert to fat, and also contain important enzymes for the body. In general, cooked starch in commercial dog foods is well digested—most come from corn, rice and wheat. Soy flour, corn-gluten meal, wheat gluten and wheat middlings are not completely digested by dogs and are therefore poor sources of usable starch. Most sources of fiber are tomato pumace, beet pulp, corn bran, oat bran and wheat bran.

A major concern about carbohydrates is that dogs digest them differently than do people. Newborn puppies have almost no ability to digest starch. However, as they get older and are exposed to highly digestible starches, the levels of the enzyme amylase increase significantly. This allows older dogs to digest starches very well after a few weeks of adapting to the new diet. In contrast to dogs being able to better digest simple sugars and highly digestible starches as they get older, they do worse with milk sugar (lactose) as they age. As puppies get older, they have more trouble digesting the lactose and few adult dogs are capable of digesting it at all.

Fiber increases the "bulk" of the food and gives dogs a full feeling. Fiber can also be used as a laxative for constipation since it absorbs intestinal fluid, making the stool softer and bulkier and stimulating the intestinal rhythm that pushes the stool through the system. Because the stool passes through the digestive tract with less effort, diets fortified with fiber are frequently used in dogs with bowel disorders.

Other benefits of fiber are only now being explored. Some types of fiber, notably pectins, guar gum, and the fibers in rolled oats and carrots, can help lower cholesterol levels in the blood. These same fiber sources may also be beneficial in helping to regulate blood sugar and insulin levels in diabetic animals. But not all fibers are equal in this regard. Bran, which contains predominantly cellulose, will not help regulate cholesterol or blood-sugar levels in dogs.

Although the fiber content of dog foods is important, there are some risks to feeding high-fiber diets. Although animals will lose weight with these diets, it has been shown that they reduce the digestibilities of protein, carbohydrate and fat. There is also some evidence that high-fiber diets might interfere with the absorption of several minerals (e.g., calcium, copper, iron, magnesium, phosphorus, and zinc) and possibly vitamin B_{12}. Thus, they should not be fed indefinitely, and not to young growing animals or any dog that is stressed or sick. High-fiber diets do have their place, but they should only be fed to dogs under strict veterinary supervision.

Excellent sources of carbohydrates for use in commercial dog foods include corn meal (not corn starch), soybean meal, whole grain rice, whole wheat, oats and bran. Ideally, most of the carbohydrate provided to dogs should be starches found in potatoes and whole grains. This would provide a sustained source of energy, and a wealth of vitamins, minerals and fiber. Unfortunately, the processing of feeds for commercial dog foods removes much of the nutritional value from the natural ingredients. Because of this, nutrients must be re-added to the finished "enriched" product and cheaper forms of fiber (e.g., beet pulp) are often used.

VITAMINS

Vitamins are organic substances that are required in the diet. They are derived entirely from plant or animal sources. One of the main differences between vitamins and other nutrients is that they are critical to life but are only required in phenomenally small amounts. The needs of vitamins are expressed in milligrams (thousandths of a gram) or even micrograms (millionths of a gram). All of the vitamins needed by a dog on a daily basis could be provided in a fraction of a teaspoon. Vitamins are one of the family of nutrients that does not contribute calories (energy) to the diet. Many, however, are important in the conversion of calories to usable energy.

Vitamins also function with other nutrients and enzymes to help the body function optimally, to help create blood cells, hormones, genetic material and special chemicals and also to promote normal function of the eyes, skin, reproductive system, heart and internal organs. Because vitamins assist in all these other processes, most are also regarded as co-enzymes, substances that help get things done.

There are many substances which have been designated as vitamins. Four of these will dissolve in fat (vitamins A, D, E, and K) and nine are soluble in water (vitamin C and eight B vitamins). These two families of vitamins are referred to as fat-soluble and water-soluble vitamins, respectively.

Vitamin A

Vitamin A is derived from animal tissue, found primarily in liver, eggs, milk and kidney. A compound related to vitamin A, beta-carotene, is found in vegetation, and can be converted to vitamin A in the body. Beta-carotene is under careful evaluation because it is an antioxidant and may have protective effects against some cancers. Vitamin A deficiency is rare in dogs but conditions that are vitamin A-responsive are more common. This may seem like a picky distinction, but some problems get better with vitamin A (vitamin A-responsive) even though blood tests may not reveal a deficiency. Since vitamin A is stored in the liver and can cause toxicity, vitamin A supplementation should only be considered when animals are directly under veterinary supervision. This toxicity is not seen with beta-carotene, but beta-carotene will not successfully manage cases of vitamin A-responsive dermatosis.

Vitamin D

Like vitamin A, vitamin D is a fat-soluble vitamin that functions much like a hormone. Vitamin D is clearly a powerful force in the regulation of calcium and phosphorus in the body. It increases the absorption rate for both calcium and phosphorus from the intestines. In this way, it maximizes the amount of calcium that can be utilized from the foods eaten. The result of this process is that vitamin D causes increased levels of calcium in the bloodstream, by increasing use of dietary calcium, preventing loss of calcium into the urine and by borrowing calcium for its storehouse in the bones. Because of this, the supplementation of a dog's diet with these nutrients can be devastating by interfering with normal regulatory activity. Not only that, but there is much evidence to suggest that vitamin D is not even needed in the diet. There is sufficient vitamin D activated in the skin to meet the body's needs, even in rapidly growing puppies. Almost all dog foods are well-fortified with vitamin D, so there is a very real risk that toxicity could result from supplementation. Although the amounts present in supplements may not seem excessive, they can generate blood levels of vitamin D hundreds of times higher than recommended. Vitamin D overload can also occur if dogs eat rat poisons that contain this vitamin; a package that contains only 0.75% cholecalciferol may seem safe enough but it provides about 10,000 times the daily recommended dosage of vitamin D, easily enough to kill a dog.

Vitamin E

Vitamin E is found in most vegetable oils, seeds, and soy but is not plentiful in most foods derived from animals. And not all forms of vitamin E are equally active. For example, safflower oil is not only a good source of linoleic acid, but

90% of the vitamin E contained is alpha tocopherol, the most potent form. Compare this with corn oil, in which only 10% of the vitamin E is present as alpha tocopherol. The vitamin E present in vegetable oils is nature's way of preventing those oils from going rancid (oxidation). Vitamin E is particularly efficient as an antioxidant, halting the damage done to body tissues. In addition to its role as an antioxidant, it is thought that vitamin E also affects the production of the prostaglandins, hormone-like substances that regulate a variety of body functions, including inflammation, blood pressure, muscle contraction and reproduction. The body's requirement for vitamin E depends on the amounts of polyunsaturated fatty acids (PUFAs) in the diet. Although we tend to think of polyunsaturates as "good fats" they do increase the body's requirement for vitamin E. Vitamin E, as you recall, stops fats from going rancid.

Vitamin K

Vitamin K is important in the blood-clotting system. The vitamin is involved in the production of prothrombin, a specific protein necessary for coagulation of blood. Deficiencies of vitamin K can lead to bleeding disorders. Most of the vitamin K that is needed for clotting comes from the diet but an adequate amount is also produced in the intestines, from bacteria in the small bowel. Many rodent poisons contain coumarins (e.g., warfarin) that exert an anti-vitamin K effect. If dogs are accidentally or maliciously exposed to these rodent poisons, they can bleed to death from inhibition of their vitamin K. The other potential risk is that vitamin K levels can be compromised in dogs maintained on long-term antibiotic therapy. The antibiotics may attack the problem-causing microbes, but may also destroy beneficial intestinal bacteria, including those that manufacture vitamin K. Vitamin K sup-plementation is only warranted when prescribed by a veterinarian for a specific purpose. There is absolutely no benefit from providing vitamin K to an otherwise healthy dog.

B Vitamins

The B vitamins do share some similarities but, for the most part, they are distinct nutrients. True, they are all water soluble and true that they are often found in the same foods but, other than that, there are marked differences between the compounds referred to as B vitamins. It is very unlikely that dogs will suffer from deficiencies of the B vitamins because they are present in so many different foods and because pet-food manufacturers supply abundant amounts in the diet. Thiamin deficiency has been seen in dogs maintained on raw fish diets.

The body has no real mechanism to store B vitamins and so they must be provided on a regular basis. Because of its unique role in amino-acid metabolism, high-protein diets increase the requirements for vitamin B_6 (pyridoxine). Therefore, the higher the protein content of the diet, the more pyridoxal must be present or a deficiency could result. A high-carbohydrate diet increases the needs for thiamin.

Vitamin C

Dogs, unlike people, are not prone to scurvy because they can manufacture ascorbic acid (vitamin C) internally from glucose. Ascorbic acid has an important role in the formation and maintenance of collagen, the foundation for the connective tissues of the body. Collagen is the supporting system for the skin, bones, tendons, ligaments, joints, blood vessels, and other tissues of the body. With the assistance of ascorbic acid, collagen is needed for the healing of wounds and the restructuring of healthy tissues. In dogs, supplementation has been recommended by some breeders and researchers for hip dysplasia, osteodystrophy and osteochondrosis. However, the likelihood of benefit has never been established for this nutrient.

MINERALS

Minerals, also known as elements, are inorganic nutrients that perform many important functions within the body. Not only do they contribute significantly to the strength of bones and teeth, but they are also intimately involved with many enzyme functions in the body.

Calcium

Calcium is the most abundant mineral in the body, and it still only makes up 2% of the body weight.

Calcium is not static within the bones and teeth; it can still move around. In fact, there is a constant exchange of calcium from the blood to the tissues and about 20% of the calcium in bone is replaced on an annual basis. The calcium in the body is maintained in normal balance by a series of hormones that work together with vitamin D. Because of this intricate balance, supplementation with calcium is not recommended in the dog. Most commercial dog foods contain many times the amount of calcium needed on a daily basis. Calcium deficiency does occur in the dog, but almost always when owners are feeding their own formulations, which have not been balanced nutritionally. These diets are often comprised predominantly of meat (e.g., hamburger, beef, pork, chicken), which is a very poor source of calcium. Not only is it difficult for owners to formulate their own diets regarding calcium content, but an additional factor that must be considered is the ratio of calcium in the diet to that of phosphorus. The ideal balance is approximately 1.3 parts calcium to 1 part phosphorus. If the ratio is much higher or lower than this, problems can result.

Phosphorus

Next to calcium, phosphorus is the most abundant mineral in the body. About 80% of the body's phosphorus is found in the bones and teeth. The remainder is scattered amongst all of the cells in the body where it is critical for a variety of metabolic processes.

Phosphorus deficiency is very rare in dogs because foods rich in protein are also rich in phosphorus. Therefore, meat, fish, poultry, eggs and organ tissues provide more than adequate amounts of phosphorus. Unfortunately, when these ingredients form the basis for a dog's diet, too much phosphorus is more likely than too little. This then interferes with calcium levels and can cause a variety of medical problems.

Magnesium

More than half of the body's stores of magnesium are found in the bones. The balance is found in muscle, heart, kidneys and body fluids. This element helps convert fats, carbohydrates and proteins into energy. Too much magnesium inhibits the proper formation of bone. Too much calcium can cause clinical signs suggestive of magnesium deficiency by impairing absorption from the intestines. Calcium and magnesium also have an important give-and-take relationship when it comes to muscle and heart function. Calcium stimulates muscles and magnesium causes relaxation of muscles. The proper balance is critical. Magnesium deficiency is probably rare in dogs fed commercial diets.

Potassium, Sodium, and Chloride

Potassium, together with sodium and chloride, help maintain the normal balance of fluids within the body and within each cell. The relationship of these minerals also permits muscles to contract, nerves to relay transmissions, and the body to maintain a normal pH balance. Sodium deficiency probably does not occur on its own, although it might be associated with starvation or chronic vomiting and diarrhea. In fact, most commercial dog foods contain many times the amount of sodium that is actually needed by dogs. Salt is frequently added to dog foods in large amounts to increase the palatability.

Zinc

Zinc is found in many different enzymes in the body and is essential for a normal functioning immune system. It also aids in normal growth and development, and the production of hormone-like prostaglandins and other proteins. Even if zinc is adequately provided in the diet, it has been shown that other nutrients such as calcium, phytates (fiber), copper, iron and tin can interfere with the absorption of zinc from the intestines. A relative zinc deficiency has been implicated in several different syndromes in dogs. One appears to be a genetic disorder involving intestinal absorption and Siberian Huskies, Samoyeds and Malamutes are predominantly affected. Another syndrome is reported in rapidly-growing pups such as Great Danes and Doberman Pinschers that may be receiving calcium supplements that interfere with the utilization of zinc in the diet. Finally, a number of dogs fed generic dog foods developed a similar condition which was referred to as generic dog food disease. Although zinc levels in these diets were adequate, it is presumed that other ingredients, such as fiber, might have created a relative zinc imbalance in affected dogs.

Copper

Copper is found in all tissues of the body, but reaches its highest concentration in the brain, heart, kidney and liver. Copper is a component of several key enzymes, including superoxide dismutase, the important scavenger of dangerous free radicals in the body and tyrosinase, the compound that helps impart color to hair and skin. Copper is also important in the maintenance of red blood cells. In some respects, resistance to infection is related to zinc and copper levels as a ratio of one another. If copper is high and zinc is low, patients are more susceptible to infections. A genetic form of copper deficiency, somewhat similar to Menke's syndrome in people, has been demonstrated in the Alaskan Malamute and perhaps the Samoyed. The Alaskan Malamutes described were dwarfed and had bowing of their legs with enlarged joints.

Copper toxicity poses a greater risk than does deficiency. Copper is stored in the liver and, under normal conditions, excesses are excreted in the bile. In the case of chronic liver and gallbladder disease, copper excretion may be reduced and toxicity could result. More troublesome is that a genetic disease exists in dogs, similar to Wilson's disease in people, in which excessive amounts of copper are deposited in the liver. Breeds at risk include Bedlington Terriers, Skye Terriers, West Highland White Terriers, and perhaps Doberman Pinschers. The treatment of dogs with copper toxicity requires some degree of chelation therapy. This therapy relies on drugs to "bind" to the mineral and help remove it from the body. This can be accomplished with penicillamine (a derivative of penicillin) or with zinc acetate.

Iron

Iron is an important constituent of hemoglobin, the oxygen-carrying part of the red blood cell. It is also found in several different enzymes and a percentage of the daily intake is stored for future use. Adequate levels of iron are needed to strengthen the immune system and to increase resistance to disease. In dogs, iron deficiency can happen with blood loss that robs the body of iron before it can be adequately replaced by the diet. Bleeding is only one way that iron-deficiency anemia can occur. A more innocuous way for anemia to occur is when pups have worms, especially hookworms. These parasites latch on to the intestinal wall to suck blood. With many parasites present, a pup might even die. With copper deficiency, iron is absorbed, but hemoglobin does not form properly and anemia will still result. Most pets' diets are heavily fortified with iron (up to 25 times the recommended amounts) because there are many other nutrients (e.g., fiber) that interfere

with iron absorption. Iron toxicity has been extensively studied in dogs and results in poor appetite, vomiting, diarrhea, intestinal upset, and weight loss. Therefore, iron should not be added to a dog's diet unless recommended by a veterinarian for medical reasons.

Selenium

Selenium is often considered a minor element but it is an important component of the immune system. It forms part of the enzyme glutathione peroxidase, which is an important antioxidant. As such, it protects the cells of the body, especially red blood cells, from the ravages of oxygen-derived free radicals. Selenium also acts in a supporting or even sparing capacity for vitamin E. Recent research has shown that adequate selenium in the diet decreases the damage caused by some cancers, arthritis and heart disease. These benefits are often enhanced by providing adequate levels of vitamin E. Studies done in people have shown that diseases such as cardiomyopathy (a heart ailment), leukemia, and cancers of the colon, rectum, breast, ovaries and lung are less likely to develop in people consuming a selenium-rich diet. Oversupplementation is not recommended because toxicities do result and can be severe. One of the best ways to naturally increase selenium levels is to add a plant-based enzyme supplement to the food (e.g., Prozyme™). This has been shown to increase selenium levels by over 30%.

Chromium

The main use of chromium in the body is to help regulate blood sugar levels by driving glucose into the body cells. Studies in people have shown that chromium salts (especially chromium picolinate) potentiate the effects of insulin and can overcome the insulin resistance seen in some diabetics. By so doing, it also reduces the risk for associated heart disease. Limited research has been done to date in dogs, but chromium picolinate supplementation will likely be an important aspect of diabetes control in dogs.

Cobalt

Cobalt is an important component of vitamin B_{12}, also known as cobalamin. As such, it is important in the formation of red blood cells and helps maintain nerve tissue and normal cell function. Cobalt is found in meats and organ meats, and dogs on strictly vegetarian diets are at risk of vitamin B_{12} deficiency (and hence cobalt deficiency). Although cobalt can be found in vegetables and fruits, it is the combined vitamin-mineral (cobalamin) that is needed to prevent anemia. Small but significant amounts of cobalamin can be found in Brewer's yeast, aloe, kelp, and algae, which should help prevent deficiencies, even in die-hard vegans.

Iodine

Most of the iodine consumed in the diet makes its way to the thyroid gland, where it is incorporated into hormones. Inadequate iodine in the diet is a rare cause of hypothyroidism in dogs (endemic goiter) but this accounts for only a very small percentage of cases. The vast majority of hypothyroid dogs have adequate intakes of iodine and their disease is most often caused by a defective immunologic mechanism, not diet. Dogs on commercial diets are very unlikely to have iodine deficiency because an iodized salt is often added to these rations. Additional supplementation is unnecessary and unlikely to provide any benefits. However, toxic reactions (iodism) are possible if supplementation is overdone.

DOG FOOD SELECTION

The best approach to intelligently selecting a commercial dog food is to understand the facts as they relate to your dog. Asking someone else for an opinion related to what they feed their dog is irrelevant in most cases. Dogs are individuals and should be treated as such.

It is very difficult indeed for anyone, even a veterinarian or nutritionist, to determine the quality of a dog food by the information provided on the label. Additional information can often be helpful and most ethical manufacturers will make this available to anyone who makes a request. Any dog food selected should have been deemed adequate on the basis of feeding trials for your dog's stage of life. The criteria have been proposed by AAFCO in the United States and by the

Canadian Veterinary Medical Association in Canada. These are not foolproof criteria but are the best options currently available.

Although there is growing concern over the wholesomeness of dog foods, it doesn't mean that "natural" dog foods are better than others. Part of the problem is that there is no legal definition for "natural" so anyone can use the term. The FDA is currently wrestling with this issue and hopefully will provide useful guidelines. Until that time it is still important to ensure that any diet fed meets AAFCO protocols, has a digestibility of at least 80% and has a nutrient profile appropriate for the dog being fed.

Don't try to compare dog foods on the basis of protein content. The percentage of protein in the diet is only a reflection of that needed to supply essential amino acids. Additional protein only turns to fat or gets excreted in the urine. Don't be fooled! It is the quality of the protein provided, not the quantity, that makes the real difference in a dog food.

Pay attention to the ingredient list provided even though it is hard to predict quality based on the terms used. For a canned product, there should be at least one animal-based protein source in the first two ingredients listed. For dry foods, an animal-based protein source should be one of the first three ingredients. Since animal-based protein sources contain a better balance of essential amino acids, this is a good clue as to how appropriately the diet has

been formulated. If meat or poultry meal is listed first on the label, but the grains have been sub-categorized (e.g., corn meal, kibbled corn, flaked corn, etc.), it is safe to assume that the manufacturer is trying to sell you a cereal-based diet but wants you to pay the price of a meat-based diet. Too high a mineral concentration (ash) is also not good and probably implies that the ration contains a lot of bone meal and poor-quality protein sources.

Buy commercial dog foods manufactured by a well-respected company that has been around for years and has contributed substantially to nutritional research in pets. These companies have the most to lose by distributing an inferior product because they have a reputation to protect. Fad diets and manufacturers will come and go but the dog food companies that intend to be around will be the ones most concerned with adequate nutrition.

Most of the information provided on the ingredient list reflects legal terms and doesn't allow for valid comparisons between different foods. Meat by-products, cereal grain products and other such terms can mean a great many things indeed. These can vary from high-quality organ meats and whole-grain cereals to cow udders and oat hulls. How can you possibly tell from the term "by-products"?

PRESERVATIVES IN DOG FOOD

The chemical preservatives used in most dog foods include ethoxyquin, butylated hydroxyanisole (BHA), butylated hydroxytoluene (BHT), proprionic acid and ascorbic acid (vitamin C). They are added to the rations to help stop the fats in the food from going rancid. It is these preservatives that allow dry dog foods to have such a long shelf life. How long would you let a mixture of hamburger and cooked corn sit on your pantry shelf without being refrigerated and without using preservatives? If a commercial dry dog food claims "no preservatives added," take it with a grain of salt unless they provide valid laboratory analysis of the finished product. Many suppliers add the preservatives before they are received by the manufacturer. The manufacturer must list only those preservatives which they put into the food, not those that were added by the supplier. Therefore, even if no preservatives were added by the manufacturer, there is no assurance that they are not in the ration.

Are preservatives harmful for dogs? There is little doubt that preservatives and other additives to dog foods may have undesirable consequences in some dogs. However, it is also obvious that dog owners want to buy dog foods that don't go rancid. The only way to avoid preservatives altogether is for dog owners to make their own dog foods at home. The other option is to feed only canned foods. Since canned dog foods are heat-sterilized in the can, no preservatives are needed to keep out bacteria and yeasts. However, remember that meat suppliers may have added

preservatives before the ingredients ever reached the manufacturer. Dry dog foods contain the most preservatives because they stand the highest risk of rancidity. Semi-moist dog foods use "humectants" as preservatives.

To be fair, dog-food preservatives present the same concerns as other food preservatives such as MSG (monosodium glutamate) or sulfites. We should not regard any preservative as being completely safe. They are often designated "generally regarded as safe," or GRAS, by regulatory agencies, which is hardly an endorsement of wholesomeness. It is best to regard preservatives as a necessary evil as long as dog owners want the convenience of buying commercial dog foods.

OBESITY

Obesity is the most common nutritional disease afflicting dogs and cats today, currently exceeding all deficiency-related diseases combined.

Perhaps the pet-food companies have done their jobs too well, but the newer foods are probably much tastier to pets than previous ones and encourage eating. Because many people leave food down all day for free-choice feeding, animals consume more and gain weight.

The incidence of obesity increases with age. It is about twice as common in neutered as in nonneutered animals of either sex and, up to 12 years of age, is more common in females than in males. The most commonly obese breeds are the Labrador Retriever, terriers, spaniels, Dachshunds, Basset Hounds and Beagles. German Shepherd Dogs, Greyhounds, Whippets, and Boxers are the least likely to become obese.

Further tying obesity to lifestyle, obesity is almost twice as common in dogs owned by overweight, middle-aged or older individuals. This increased incidence is

nutritionally balanced, reduced-calorie diet that has been specifically formulated for the high-risk, obesity-prone animal. Weight reduction in most animals can be accomplished with a medically supervised program of caloric restriction. This requires the genuine, long-term commitment by the pet owner to alter poor feeding habits and provide adequate exercise.

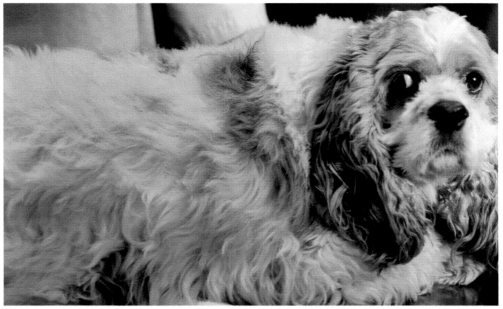

Obesity is the most common nutritional problem seen in pets.

attributed to reduced physical activity and a greater tendency to feed table food, treats, and snacks. Dogs fed these items are 50% more likely to be obese than those fed only prepared pet foods.

Recent studies indicate that even moderate obesity can significantly reduce both the quality and the length of an animal's life. Fortunately, it is a situation that can be remedied.

Neutered animals should be fed a

Currently, more than one quarter of dogs and cats weigh greater than 15% above their optimum body weight. Studies indicate that these animals are at a greatly increased risk of life-shortening illness. Help your pet overcome these problems; it will lead a longer and more enjoyable life.

NUTRITIONAL SUPPLEMENTATION

Nutritional supplementation is a common practice amongst pet owners in North America. Therefore, there must be a perceived need that pets are not receiving complete nutrition in their diets. Many others supplement to gain a desired effect, such as a glossy coat. Most experts in the field of pet nutrition agree that normal animals on a good basic plane of nutrition achieve little benefit from supplementation; most commercially prominent diets provide considerably more of all the known requirements for vitamins and minerals than needed by our pets on a daily basis.

However, there are also some compelling reasons to consider supplementation. Some dogs do respond to supplements even if there is no dietary deficiency. This is because some nutrients have positive benefits apart from their nutritional claims. For instance, vitamin C does much more than just prevent scurvy in people; fiber has beneficial effects even though there is no dietary requirements for fiber. There is therefore quite a bit of difference between providing nutrients at a level that prevents deficiencies and providing nutrients with a goal in mind.

It is this concept of "nutritional therapeutics" that often creates a brick wall between conventional medicine and those practitioners who seek out more natural alternatives. Of course, there need be no wall at all. There is more than enough room in health care for both perspectives. Nutritional therapies should not necessarily replace drug therapy but both might work better together than either one alone. And,

if nutritional therapies even help us to reduce the dosages of prescription items needed, they've more than done their job.

SINGLE-NUTRIENT SUPPLEMENTS

Calcium

Calcium is a commonly used supplement by breeders but it carries many more risks than benefits. Calcium should not be added to the diets of most dogs, especially those that are growing rapidly or are pregnant; these, however, are usually the ones given excess amounts of calcium by their owners. The fact is that calcium levels in the body are carefully regulated by hormones (such as calcitonin and parathormone) as well as vitamin D. Supplementation disturbs this normal regulation and can cause many problems. It has been well documented that calcium supplements given to rapidly growing pups can interfere with cartilage and bone formation. It has also been shown that calcium supplementation can interfere with the proper absorption of zinc from the intestines.

In short, there is no reason to supplement the diet with calcium, unless instructed to do so by a veterinarian. In truth, this is very rarely required, even in breeding bitches. The lesson to be learned— not all supplements are good for your pet!

Zinc

Zinc is a phenomenally important mineral that serves many useful

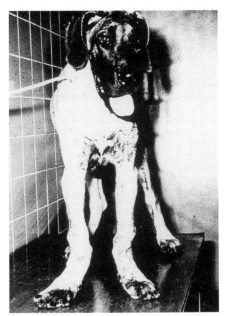

A five-and-a-half-month-old Great Dane with short stature and leg deformities caused by calcium supplementation. This dog was completely recovered by 18 months of age by discontinuing the supplements. Courtesy of Dr. Paul Poulos, Poulos Veterinary Imaging, Davis, California.

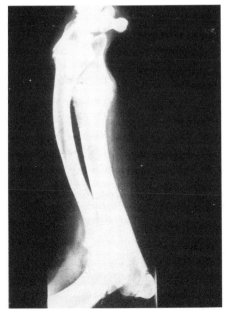

Radiograph of the Great Dane pup showing the curves radius, the open growth plates, and retained cartilage cones. Courtesy of Dr. Paul Poulos, Poulos Veterinary Imaging, Davis, California.

functions in the body, including promoting normal immune functions. Some ingredients in dog foods (e.g., phytates), as well as supplements containing calcium, iron, tin and copper, can decrease zinc absorption. As we have learned, there are many other situations that can impair the utilization of zinc and which warrant supplementation.

It is known that there are certain skin diseases that clear entirely with zinc supplementation. This is referred to as zinc-responsive dermatosis. Most of the affected animals are sled-dog breeds: Siberian Huskies, Malamutes and Samoyeds. It was felt that they might have a genetic defect that results in a decreased ability to absorb zinc from the intestines.

Many other problems associated with zinc are secondary in nature. Cheap diets with a high cereal content can interfere with zinc absorption. Similarly, zinc absorption can be impaired if owners give their dogs calcium supplements.

Zinc alone may be a useful supplement when an animal has chronic skin problems or some immune deficit. And it may be helpful, even when there is no deficiency. That's because zinc levels can be lowered by diarrhea, kidney disease, liver disease or diabetes that might not be linked to any nutritional problem, and because of zinc's beneficial effects on the immune system. Zinc acetate has also been used to treat copper toxicity. This condition is seen as an

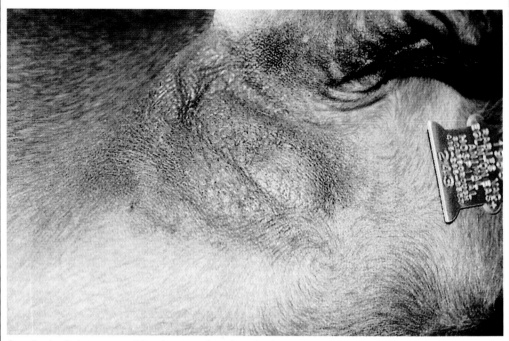

Acanthosis nigricans, a condition that sometimes benefits from administration of vitamin E.

reduce the risk of heart disease by up to 40%. The Health Professionals Follow-up Study of 51,529 men taking vitamin E for two years found 37% fewer cases of heart disease than those not taking vitamin E. The Nurses Health Study of 87, 245 women found a 40% reduction in heart disease among those taking vitamin E supplements. The benefit was thought to be from slowing down the process of atherosclerosis. These benefits may or may not be seen in dogs since high cholesterol and atherosclerosis are not as common causes of heart disease in canines as they are in people.

The body requires adequate levels of zinc to maintain proper levels of vitamin E in the blood. Vitamin E is very safe but large doses should be used cautiously in dogs with overactive thyroids (i.e., hyperthyroidism), high blood pressure or diabetes.

L-carnitine

L-carnitine is an amino acid that is not currently described as being an essential nutrient for pets but it is directly involved with energy metabolism. Recent studies have indicated that carnitine may be limited or inadequate in certain dogs.

L-carnitine has been associated with cardiomyopathy, a heart ailment, in certain breeds of dogs. These dogs have deficiencies of this amino acid in their heart muscle, but not in their bloodstream. This complicates diagnosis because currently a heart muscle biopsy is needed to confirm the diagnosis. Although the underlying cause of

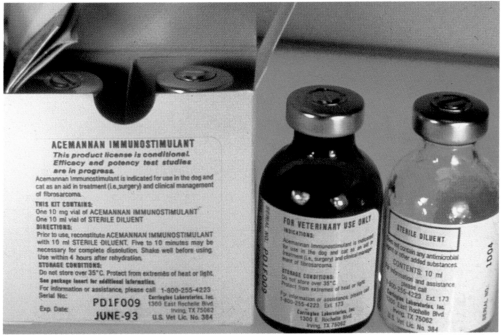

Acemannan, the immune stimulant derived from Aloe. Courtesy of Carrington Veterinary Medical Division, Dallas, Texas.

In scientific studies, neither brewer's yeast nor garlic has been shown to repel fleas. Courtesy of Fleabusters, Rx for Fleas, Inc., Ft. Lauderdale, Florida.

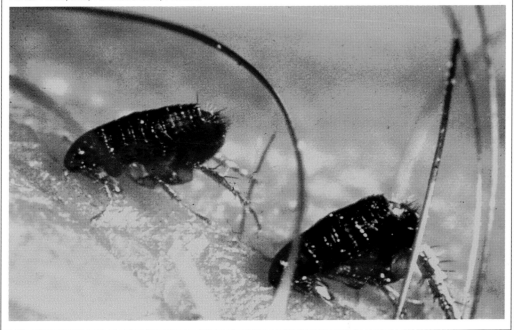

dilated cardiomyopathy in dogs remains unknown, an inherited defect resulting in carnitine deficiency of the heart muscle may be important, especially in Boxers. Whether or not this is true in other breeds has yet to be determined.

Since carnitine does not appear to have any side effects, it would be reasonable to use it as a supplement for any dog with dilated cardiomyopathy. Carnitine is available without a prescription from health food stores, but, because of the serious nature of the ailment, all treatments should be under the supervision of a veterinarian.

Aloe Vera

Aloe vera is derived from members of the Aloe plant and it has been advocated as a natural remedy for over a thousand years. The scientific study of aloe vera has indeed confirmed that it increases the rate of healing of burns and cuts.

Recently, a complex carbohydrate derived from aloe called acemannan has been found to be a potent stimulator of the immune system. It has been used experimentally in the treatment of infectious diseases, immunologic diseases, periodontal disease and some cancers. Recently, a commercial acemannan product has been licensed for the treatment of a malignant cancer (fibrosarcoma) in dogs and cats.

Brewer's Yeast

Brewer's yeast has been advocated as a nutritional supplement as well as a safeguard against fleas. It does contain some useful nutrients, including most of the B vitamins, but it is a poor supplier of others, including vitamins A, C, and E. Scientific studies of Brewer's yeast have not shown it to be of any real benefit in controlling fleas, although some owners still aren't convinced.

Brewer's yeast is considered a safe supplement but, because it contains large amounts of phosphorus, it should be used cautiously in young pups and in elderly dogs. Brewer's yeast should be used cautiously in dogs with recurrent yeast infections as sensitivity (allergy) may become a problem.

Kelp

Kelp is a type of seaweed (e.g., *Ascophyllum nodosum*) which is a rich source of vitamins, minerals and trace elements, and is particularly rich in iodine. Kelp has been advocated for the treatment of a variety of skin problems and, because of its iodine content, for the management of patients with marginal thyroid function. However, these claims are difficult to defend.

Iodine is not a good treatment for dogs because hypothyroidism in this species is almost never due to iodine deficiency. Certainly less than 1% of hypothyroid cases may have iodine deficiency. Kelp may be a good general supplement to provide vitamins, minerals and trace elements but it should not be relied upon to be nutritionally complete on its own. It should be administered cautiously to animals that are already receiving more than adequate levels of iodine or toxicity could result.

Garlic

Garlic is probably the most prescribed herbal remedy and acts as a natural antibiotic, immune stimulant, regulator of digestion, and detoxifier. Contained within the garlic bulb are numerous chemicals, including unsaturated aldehydes, volatile oils, vitamins and minerals. Research in people suggests that garlic might lower cholesterol and triglycerides as well as block the ability of cancer-causing chemicals (carcinogens) to turn normal cells into cancerous ones. Breeders have advocated garlic supplements for flea control but there is no scientific evidence to support these claims.

Garlic is an excellent supplement to give pets with immune problems, digestive upsets or recurrent infections. Newer versions even lack the odor which has plagued garlic use for centuries.

MULTI-NUTRIENT SUPPLEMENTS

The most common supplements to be used in dogs are multi-nutrient supplements that contain a variety of vitamins, minerals, and other nutrients. These can be seen lining the shelves of pet supply outlets across the country.

Multi-nutrient supplements are most appropriate when they are well researched and provide nutrients for specific purposes. A general coat-care supplement that

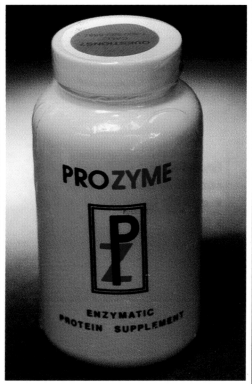

Prozyme™, a plant-based enzyme supplement.

contains fats and cheap vegetable oils probably achieves little benefit. It is always advisable to supplement a pet with individual ingredients rather than a potpourri of nutrients unless they have been formulated for a specific purpose.

DIGESTIVE ENZYMES

Digestive enzyme preparations are commercially available for dogs and include pancreatic enzymes as well as plant-derived enzymes. The plant-derived enzymes are available without a prescription (e.g., Prozyme™) and are used to increase the absorption of nutrients from the diet being fed. Preliminary research conducted on the Prozyme™ product suggests

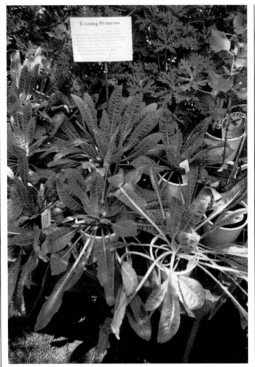

Evening primrose plants. Photo taken at Penny Royal Herb Farm, Bundaberg, Queensland, Australia.

that it increases the amount of zinc, selenium, linoleic acid, and some other nutrients from food.

Breeders have recommended using these plant-based digestive enzymes in geriatric pets and in dogs with skin disease, digestive ills and arthritis. These conditions might well benefit from the increased utilization of nutrients in the diet and studies are underway to investigate these claims.

Most enzyme supplements are designed to be applied to the food before it is eaten, not given directly to the dog. The enzymes should be applied to the food for several minutes before feeding so that they have an opportunity to digest the proteins, carbohydrates and fat in the meal before it is consumed.

FAT SUPPLEMENTS

Fat supplements are probably the most common supplements purchased from pet-supply stores. They frequently promise to add luster, gloss, and sheen to the coat, and consequently make dogs look healthy. There are two reasons to add fat supplements to the diet and both are worth understanding.

To add gloss to the coat, dogs might indeed benefit from fatty acid supplementation. However, the only fatty acid that is essential for this purpose is cis-linoleic acid, which is found in flaxseed oil, sunflower seed oil, and safflower oil. Corn oil is a suitable but less effective alternative. Most of the other oils found in retail supplements are high in saturated and monounsaturated fats and are not beneficial for shiny fur or healthy skin.

For dogs with allergies, arthritis, high blood pressure (hypertension), high cholesterol, and some heart ailments, other fatty acids may be prescribed by a veterinarian. The important ingredients in these products are gamma-linolenic acid (GLA), eicosapentaenoic acid (EPA), and docosahexaenoic acid (DHA). These products are very different from the fatty acids used to add sheen to the coat; they have gentle and natural anti-inflammatory properties. But don't be fooled by imitations. Most retail fatty-acid supplements do not contain these functional forms of the essential fatty acids—look for gamma-linolenic acid, eicosapentaenoic acid, and docosahexaenoic acid on the label.

Fatty-acid supplementation should not be done indiscriminantly. The use of polyunsaturated fatty acids in the diet increases the need for vitamin E. They can also cause diarrhea and vomiting if overdone. When purchasing these supplements, select opaque containers since exposure to light renders the essential fatty acids useless. Also, tightly re-seal the container after use because exposure to air also decreases the effective fatty acid content.

DAILY ALLOWANCE SUPPLEMENTS

There are many supplements in the marketplace that provide a combination of vitamins and minerals meeting the daily nutritional requirements of dogs. If dogs are receiving a well-balanced diet which includes some exposure to fresh vegetables and grains, a daily vitamin/mineral supplement is probably not required.

These vitamin/mineral supplements are not likely to be useful in managing any health care problems, even though they may contain nutrients that should be helpful. The reason is that there is a big difference between the amount that will prevent deficiencies and the doses often used to treat problems. For example, the recommended daily allowance for vitamin E for a 20-pound dog is about 10 IU, and yet during treatment we may use 200 IU two to three times daily in the same animal to get the desired effect. Therefore, it is very unlikely

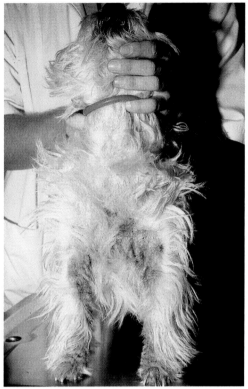

An allergic dog that might benefit from administration of omega-3 and omega-6 fatty acid combinations.

that the dosages in a daily vitamin/mineral supplement will help an animal with a specific medical problem.

However, specific combinations of nutrients are the practical way to approach many health care problems. If they have been intelligently formulated, they should contain nutrients in the correct balance and proportion to best manage the problem for which they are intended. For example, elderly pets would benefit from supplements that take into account the changing dietary needs of this stage of life. Dogs with kidney disease also benefit from some intelligent nutritional supplementation. Skin diseases are probably the most common condition for which nutritional supplementation is sought but it is difficult to predict whether retail products have been effectively formulated.

PROTEIN SUPPLEMENTS

Protein supplements are also commonly purchased by dog owners but there is little evidence that they have any real benefit. Remember, dogs do not have a requirement for protein in their diet; they need specific amino acids.

Since most commercial pet foods have more than adequate amounts of protein, protein deficiency is rare in animals and only seen in individuals fed a poor-quality diet or those animals which are ill and unable to take adequate feedings. Changing to a better quality diet is more realistic than trying to supplement a poorly formulated homemade or commercial diet.

ADDITIONAL READING

Ackerman, L: Nutritional facts, fads, and fallacies. *Pet Focus*, 1991; 24-26.

Ackerman, L: Nutritional supplementation for skin conditions. *Pet Focus*, 1990; 2(4): 51-54.

Ackerman, L: *What Every Dog Owner Should Know About Nutrition*. Alpine Publications, 1995.

Alexander, JE; Wood, LLH: Growth studies in Labrador Retrievers fed a caloric- dense diet: time restricted versus free-choice feeding. *Canine Practice*, 1987; 14(2): 41-47.

Barrette, DC: Calcium and phosphorus for cats and dogs. *Canadian Veterinary Journal*, 1988; 29: 751-752.

Blomhoff, R; Green, MH; Norum, KR: Vitamin A: Physiological and biochemical processing. *Annual Review of Nutrition*, 1992; 12: 37-57.

Brewer, GJ: Use of zinc acetate to treat copper toxicosis in dogs. *Journal of the American Veterinary Medical Association*, 1992; 201(4): 564-568.

Brown, RG: Gastrointestinal upsets with high performance diets. *Canadian Veterinary Journal*, 1987; 28: 419-420.

Brown, RG: Protein in dog foods. *Canadian Veterinary Journal*, 1989; 30: 528- 531.

Brown, RG: Vitamin and mineral supplements. *Canadian Veterinary Journal*, 1987; 28(11): 697-698.

Buffington, CA: Therapeutic use of vitamins in companion animals. *Current Veterinary Therapy X*, edited by Kirk & Bonagura. W.B. Saunders Co., Philadelphia, 1989; 40-47.

Donoghue, S: Providing proper nutrition for dogs at different stages of the life cycle. *Veterinary Medicine*, 1991; July: 728-733.

Folkers, K: A renaissance in biomedical and clinical research on vitamins and coenzymes. *Journal of Optimal Nutrition*, 1992; 1(1): 11-15.

Hazewinkel, HAW; Goedegebuure, SA; Poulos, PW; Wolvekamp, WThC: Influences of chronic calcium excess on the skeletal development of growing Great Danes. *Journal of the American Animal Hospital Association*, 1985; 21: 377-391.

Hilton, JW: Potential nutrient deficiencies in pet foods. *Canadian Veterinary Journal*, 1989; 30: 599-601.

Hilton, J: Carbohydrates in the nutrition of the dog. *Canadian Veterinary Journal*, 1990; 31: 128-129.

Hilton, JW: Feed energy (caloric density): Determination and significance in pet foods. *Canadian Veterinary Journal*, 1989; 30: 183-184.

Houston, DM; Hulland, TJ: Thiamine deficiency in a team of sled dogs. *Canadian Veterinary Journal*, 1988; 29: 383-385.

Huber, TL; Laflamme, DP; Medleau, L; et al: Comparison of procedures for assessing adequacy of dog foods. *Journal of the American Veterinary Medical Association*, 1991; 199(6): 731-

Huber, TL; Wilson, RC; McGarity, SA: Variations in digestibility of dry dog foods with identical label guaranteed analysis. *Journal of the American Animal Hospital Association*, 1986; 22(5): 571-575.

Keene, BW: L-carnitine supplementation in therapy of canine dilated cardiomyopathy. *Veterinary Clinics of North America, Small Animal Practice*, 1991; 21(5): 1005-1009.

Kronfeld, DS: Protein quality and amino acid profiles of commercial dog foods. *Journal of the American Animal Hospital Association*, 1982; 18(4): 679-683.

Maki, PA; Newberne, PM: Dietary lipids and immune function. *Journal of Nutrition*, 1992; 122: 610-614.

McCarty, MF: The case for supplemental chromium and a survey of clinical studies with chromium picolinate. *Journal of Applied Nutrition*, 1991; 43(1): 58-66.

Norris, D: Zinc and cutaneous inflammation. *Archives of Dermatology*, 1985; 121: 985-989.

Olson, WG; et al: Iodine: A review of dietary requirements, therapeutic properties and assessment of potential toxicity.

Compendium for Continuing Education for the Practicing Veterinarian, 1980; 2(10): S164-S167.

Rath, M; Pauling, L: Vitamin C and lipoprotein (A) in relation to cardiovascular disease and other diseases. *Journal of Optimal Nutrition*, 1992; 1(1): 61-64.

Sherman, AR: Zinc, copper, and iron nutriture and immunity. *Journal of Nutrition*, 1992; 122: 604-609.

Sousa, CA; et al: Dermatosis associated with feeding generic dog food: 13 cases (1981-1982). *Journal of the American Veterinary Medical Association*, 1988; 192(5): 676-680.

Sternlieb, I: Copper and the liver: Comparative aspects in man and animals. *Proceedings of the 10th American College of Veterinary Medicine Forum*, May, 1992. pp. 49-52.

Skin Disorders in D

Skin problems are the most common reason for pet owners to take their dogs to the veterinarian. Did you know that dogs get many of the same skin problems that people do? Well, we don't treat many dogs for acne or psoriasis but we do see a variety of other problems, including allergies, infections, hereditary problems and autoimmune diseases. Dogs even get a variety of skin cancers.

The problem with many skin problems is that a lot of them look alike. A rash looks like a rash. A dog scratching from allergies looks very much like a dog scratching from fleas. It is therefore often difficult to just look at a dog with skin problems and know for certain what the problem is—very often we need to do tests first.

When it comes to treating skin problems, it is very important we know what we are treating. This may sound obvious but many owners request shampoos, ointments, sprays and powders to treat a rash or eczema or sores. If you don't know what you are treating specifically, don't expect these treatments to work consistently.

Because of the wide range of skin problems affecting dogs, it should not be surprising that there are specialists, veterinary dermatologists, to help with difficult skin problems. These specialists will work with your regular veterinarian to get t bottom of the problem, get a proper diagnosis, and start appropriate treatment. If you need the help of a veterinary dermatologist, your veterinarian can provide a referral.

HEREDITARY SKIN DISORDERS

There are many different skin problems that tend to have a hereditary nature. This discussion, however, will only concern itself with those conditions for which the pattern of inheritance has been documented. Many other conditions have breed tendencies or predilections but the exact nature of the heritability remains unknown in most cases.

The Institute for Genetic Disease Control in Animals (GDC) is a nonprofit organization that maintains an open registry for several hereditary conditions. In July of 1992, the GDC established the skin disease registry for inherited sebaceous adenitis. The GDC represents the first open registry of hereditary diseases in North America that aids in genetic selection of breeding stock and supports research for the control of genetic diseases of dogs. GDC also offers professional genetic evaluation and scientific support services. For more information, contact the Institute for Genetic Disease Control in Animals (GDC), P.O. Box 222, Davis, CA 95617, Phone and FAX (916) 756-6773.

Acrodermatitis

Acrodermatitis is a fatal disorder seen in Bull Terriers and is inherited as an autosomal recessive trait. That means that a defective gene must be inherited from both parents. The difficulty is that the parents appear clinically normal.

Affected pups do not grow properly and develop infections of their feet and face, as well as diarrhea, pneumonia, and abnormal behavior, before dying before a year and a half of age. Affected pups often have a lighter coloring than normal littermates, which becomes accentuated with time. Pups that are only mildly affected may survive longer.

We don't know the exact reason why these pups don't survive but many theories have been proposed, including a relative zinc imbalance or an abnormal thymus gland (important for the immune system).

Treatment to date has been unsuccessful in most cases. These dogs do not respond to zinc supplementation and eventually die because of overwhelming infection, usually pneumonia. It is important that neither parent be used in breedings. Recently, treatment has been reported with ketoconazole, a drug used to treat fungal infections, and some success has been realized. Etretinate, a synthetic vitamin A derivative, is also being evaluated and may be of some benefit.

Color Dilution Alopecia

Color dilution alopecia, also known as color mutant alopecia, describes the patchy, poor haircoat that develops in animals bred for abnormally colored hair. The principal breeds involved include blue Doberman Pinschers, Great Danes, Dachshunds, Whippets, Chow Chows, Italian Greyhounds and Standard Poodles. Red Doberman Pinschers and Fawn Irish Setters may have milder forms of the disorder. The condition has also been described in gray-blue Yorkshire Terriers, tricolor Salukis and a blue-and-white mixed-breed dog. It is supposed that an abnormal gene (allele) on the d (dilution) locus is responsible for the problem. These animals are born with normal coats but later suffer from hair loss, dry skin and bacterial infections. If one looks closely, the skin disease is confined only to abnormally colored hairs.

Color dilution alopecia can be suspected based on clinical examination but confirmation requires biopsy or examining plucked hairs microscopically. Because the hair follicles actually develop abnormally, there is no cure for this disorder. Medicated shampoos are normally prescribed to remove the prominent scale that forms on the skin surface and emollients and moisturizers are often given for the dry skin. Hair does not regrow with thyroid medication or zinc supplementation. Therapy should be considered lifelong and affected animals should not be used for breeding. If the abnormal allele on the d locus is eventually identified, a prevention program should be possible.

Cutaneous asthenia

Cutaneous asthenia (Ehlers-Danlos syndrome) is a biochemical disorder that causes the skin to be overly fragile and stretchable. These animals are the rubber men of the dog world. When the skin of affected dogs is pulled, it stretches excessively to the point where it can even tear. Affected breeds include the Beagle, Dachshund, Boxer, St. Bernard, German Shepherd Dog, English Springer Spaniel, Greyhound, Schnauzer and mongrels. The genetic nature of the condition is complex, but there is much evidence to suggest a dominant trend.

The condition is usually easily diagnosed but if there is any question a series of measurements can be taken that constitutes a skin extensibility index. Biopsies are sometimes helpful but are not diagnostic in all cases.

There is no specific treatment for cutaneous asthenia because there is no method to overcome the inherited collagen defect. Large doses of vitamin C (vitamin C is a cofactor in collagen synthesis) may be given but this will not correct the problem. These animals should definitely not be bred. Further, it is usually not safe for them to undergo surgery, even neutering.

Canine cyclic hematopoiesis (Gray Collie Syndrome)

Some Collie pups born with a silver-gray haircoat may be smaller and weaker than their normal littermates, and may have a light-colored nose. It appears to be transmitted as an autosomal recessive trait. By eight to twelve weeks of age, they start to develop problems such as fever, diarrhea, eye infections, painful joints (arthralgia) and abnormalities of their white blood cells. This syndrome has also now been reported in Pomeranians and Cocker Spaniels.

When blood samples are collected daily over a two-week period, it can be seen that the neutrophils, a type of white blood cell, fluctuate from high to low over an 11–14-day cycle. When the neutrophils are at their lowest point, these pups are very susceptible to overwhelming infection and usually die during these periods.

Diagnosis can be confirmed by sequential blood counts over a 14-day period. Therapy is invariably unsuccessful and most animals succumb during periods of low neutrophil counts. Parents and littermates should not be used for breeding.

Dermatomyositis

Dermatomyositis is seen mostly in Collies, Shetland Sheepdogs and their crosses, and is a disease that affects skin and muscle. Recently, cases of dermatomyositis have also been reported in Australian Cattle Dogs and Pembroke Welsh Corgis. If one reviews the literature, it is likely that the condition originally was diagnosed as epidermolysis bullosa simplex (EBS) but we now suspect that most, if not all, of those early cases were really

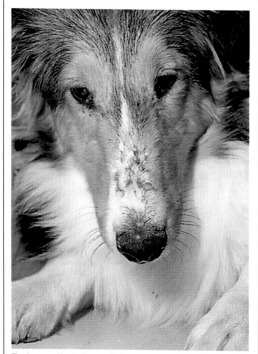

Early manifestations of dermatomyositis. Courtesy of Dr. Thomas Lewis, Dermatology Clinic for Animals, Albuquerque, New Mexico.

dermatomyositis. The exact cause of the disorder is still a matter of debate. It is known to involve the immune system and likely has hereditary (and possibly infectious) components.

Animals first begin to show signs at about 12 weeks of age which may look like scrapes on the face, ears, elbows, hocks and other friction points. Hair may also be lost from the tip of the tail. In later stages, muscle wasting may also be seen, especially on the top of the head (temporalis muscles) and over the hindquarters. In Pembroke Welsh Corgis, it appears that the ears and face are predominantly affected .

The condition is inherited as an autosomal dominant trait with variable expressivity. This means that if one parent is affected, most of the pups will be affected. This is an important consideration, since parents may only be mildly affected themselves but should be closely scrutinized if they produce affected young. There is also speculation that a virus may be involved in the condition, since virus-like particles are occasionally observed in biopsies. It is thought that a virus could induce clinical signs typical of the disease in genetically predisposed dogs.

There is no blood test to identify carriers, and not enough data have been collected to permit pedigree analysis to select good breeding stock. Most cases are diagnosed on the basis of the history, clinical signs, electromyography and biopsy. Well-chosen biopsies often reveal characteristic changes and electromyographic (EMG) studies may show abnormalities in the muscles as well.

Therapy is only symptomatic. Both vitamin E and corticosteroids have been used to relieve scaling and scarring but neither will cure the condition. Pentoxifylline is currently being investigated experimentally to see if it holds any promise for the treatment of dermatomyositis.

The disease usually determines its own path around the time of puberty, when some animals deteriorate further or recover spontaneously. Recovered animals should definitely not be bred, since offspring will undoubtedly be affected, at least to some extent.

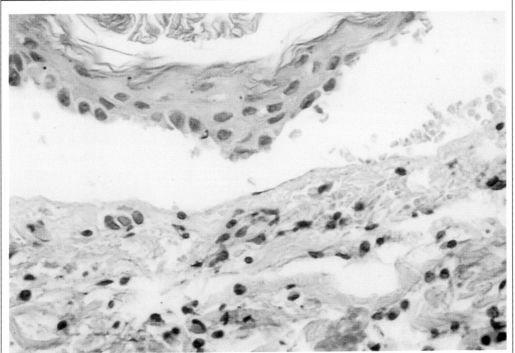

Clefting evident between the epidermis and dermis in a case of dermatomyositis. Courtesy of Dr. Thomas Lewis, Dermatology Clinic for Animals, Albuquerque, New Mexico.

Electromyographic (EMG) tracing showing abnormalities in a dog with dermatomyositis. Courtesy of Dr. Don Levesque, Veterinary Neurological Center, Tempe, Arizona.

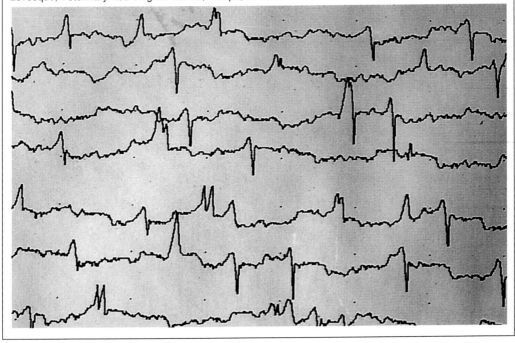

IgA Deficiency

IgA deficiency refers to a lack of a specific family of antibodies known as immunoglobulin A, or IgA for short. This antibody family is important in protecting the body surface, especially the skin, respiratory tract, digestive system, and reproductive system. This condition is most commonly seen in the Chinese Shar-Pei, Beagle, and German Shepherd Dog breeds but has been recorded in several other breeds as well.

The clinical pattern is one of recurrent infections of the respiratory tract, urinary tract, and skin. Chronic ear infections are not uncommon with this problem.

The diagnosis is made by running immunoglobulin levels on suspected dogs. These samples need to be sent to specialized laboratories capable of running the tests. Serum levels of IgA are undetectable or very low, whereas other immunoglobulins and T-cell functions are normal. Respiratory infections in these dogs are attributed to inadequate secretory IgA levels at mucosal surfaces.

Nodular Dermatofibrosis

Nodular dermatofibrosis is a condition most commonly seen in German Shepherd Dogs and has been recognized since 1967. This condition evolves as a series of lumps most often seen involving the areas between the toes and on the legs but capable of becoming generalized. The lumps are considered painless, but may become ulcerated and interfere with movement, depending on their location.

The significance of this condition is that, although the skin problems themselves do not usually affect the health of the animal, these animals invariably later develop a specific type of malignant kidney tumor (cystadenocarcinoma) and bitches may also develop cancers of the uterus.

Any German Shepherd Dog having lumps on its legs should be evaluated for the possibility of nodular dermatofibrosis. No dogs with this condition should be used for breeding, and all should be screened for the presence or future development of kidney or uterine tumors. Affected animals should be evaluated at least every three months since with early recognition, the kidney tumors may be surgically removed before the cancer has had time to spread.

Sebaceous Adenitis

Sebaceous adenitis, also known as periappendageal dermatitis, is a recently described problem in which there is inflammatory damage of the hair follicles and the sebaceous glands that supply them. It is most commonly seen in the Standard Poodle but has also been reported in many other breeds, including the Vizsla, Samoyed, Irish Setter, Akita, Collie, Golden Retriever, Old English Sheepdog, Doberman Pinscher, Springer Spaniel, Basset Hound, Scottish Terrier, German Shepherd Dog, Miniature Poodle, Miniature Pinscher, Chow Chow, Weimaraner, Lhasa Apso,

Dalmatian, Dachshund and some mixed breeds.

Most animals are in young adulthood when first affected and develop flaking of the skin and then a loss of hair. In general the condition is not itchy or irritating unless the dogs have managed to develop infection in these sites. Other than these changes, the dogs appear in good health.

It may very well be that different breeds actually have different disorders but, at present, we are using the term sebaceous adenitis as a description rather than a diagnosis until we understand the disease better. A new classification divides most long-haired breeds (e.g. Standard Poodle, Old English Sheepdog, Samoyed, Akita) into a Type I description which progresses rapidly and responds to symptomatic therapy only. Type II is seen in the Viszla and other short-coated breeds, slowly progresses and responds best to retinoids and cyclosporine.

For proper diagnosis, biopsies are required and they should be sent to veterinary pathologists with expertise in skin disorders. In the Standard Poodle, normal-appearing carriers can sometimes even be predicted by early biopsies. Animals that appear normal but that have more than two hair follicles affected out of two 6mm punch biopsies are classified as subclinical and should not be used for breeding. These biopsies are usually taken from the topline between the head and the shoulder blades. For breeds other than the Standard Poodle, two 6mm biopsies should be taken from affected areas early in the course of the disorder, when changes are most likely to be evident.

Therapy of early cases is often attempted with corticosteroids, which are derivatives of cortisone, but there is much variability in the chances of success. Some preliminary work has been done with isotretinoin, a synthetic form of vitamin A used in the treatment of acne, and continued research will undoubtedly provide additional options. This is more effective in the Vizsla and Standard Poodle than in other breeds. Etretinate, another form of synthetic vitamin A, is more effective in the Akita, which generally responds poorly to all forms of therapy. Antibiotics are usually also helpful for Akitas because they tend to have more bacterial complications than the other breeds. Essential fatty acid supplements are indicated for all cases because they are mildly anti-inflammatory and have few or no side effects.

Topical treatment is important because the skin becomes very dry and scaly. This means frequent shampooing with products that help remove surface scale (e.g. tar, sulfur, salicylic acid, selenium sulfide) and improving the moisture content of the skin with rinses of 50% propylene glycol and various other moisturizers, emollients and humectants. Human products that utilize lactic acid, urea or hot oil treatments may be helpful but require intensive owner commitment.

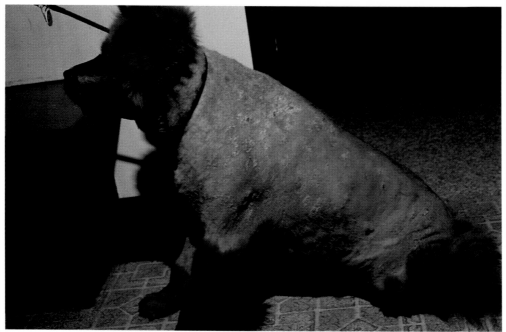

Hair loss associated with sebaceous adenitis.

ALLERGIES

Allergies are as common in dogs as they are in people. Most allergies are caused by substances that we breathe in, that we ingest, that bite us or otherwise contact our skin. Not surprisingly, dogs are no different. Some of the most common allergies in dogs have to do with inhalants (hay fever), flea bites, and foods.

Inhalant Allergies

Allergic inhalant dermatitis (atopy, hay fever) is one of the most common skin problems that dogs get. In the past it has been mislabeled as "grass itch," "grass fungus" and eczema, but now we know the problem is caused by dogs breathing in various pollens, molds and housedust. Unlike people, however, dogs don't usually sneeze with inhalant allergies; they lick, chew and scratch. Inhalant allergies may therefore be confused with other itchy skin conditions, especially fleas.

Breeds with a particularly high incidence of allergies include terriers (especially the West Highland White Terrier, Skye Terrier, Scottish Terrier and Boston Terrier), Golden Retrievers, Poodles, Dalmatians, German Shepherd Dogs, Chinese Shar-pei, Bichons Frises, Shih Tzu, Lhasa Apsos, Pugs, Irish Setters and Miniature Schnauzers. Any animal, however, purebred or mutt, may be affected by inhalant allergies. Although we recognize that these breeds have more allergies than others, it is important to realize that the genetics of allergy are not obvious—allergies run in families in

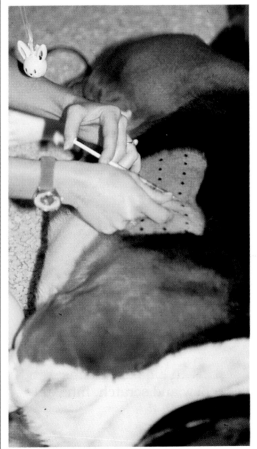

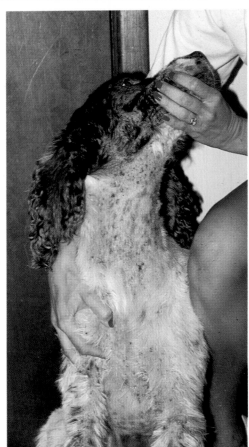

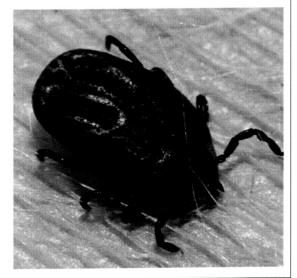

Above left: Performing intradermal allergy testing.

Above right: Severe inhalant allergies can result in secondary bacterial infections.

Right: A housedust tick. Courtesy of Greer Laboratories, Inc., Lenoir, NC.

Guide to Allergenic Trees, Weeds, and Grasses in the U.S.

Degree of importance: • minor; •• moderate; ••• major

Common Name / Latin Name (Genus)	Some Important Species	North-East	Mid-Atlantic	South-East South Cent.	Mid-West	Great Plains	Cent. Texas OK	Desert South-West	Inter-Mtn.	South CA	West Coast Alaska	So. FL Hawaii Carib.
TREES												
ASH — *Fraxinus* spp.	White, Arizona, Green Ash	••	••	••	••	•		•••	•	•	•	
BIRCH — *Betula* spp.	White, Paper, Red, Sweet, Spring Birch	•••	••	••	••	•	•		••	•	•	
CEDAR — *Juniperus* spp.	Mountain, Red, Rocky Mtn. Cedar, Western Juniper	•	•	••	•	•	•••	••	••	•	••	••
ELM — *Ulmus* spp.	American, Chinese, Fall Blooming Elm	••	••	••	•••	••	••	•	•	•	•	
MAPLE — *Acer* spp.	Sugar, Red, Silver Maple, Box Elder	••	••	•	•	••	•		••	•		
OAK — *Quercus* spp.	White, Red, Black, Scrub, Live, Post, Calif. Live Oak	•••	•••	•••	•••	•••	•••	••	••	••	••	••
PECAN — *Carya* spp.	Pecan, White Hickory, Shagbark Hickory	••	••	•••	•	•	••	•		•	•	••
WALNUT — *Juglans* spp.	Black, English, Hinds, Calif. Black Walnut	•	•	••	•	•	•		•	••	•••	
SYCAMORE — *Platanus* spp.	Eastern, Western Sycamore, Plane Tree	••	•••	••	•••	••	•••		•	•	••	
WEEDS												
COCKLEBUR — *Xanthium* spp.	Common, Spiny Cocklebur	•	••	•••	•••	•••	•••	••	••	•		•
ENGLISH PLANTAIN — *Plantago lanceolata*		••	••	••	••	••	••	•	•	••	•	•
KOCHIA — *Kochia scoparia*					••	•••	•	•	•••	•	•	
LAMB'S QUARTERS — *Chenopodium* spp.	Mexican Tea	••	••	••	••	••	••	••		•		•
PIGWEED — *Amaranthus* spp.	Redroot, Spiny Pigweed	•	••	•••	•••	•••	•••	••	••	•		••
RAGWEED, TALL — *Ambrosia trifida*		•••	•••	•••	•••	••		•				
RAGWEED, SHORT — *Ambrosia artemisiifolia*	Western, Southern Ragweed	•••	•••	•••	•••	•••	•••	••	••	•		••
RUSSIAN THISTLE — *Salsola kali*			•	•	•	•••	•••	••	•••	•	••	•
SAGE — *Artemisia* spp.	Mugwort, Wormwood, Sagebrush, Carpet & Pasture Sages	••	••	•	•	•••	•	•••	•••	••	••	
GRASSES												
BERMUDA GRASS — *Cynodon dactylon*		•	••	•••	•	•	•••	•••		•••	•	•••
BLUE GRASS — *Poa* spp.	Kentucky (June), Canadian, Annual Blue Grass	•••	•••	•••	•••	•••	•••	••	••	•••	••	•
JOHNSON GRASS — *Sorghum halepense*		•	•	••	•	•	•••	••	•	••		••
ORCHARD GRASS — *Dactylis glomerata*		•••	•••	••	•••	••	•		•		•	
RYE GRASS — *Lolium* spp.	Perennial, Italian Rye Grass	•••	•••	•••	•••	•••	•••	••	••	•••	•••	•
TIMOTHY GRASS — *Phleum pratense*		•••	•••	••	•••	•••	••	••	••	••	••	•

people and the same is true about dogs. If a dog is allergic, there is a very good chance that at least one of the parents is allergic as well.

CLINICAL SIGNS

The dog with inhalant allergies usually isn't itchy from birth. On average, the clinical signs start to appear between six months of age and three years of age. The symptoms may be year 'round or seasonal, depending on what the allergies are to. Most pollen allergies are seasonal but housedust and mold allergies are usually present throughout the year.

The allergic dog is usually especially itchy in areas of sensitive skin. Therefore, most spend time licking and chewing at their feet and may also have problems with their armpits, groin, flanks, face and ears. In time, the skin gets red and warm, darker in color, greasy and infected. When a patch of skin gets very inflamed and becomes traumatized, it is called a "hot spot." Hot spots occur most frequently with inhalant allergies, food allergies or flea allergies.

DIAGNOSIS

Because many allergic skin diseases look alike, special testing is often necessary to make a diagnosis. Inhalant allergies are identified in dogs not so differently from the procedure in people in which a variety of substances are

Facing page: Guide to Allergenic Trees, Weeds & Grasses of the United States. Center Laboratories, Div. EM Industries, Inc. Reprinted with permission.

injected into the skin and the results evaluated shortly thereafter. In fact, the whole test, from start to finish, takes less than an hour, and the results are all available at that time. The testing is often done by dermatologists and may require referral to a specialty center. To perform the test, we shave a rectangular area on their side for the test site and the potentially allergy-causing substances (allergens) are injected individually. It is not unusual to test for 40 or more allergens during an allergy test, and the site has to be large enough to accommodate one injection for each allergen. The procedure is relatively painless since only a very tiny amount is actually injected, with a very small needle, and only into the very uppermost layers of the skin.

Recently, blood tests with names like RAST (radioallergosorbent test) and ELISA (enzyme-linked immunosorbent assay) have been developed to help diagnose allergies but, at present, they are not as good as skin tests. If you have the choice, it is best to have skin testing done by a specialist. Blood tests are not the best option but make sense if they are the only option available. Research suggests that these blood tests tend to overestimate the extent and nature of allergies and that they are not very specific.

THERAPY

The treatment of inhalant allergies is very much like that of hay fever in people. Allergy shots

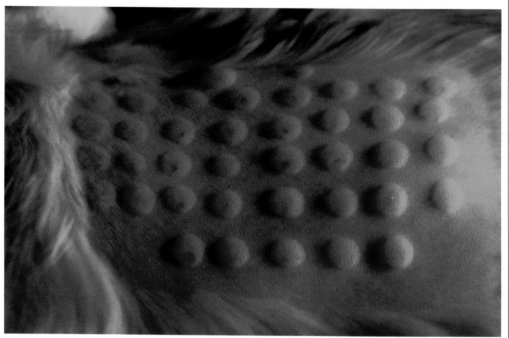

Results of intradermal allergy testing.

(immunotherapy), antihistamines and special fatty-acid supplements are available to help control symptoms. Cortisone-based preparations often help relieve itching, but, because of their potential for side effects, should only be used sparingly. The goal is to make the pet more comfortable while not complicating the picture too much with drugs.

One of the quickest ways to comfort an allergic pet is with a relaxing bath. The effect doesn't last long but it does help to relieve itchiness. The bath water should be cool rather than hot since hot water can actually make the itchiness worse. Adding colloidal oatmeal powder or epsom salts to the bath water makes it even more soothing, and a variety of medicated shampoos available from veterinarians will also improve the situation. It is unlikely that a medicated bath will reduce itchiness for more than a couple of days, but it is a safe way to give your allergic pet some relief and it can be repeated frequently. Some newer forms of allergy shampoos even incorporate safe corticosteroids (e.g., FS Shampoo™, Dermagard™) that help provide symptomatic relief of itching. There are many safe sprays available from your veterinarian that can also give some temporary relief. If the allergies are complicated by infection, the infection may also be itchy; antibiotics are sometimes required.

Immunotherapy (allergy shots, hyposensitization, desensitization) is one of the best treatment options for allergic dogs, as it is in people.

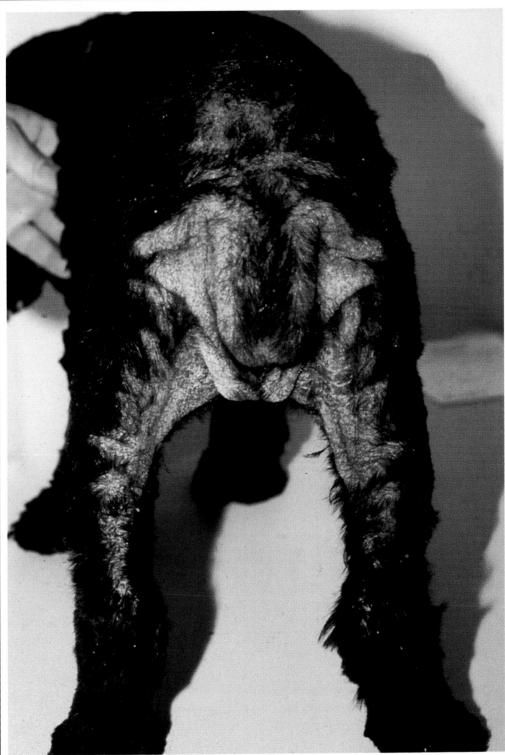

Clinical flea bite hypersensitivity (FBH) in a dog.

The main advantage is that it is very safe. The injections are given according to schedule and serve to increase the tolerance of pets so they become less sensitive to their allergies over time. Allergy shots work in the majority of cases, but not all, and it takes time for them to start working, usually six to eight months. In the meantime, it is often helpful to use other products to help give some relief.

Cortisone-based products, antihistamines and fatty-acid supplements help reduce the itchiness of allergies. Corticosteroids, which are cortisone-like compounds, are very helpful at reducing itchiness but they have a number of side effects when used long-term. Even cortisone-containing ointments and creams can be dangerous if used for more than about a week at a time. This is unfortunate because corticosteroids are very effective at treating the symptoms of allergy. Corticosteroids such as prednisone and triamcinolone can be used safely, but pets should be regularly monitored by their veterinarian when on treatment long-term. Most dogs on corticosteroids will have increased thirst, increased need to urinate and increased hunger; behavioral changes are not unusual and can be alarming. Long-term use may result in more widespread problems.

Antihistamines are sometimes useful in the treatment of inhalant allergies in dogs but they don't work well in the majority of cases. It appears that about one-third of allergic dogs may receive some benefit from antihistamines.

Combinations of omega-3 and omega-6 fatty acids are also sometimes effective and work for about one-fifth of total dogs. They are derived from fish oils and vegetable oils and are not the same products used to increase luster. They are predominantly available from veterinarians. Although neither antihistamines nor fatty acids work in the majority of cases, they are often combined and given as part of an allergy-treatment regimen, including allergy shots. The reason they're often used is a simple one—compared to corticosteroids, they are both incredibly safe.

One of the best things we could do for our allergic pets is to help them avoid the things they're allergic to. Unfortunately, this is rarely possible. We can use air cleaners and other equipment to make the air as clean as possible but it won't solve the whole problem. Individuals that are allergic need only inhale very small amounts of allergen to cause symptoms. When you consider that a simple ragweed plant can produce one billion pollen grains and that most pollens and molds can travel 30 miles in the wind, you can appreciate the problem. Our goal should therefore be to reduce, but not eliminate entirely, the airborne products that are causing our pets' problems. Because a home heating and cooling system can trap much dust, ducts and filters should be periodically cleaned. High-efficiency particulate air (HEPA) filters can clear over 95% of pollens, molds, yeasts, bacteria, and viruses in the air, and when coupled with a charcoal filter can remove most of the dust.

So, inhalant allergies are very common in dogs and there are many options for diagnosis and treatment.

Flea Allergy

Flea allergy, also known as flea bite hypersensitivity, is an allergic reaction to flea saliva. Not all dogs with fleas have flea allergy and, in fact, dogs most at risk are those that are only periodically exposed to fleas. There's a good chance that you'll never even see a flea on a truly flea-allergic dog!

CLINICAL SIGNS

In the flea-allergic dog, the bite of one flea every five to seven days will give you a continual problem. If you also keep in mind that for every flea you see on the dog, there's likely 100-300 nearby that you didn't see, you can appreciate the problems. It is thought that these dogs get so itchy from the flea bites that they tend to groom themselves meticulously by biting and chewing at themselves. This quickly removes the fleas so that they are difficult to find. Unfortunately, once the flea has bitten, the damage is already done even if it is immediately removed.

DIAGNOSIS

Even if you never see a flea, a diagnosis can be rendered with an appropriate allergy test. Rather than injecting pollens and molds, the test can be done with flea antigen and read in 15 minutes, then again in 48 hours.

THERAPY

Flea control in the flea-allergic dog is a real effort because even one flea bite can cause problems for up to one week. Killing the fleas with sprays, shampoos, and powders after it has already bitten the dog does not solve anything. We need to prevent the dog from being bitten in the first place.

Prevention can be attempted with a variety of insecticides and natural products, but the ideal way is to not let your dog contact any other animals that might be carrying fleas. This is possible if your pet is a house dog but very difficult if your dog is at all sociable with other animals.

Natural flea repellents include citrus oils, pennyroyal and eucalyptus, and these can be made into powders or sewn into cloth collars. They are not effective in all cases and just because they are natural does not mean they can be used without risk; poisonings have been reported with these products but are less common than with insecticides. A simple citrus preparation can be made at home by adding sliced lemons to a pot and steeping the concoction for at least 12 hours and then sponging the solution on the pet on a daily basis as needed. Although the use of garlic, sulfur and Brewer's yeast has been touted for generations as a natural repellent for parasites, this has never been demonstrated in scientific studies. Worse yet, these natural compounds hold risks of their own. Electronic flea collars promise high-tech flea control but reliable scientific studies have never shown them to be effective.

Some insecticides are better flea repellents than others and you should check with your veterinarian for recommendations. Most flea collars do not come close to meeting their claims as flea repellents. They work best when pets don't actually have fleas and may be sufficient control when contact with fleas is only intermittent. Unfortunately, if a flea bites a dog and then dies because of the insecticide in the collar, the damage has already been done.

Flea shampoos only kill fleas on the dog at the time of the bath and can not be relied upon to be helpful in case of flea allergy.

Allergy shots (immunotherapy) with flea antigen are a safe treatment option, but at present are helpful less than half the time. The reason is that current commercial sources are crude extracts; when a purified extract is available, immunotherapy for flea allergy will be a more rational approach.

Food Allergies and Food Intolerance

Food allergies account for about 10% of allergies in dogs and few topics in veterinary dermatology spawn as many misconceptions. Many people have difficulty believing that their dog could be allergic to a food that they have

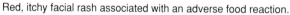
Red, itchy facial rash associated with an adverse food reaction.

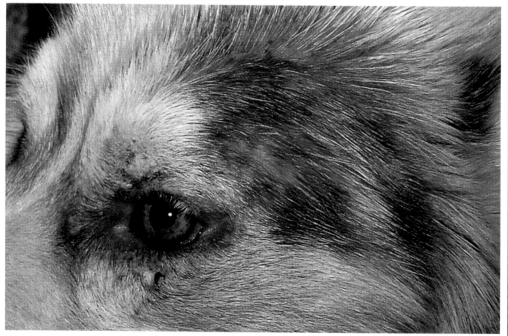

been feeding for years without problems. They find it difficult to believe a food allergy is possible because they feed only a premium dog food. Or, they may assume (wrongly) that it can't be a food allergy because their dog really likes that food. Many others test the theory by changing to another brand of dog food and, if the condition does not improve, conclude (wrongly) that the problem couldn't be food allergy. Finally, some don't believe their dog could be food allergic because they are feeding one of the new lamb-containing diets and they heard they were supposed to be good for allergic dogs.

Why all the confusion? Well, food allergies usually occur in dogs fed the same food for months or years and the problems often don't seem to coincide with mealtime. Food-allergic dogs react to beef or soy or corn or milk by-products and not to a brand name of food. Therefore, if your dog is allergic to corn and you change from Brand X to Brand Y, and both contain corn, don't expect to see a difference.

CLINICAL SIGNS

Most reactions to foods cause itchiness rather than diarrhea. In an itchy dog, it becomes extremely difficult to tell the difference between food allergy, inhalant allergy, and the effect of fleas, ticks or mites just by looking. One helpful clue is that the majority of food-allergic dogs have problems year 'round. If the problem only happened at certain times of the

year, inhalant allergies or parasite problems would be more likely.

Although this discussion concerns food allergy, you should be aware that there is a difference between food allergy and food intolerance. Many dogs, and people, have intolerances which don't allow them to properly digest foods such as milk or soy. This may result in diarrhea, flatulence or cramping but usually doesn't cause itchiness.

DIAGNOSIS

There is no easy way to prove a food allergy. The best way is with a hypoallergenic diet trial. The goal is to feed a diet, for a minimum of four weeks, to which the pet will not be allergic. How do we know which foods won't cause allergy? Well, the rule is that you can't be allergic to something you've never eaten before. Remember, we're talking ingredients, not brand names. If a dog has never eaten lamb, it can't be allergic to it. But, that doesn't mean that lamb is good for allergies. If your pet eats a lamb-based diet, it can develop allergies to the lamb as easily as to beef or any other ingredient. However, if the pet's condition improves on a reliable food trial, this implicates a problem in the diet. If improvement is not seen, the problem is unlikely to be food-related.

The most common way to do a food trial is to prepare a homemade diet with fresh ingredients, no colorings, no preservatives, and no other ingredients that we don't want. Lamb, rabbit and venison are commonly considered hypoallergenic protein sources, since they are not commonly found in commercial diets. There is nothing magical about lamb, rabbit or venison—we only consider them hypoallergenic if a dog has never been exposed to them before. Chicken, fish, pork, corn, and beef are all commonly used in many commercial foods and are therefore not helpful in a hypoallergenic diet trial.

The meal is prepared by mixing one part lamb, rabbit or venison (or other protein source to which the dog has never been exposed) to two parts rice and/or potatoes. All ingredients should be served boiled and fed in the same total volume as the pet's normal diet. Once cooked, the meal can be packaged in individual portions, frozen and then thawed as needed, greatly decreasing the need for cooking daily. During the trial, hypoallergenic foods and fresh, preferably distilled, water must be fed exclusive of all else. Remember, this diet is not to be fed long-term. It is not nutritionally balanced to be a regular diet. It is only fed for one to two months as a "test" diet.

Absolutely nothing else must be fed, such as treats, snacks, vitamins, chew toys and even flavored heartworm preventive tablets. Access must also be denied to food and feces of other dogs and cats in the household. If you are going to do the test, do it right so that you don't have to repeat it in the future.

Isn't there a simpler way of doing this? I heard something about blood tests. How about just feeding the new lamb-based diets available from food outlets? Sorry. The blood tests are terribly inaccurate when it comes to food allergies and the commercial lamb and rice diets only allow you to be 80% sure about the diagnosis. A full 20% of actual food-allergic dogs are just as bad on the commercial lamb diets as they are on their original food.

THERAPY

The treatment of choice for adverse food reactions is to feed a diet that does not contain the ingredient(s) that seem to be causing the problem. Commercial lamb, rabbit, venison, or egg-based diets are only worthwhile if an animal improves greatly during the homemade hypoallergenic diet trial. If not, they are no better than any other diet. Another alternative is to "challenge feed" your food-allergic dog with individual ingredients (e.g., beef, liver, pork, chicken, fish, corn, soy, wheat, milk, egg), one at a time, for five to seven days each, to determine which items are actually causing the problems.

Fortunately, food allergies do not seem to be inherited in the same fashion as inhalant allergies. However, be aware that some animals with intolerances, such as German Shepherd Dogs, Irish Setters, Schnauzers and Chinese Shar-Pei, may have problems (non-allergic) that they can pass on to future generations.

Contact Eruptions

Contact eruptions can be due to actual allergies, or more commonly, to irritants. Contact irritation can be caused by many different substances, from flea collars to shampoo ingredients. Other common causes are disinfectants, lawn chemicals, and salt on roadways.

Contact hypersensitivity (allergy) results when an ingredient contacts the skin and results in an immunologic reaction. In people, one of the most common examples is Rhus (poison ivy, poison oak) hypersensitivity. In general, dogs are less prone, because they have fur covering their bodies. Contact eruptions can only occur on those parts of the body that are sparsely covered with hair, such as the belly, scrotum, muzzle, and ears.

The causes of contact allergy are many and varied and don't occur to most people. For example, cement allergy has been reported in dogs (and people) and usually occurs due to a sensitivity to dichromates and nickel. Plants (e.g. Wandering Jew, Asian Jasmine, Oleander) may also be the cause of contact eruption in dogs. Other causes are medicated shampoos, rubber, plastics, dishwashing liquid, carpet deodorizer, cedar wood chips, leather, and insecticides.

CLINICAL SIGNS

Like many forms of allergy, contact eruptions cause a rash. Often, the rash is restricted to the area where the culprit contacted the skin. Therefore, there may be redness seen on the sparsely haired parts of the body if fabrics or foliage are involved. A flea collar contact eruption is typically seen as a ring around the neck where the flea collar was applied. Sometimes shampoos and other topicals can cause more widespread reactions because they can soak through the fur to the skin.

DIAGNOSIS

Contact eruption is difficult to diagnose in dogs because it is rarely suspected as a likely cause of skin problems. Also, the patch tests that are routinely used for people are hard to apply to dogs. A variety of these ingredients need to be applied to a shaved area of skin under a gauze bandage and evaluated in 48 and 96 hours. It is often difficult to stop dogs from removing the patch during this interval.

THERAPY

There is only one sensible treatment for contact eruption—avoid the problematic substance. If a dog has a reaction to a shampoo, dishwashing liquid, or flea collar the treatment is relatively easy. However, if a dog is allergic to a ground cover plant, or cement, and this is its normal environment, treatment can be difficult. These dogs benefit from frequent shampooing to remove contact allergens, and minimizing exposure as much as possible. Most drugs (including corticosteroids) do little to relieve the symptoms of contact eruption.

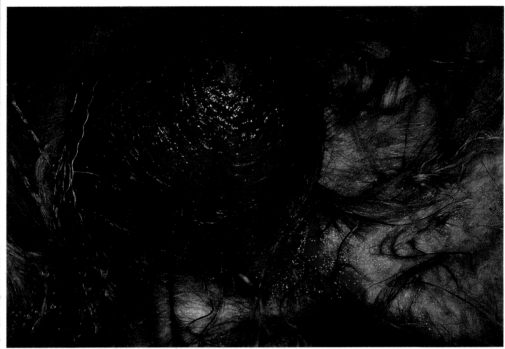

Contact eruption on the scrotum of a dog.

Bacterial infection (folliculitis) in a dog.

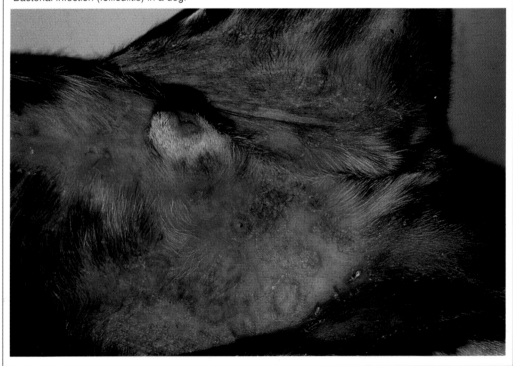

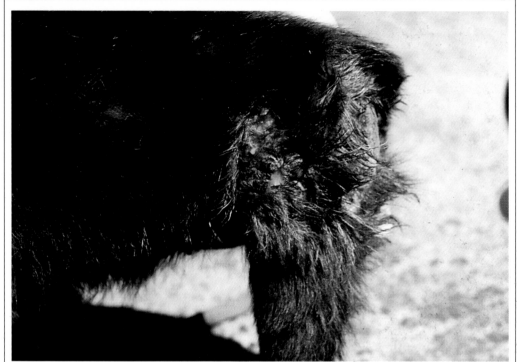

Deep bacterial infection (pyoderma) in a dog.

Bacteria (*Staphylococcus*) growing on a Pyo-Dermplate. Courtesy of Bacti-lab, Mountain View, California.

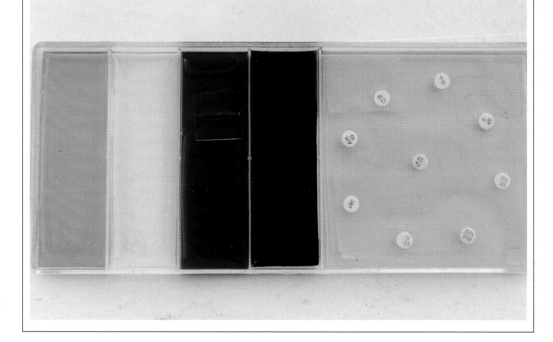

Bacterial Infections

Most bacterial infections in dogs are caused by a bacterium called *Staphylococcus*, or "Staph" for short. It is important to realize that this microbe is present on normal animals and is not really contagious. Thus, animals which have a problem with this organism have an underlying problem which allows the microbes to flourish on the skin surface. These bacteria are not contagious to other dogs or to people. When dogs get recurrent Staph infections, we have to ask an important question—"Why does Staph cause problems in this dog and not in most others?" The answer that is correct most of the time is that the Staph needs help to cause problems. Something else needs to be causing problems in this dog that interferes with its own ability to keep the bacteria under control. Some of the more common reasons for recurrent infections are underlying allergies, immune problems, hormonal problems, seborrhea and parasites. Unless these underlying problems are sorted out, the bacterial infections are likely to clear with an appropriate antibiotic but recur shortly after the drug has been discontinued.

Most dogs that develop Staph infections develop a condition that is often referred to as "pyoderma." Pyoderma really doesn't mean much other than there might be pus production. Folliculitis only means that the infection involves the hair follicles. Similarly, dermatitis only means that there is inflammation in the skin. We know this. What we really want to know is ...why?

CLINICAL SIGNS

Bacterial infections can be present in many different ways. There may be pimples on the sparsely haired regions of the belly. There may be cyst-like structures between the toes. The ears may be red and inflamed. There may be deep, oozing tracts and firm lumps in the skin. There may be localized inflamed patches of skin that are often referred to as "hot spots." We can use many terms to describe all of these presentations, but the most important thing we can do is uncover why they are happening at all. A normal dog with a normal immune system is very resistant to Staph infections.

DIAGNOSIS

Any recurrent Staph infection warrants a thorough workup to look for underlying problems that might be contributory. Inhalant allergies and food allergies are common underlying causes, as are inherited immune problems, seborrheic skin conditions and hypothyroidism. We can usually treat the infection with appropriate antibiotics but, if we haven't figured out why it happened in the first place, we should expect the infection to return when the drugs run out. The more times we use antibiotics, the more likely we are to develop resistance or have drug-related side effects.

Diagnosis of pyoderma appears straightforward—just culture the skin and see what grows. This is not as easy as it sounds because there are normally all kinds of bacteria on the skin surface, including Staph, and just because something grows does not mean it's the root of the problem.

Chronic, recurring infections require careful veterinary examination and, if long-term, a referral to a dermatology specialist. Many tests may be indicated to try to uncover the "real" problem. This is not always an easy task. Testing for inhalant or food allergies may be necessary, but often the first tests involve scraping the skin, examining the stool for possible parasites and running some basic blood tests to make sure that everything is functioning normally inside. Specific tests for thyroid and immune function may also be needed. Certain breeds are at risk for certain specific disorders and so these are usually selected as the individual case warrants.

THERAPY

The treatment for recurrent Staph infections can be easy or difficult, depending on what the underlying cause is and whether it can be corrected or controlled. For instance, a dog with infection because of a thyroid-hormone deficiency should recover entirely when supplemented with the appropriate thyroid hormone. An allergic dog with recurrent infections will recover when the allergies have been controlled.

If an underlying problem has not been identified, the options are limited. Some dogs are maintained on long-term antibiotics, but this is not desirable because of the possibility of resistance and the expense of most antibiotics. Antiseptic shampoos are an excellent option to help decrease the bacterial population on the skin surface but must be used frequently (once to twice per week) to be effective. Another option is to try to "boost" your dog's immune system with immune stimulants. Most of these are given as a series of injections, like allergy shots, but some tablets are available as well that might help. If you keep in mind that no form of treatment will make your dog's skin sterile, and that it was never intended to be so, you will appreciate how important it is to determine the ultimate cause and select the most appropriate treatment.

The Non-pyodermas

There are many conditions in dermatology that we see diagnosed as pyoderma, implying a bacterial cause, that really aren't bacterial at all. You might find this confusing, but many problems originally believed to be due to infection have been found to be due to other causes.

Interdigital pyoderma or interdigital cysts, in which sores are found between the toes, have never seemed to respond well to antibiotics, and we never really knew why. It now appears that few if any of these are actually cysts, and that bacteria may not even be the primary problem. Although the exact cause is still a matter of debate, many of these cases respond better to anti-inflammatory therapy than to antibiotics. Additional research is definitely needed.

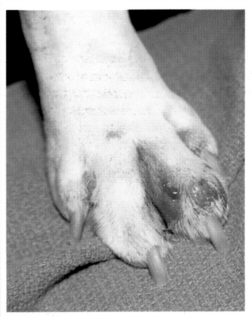

Interdigital pyoderma due to sterile pyogranuloma syndrome. Courtesy of Dr. Thomas Lewis, Dermatology Clinic for Animals, Albuquerque, New Mexico.

Perianal fistulae in a German Shepherd Dog.

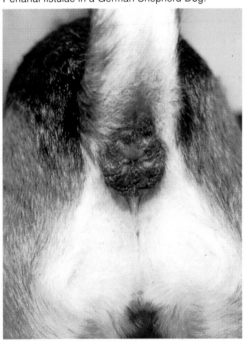

Nasal pyoderma refers to an infection on the bridge of the nose. It was often blamed on "rooting" behavior in dogs with long noses (Collies, German Shepherd Dogs) but the condition responds only poorly to antibiotics. Although the exact cause is not known, immune disorders are often suspected.

Acne, in dogs as in people, is not simply a bacterial problem. Certain breeds, such as the Great Dane, Doberman Pinscher, Bulldog and Bull Terrier, are particularly at risk, but any animal may be affected. Treatment should involve frequent scrubbing of the area with antiseptics; the condition often improves somewhat when animals reach about three years of age.

Callus pyoderma is an infection of the hard calluses that develop on the elbows and hocks of some large breeds of dogs, including the Great Dane and St. Bernard, and on the chest of other breeds, including the Dachshund and Doberman Pinscher. They result from repeated impact as dogs drop onto a hard surface, usually when lying down. The best results are achieved when these areas are protected or "cushioned" and when antiseptics are used to cleanse the areas affected.

Perianal pyoderma, also known as perianal fistulae, is most commonly seen in German Shepherd Dogs and Irish Setters and involves the presence of draining tracts around the anus. The lack of lasting response to antibiotics has led most researchers to the conclusion that

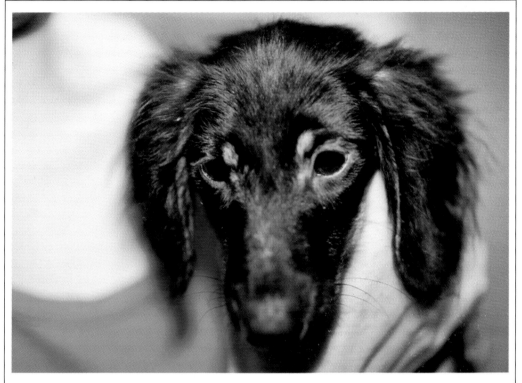

Above and below: Scaling and hair loss in a young dog with dermatophytosis (ringworm).

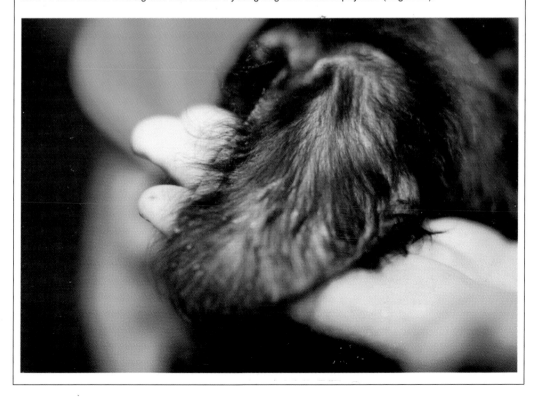

the problem is not wholly the result of bacteria. Different surgical techniques have been employed to remove the affected tissues, with only marginal success. No doubt once the condition is better understood, improved forms of therapy will become available.

FUNGAL INFECTIONS

Dermatophytosis (Ringworm)

Ringworm is an old term for a superficial fungal infection caused by certain microbes. Considering the fact that there are no worms involved at all, and that the pattern of infection is rarely one of a ring, it is surprising that the name "ringworm" has held on as long as it has. The more correct term for this infection is dermatophytosis.

Dermatophytosis means infection with dermatophytes; dermatophytes (which means "skin fungi") refers to special fungi that are capable of causing problems in animals and people. Not just any fungus can cause dermatophytosis; in dogs and cats, three species, *Microsporum canis*, *Microsporum gypseum*, and *Trichophyton mentagrophytes* account for over 95% of all cases. All of these are contagious between people and pets.

CLINICAL SIGNS

Dermatophytosis is often a difficult diagnosis to make in dogs unless owners have the characteristic rash. The fact is that many people do not develop any rash when exposed to dermatophytes.

Similarly many dogs and cats can be carriers of dermatophytosis yet show no symptoms themselves. Dermatophytosis may cause no problem whatsoever, or display changes that vary from hairless patches to scaling, to an inflamed rash, to actual lumps. These differences reflect the activities of the immune system. Those animals with the fewest symptoms likely have the most fungi.

Dermatophyte infections may resolve on their own over months to years, but, since spores released into the environment may last for 18 months and are contagious to people, it is important to identify and treat animals quickly. Any building or room in which infected animals have been housed could potentially be a source of infection. Brushes, bedding, transport cages, and other paraphernalia are all potential sources of infection or reinfection. Fungi have even been cultured from dust, heating vents, and furnace filters.

DIAGNOSIS

Fungal culture is the most accurate way to diagnose dermatophytosis in animals although it may take up to three weeks to recover the organisms. Wood's lamp evaluation with a special ultraviolet light is more helpful in people and identifies infection in animals less than 50% of the time. When it does work, however, it does give a quick answer. All suspect cases should be cultured to help determine how the infection was acquired, because

Wood's lamp diagnosis is often wrong.

Fungal culture is the most reliable method of confirming dermatophytosis. It may take as long as three weeks to identify fungi by this method. Anything that grows on the culture plate should be identified by microscopic examination. Most samples are collected by plucking suspicious hairs for culture, but, when there are no symptoms at all, we might use a sterile toothbrush to comb through the haircoat and then touch the bristles to the culture surface.

THERAPY

The significance of dermatophytosis may vary from a mild inconvenience to major skin disease. Treatment depends on a number of criteria and varies with the individual animal. Mild infections are self-limiting and may spontaneously regress; others are chronic, debilitating and poorly responsive to therapy. The aim of treatment is to clear the infection, prevent the spread of infection to other animals and people, and decontaminate the environment to prevent future infections.

It is advisable to clip the haircoat as short as possible (the fungi are located in the hair follicles) and to use antiseptic cleansers twice weekly. Preferred ingredients include chlorhexidine, iodine, lime sulfur, and clotrimazole. It is important to treat all animals in the household once to twice weekly until the problem is controlled (at least six weeks). In Europe, enilconazole (Imaverol-Janssen) can be used as a wash, in a dilution of 1:50 on four occasions at three-day intervals.

When stronger measures are needed, we often rely on oral medicines designed to kill fungi from the inside out. Griseofulvin is the most common medication used, and treatment must go well beyond apparent clinical cure (at least six weeks). Griseofulvin can cause birth defects and should not be given to pregnant animals. Ketoconazole is sometimes used in very chronic or resistant cases.

It is relatively easy to kill dermatophyte fungi on hard surfaces and a 1:10 dilution of household bleach will kill these organisms on contact. This is suitable for kennels, cages, litterboxes, floors, and walls. Cages should be cleaned once daily with a 1:4 dilution of chlorhexidine solution, which is available from veterinarians. Brushes, bedding, combs, and toys should be disinfected or destroyed.

The biggest problem of premise disinfection is dealing with contamination of carpets and furniture. Remember that hairs shed into the environment that contain fungal spores may be infectious for up to 18 months. Carpeted areas and furniture should be vacuumed at least once weekly, and the vacuum bag should be discarded after each use. Steam cleaning carpets will not eliminate fungi unless combined with an antifungal disinfectant.

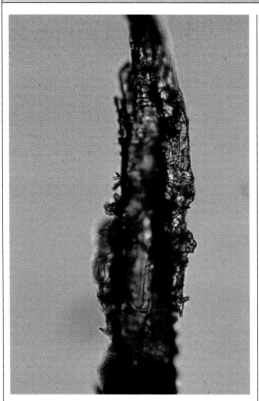

All heating and cooling vents should be vacuumed and disinfected. Furnaces should be cleaned by a commercial company with high-power suction equipment and filters should be changed frequently.

A new compound, enilconazole (Clinafarm-Janssen) has recently become available in Europe for environmental cleaning of dog kennels. This would be a sensible approach for kennel facilities, when the product is available in North America.

Left: Microscopic view of a hair parasitized by dermatophytes. The hair shaft has been distorted by the presence of fungal spores and hyphae.
Below: Dermatophytes grow as white fluffy colonies. Here is *Microsporum canis* growing on a Sab-Duet plate. On the left is Dermatophyte Test Medium (DTM) and on the right is Sabouraud's agar. Courtesy of Bacti-lab, Mountain View, California.

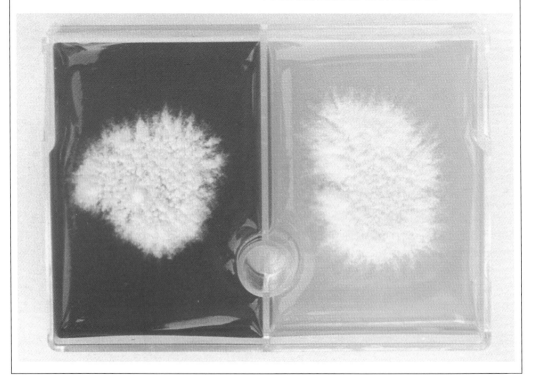

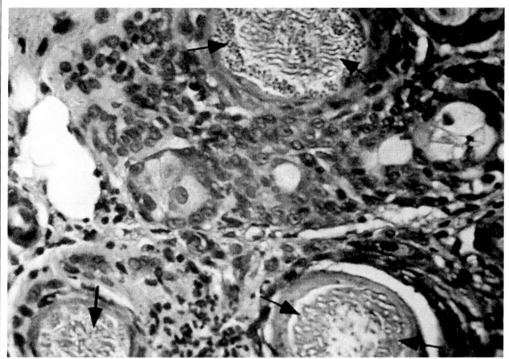

Biopsy specimens showing fungal spores (arrows) within hair follicles.

At the center of the picture are a pair of Blastomyces organisms, the cause of blastomycosis.

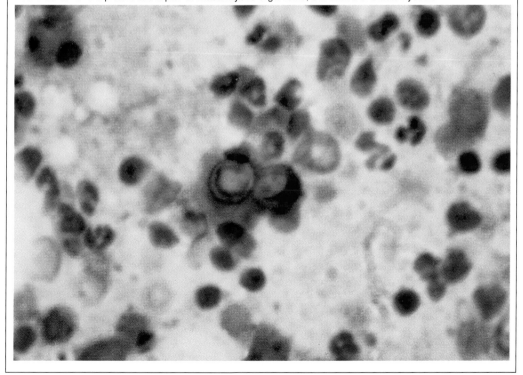

VACCINES

There may be a new option on the horizon for helping to prevent dermatophytosis. Recently a ringworm vaccine has been marketed for use in cats (Fel-O-Vax: Fort Dodge). This particular vaccine is an inactivated (killed) preparation of *Microsporum canis*, the most common cause of ringworm in both dogs and cats. The product is so new that the results are only preliminary. The company claims that the incidence of ringworm decreases significantly in infected catteries following vaccination but this has not been verified by independent sources. At present, the vaccine is only licensed for use in adult cats and is not intended for use in dogs.

Yeast Infections

Yeast infections have become a popular topic in veterinary dermatology. Whereas humans are primarily plagued by *Candida albicans*, the yeast most commonly recovered from dogs is called *Malassezia pachydermatis*. Prior to 1991, a diagnosis of Malassezia dermatitis was rarely made in dogs.

The reason why some dogs should get yeast infections while most don't is the subject of much debate. Most cases are seen in dogs of certain breeds, and those with keratinization disorders (seborrhea), allergies, or those that received long-term antibiotic therapy. Breeds at particular risk are West Highland White Terriers, Basset Hounds, and Dachshunds. The yeasts are thought to cause skin problems by several different mechanisms and some dogs may even develop hypersensitivities (allergies) to them.

CLINICAL SIGNS

Malassezia dermatitis usually presents an itchy condition that only partially respond to antibiotics or corticosteroids. Affected areas of the skin are either dry or oily and may be red, dark, thickened and/ or hairless. The areas most commonly affected are the face, neck, armpits (axillae), groin, legs, and feet. Greasy infected ears are also frequently reported. Thus, most cases are commonly misdiagnosed as allergies or keratinization disorders (seborrhea).

DIAGNOSIS

The yeast organisms can be demonstrated on biopsy or cytologic "yeast preps." Swabs taken from the skin, impression smears, or skin scrapings can be prepared and appropriately stained to reveal the peanut-shaped yeasts.

The presence of yeasts alone does not confirm a diagnosis because small numbers of yeasts can be found on most normal healthy dogs, especially in the ear canals. In those cases in which yeast is believed to be clinically important, large numbers of organisms are typically recovered.

THERAPY

The treatment of these yeast infections in dogs are typically accomplished with oral antifungal medications, special shampoos, and topical creams and ointments.

Ketoconazole, the drug used to treat deep fungal infections, is often effective in controlling Malassezia dermatitis. The doses required for this purpose are lower than for deep fungal infections but typically need to be given for 30-60 days.

Several new shampoo therapies are available for treating this condition. Most contain one of the following: ketoconazole, miconazole, chlorhexidine, selenium sulfide, or povidone/iodine. Whichever shampoo is chosen, it needs to be used two or three times a week allowing for ten minutes of contact time before being rinsed off.

Spot treatment is sometimes sufficient for localized infections, especially those of the ear canal. Creams and ointments for this purpose usually contain miconazole, clotrimazole or ketoconazole. They are used once to twice daily, often for one-to-two months.

Regardless of the therapy used, recurrences are common because the organism is a normal inhabitant of dog skin and is difficult to eliminate. The best chance to prevent a relapse is to determine the underlying cause (keratinization disorder, allergy) and correct it.

Deep Fungal Infections

Dermatophytosis only involves the most superficial aspects of the skin, but several fungi can involve a variety of internal organs and can be life-threatening.

Most of these deep fungal infections are not contagious between animals and people but are picked up as spores from the environment. Most of these infections are caused by inhaling spores from the ground into the lungs and from there the infection can move to other tissues.

Five of the most dangerous fungal infections dogs can pick up from the environment include: blastomycosis, coccidioidomycosis, cryptococcosis, histoplasmosis and sporotrichosis. Blastomycosis is more common in areas drained by rivers in the eastern United States and Canada. Coccidioidomycosis (valley fever) is more common in the southwestern United States and Central and South America. Histoplasmosis is most prevalent around the Great Lakes and the Mississippi, St. Lawrence and Ohio River Valleys. Cryptococcosis is often spread in pigeon droppings and both it and sporotrichosis have no regional preference.

CLINICAL SIGNS

Most of the deep fungal infections cause respiratory infections such as pneumonia because they are contracted by breathing in infectious spores. The infections might seem mild at first, but in time the condition tends to worsen.

Although we tend to concentrate on the respiratory symptoms associated with these conditions, there are many other clinical signs that might occur. For instance, many dogs with coccidioidomycosis may have problems with lameness because this organism tends to concentrate in the bones. Dogs with blastomycosis may have eye problems because the fungal organisms may target this tissue as well as others. Histoplasmosis often causes digestive disorders because it tends to concentrate on the intestines. Cryptococcosis may cause neurological problems because it tends to congregate in and around the brain, spinal cord, and other nervous tissues.

Animals with systemic fungal infections may have a fever and it is not uncommon that they be lethargic and tend to lose weight. Often the lymph nodes increase in size as the body tries to combat the infection on its own.

All of the deep fungal infections can cause skin problems, most noticeably lumps and bumps that might tend to discharge pus and fluid. Of the four principal organisms that cause systemic disease, blastomyces and coccidioides are more likely to cause skin problems in dogs than cryptococcus or histoplasma.

DIAGNOSIS

The only way to absolutely confirm a diagnosis is to find organisms present. This is accomplished by biopsying suspicious areas or by collecting material from discharging lumps and examining it with a microscope for evidence of the fungi. There are many different ways that samples can be collected for assessment. Biopsies take actual chunks of tissues that pathologists can then prepare and evaluate. Needle biopsies can be used to sample tissues from diseased bone and internal organs. Or, if animals have skin problems, discharge can be applied directly to a microscope slide, stained to highlight organisms, and evaluated without delay.

In many instances, actual organisms cannot be found or it is not possible to collect tissues for analysis. In these cases, blood tests and chest radiographs (x-rays) are taken to help support a diagnosis. Often, affected animals have some degree of pneumonia with some characteristic changes that might help confirm the diagnosis.

There are blood tests which can be used to screen for the systemic fungal infections. The most specific tests are often the agar gel immunodiffusion tests, which have a high degree of accuracy. The more commonly used, and less expensive, complement-fixation tests are often suggestive, but not without their own problems. For example, with complement fixation tests, there are cross reactions between blastomycosis and histoplasmosis. Also, about 25% of dogs have blood on which this test cannot be properly evaluated (anticomplementary).

Blood tests are convenient but must be interpreted with some caution. One test alone only provides a small piece of the puzzle. For example, in dogs with valley fever (coccidioidomycosis), the agar gel immunodiffusion test (AGID) is usually positive early in the course of infection, and the complement fixation (CF) test at this time is usually negative. Later on, during active infection, both tests tend to be positive. However, later in the disease the AGID test tends to become negative while the CF test remains positive for many months. This is why veterinarians like to run a battery of tests to get the most information possible. A single test may provoke more questions than answers.

THERAPY

The newer treatments for these infections are quite effective but it still may take months or years to overcome infection. Ketoconazole is generally regarded as the drug of choice although newer derivatives are constantly being explored. The old treatment was amphotericin B which needed to be given intravenously. Although it was successful in many cases, it was also profoundly toxic for the kidneys and liver. All treatments have some side effects of their own and this must be considered as well.

KERATINIZATION DISORDERS (SEBORRHEA)

Seborrhea is not a specific diagnosis in dogs but rather a descriptive term, like rash, eczema or dermatitis. Any dog that has greasy, dry or smelly skin can be called seborrheic, but that doesn't tell you anything about the cause

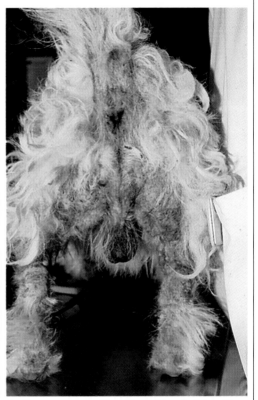

Scaling associated with epidermal dysplasia in a West Highland White Terrier.

of the condition. You should be aware that dozens of different skin diseases can result in seborrhea and, unless you identify the correct course, treatment is likely to be disappointing.

A better term than seborrhea is "keratinization disorder" which correctly identifies the problem as a disorder of the keratinization process, not of sebum. One of the main reasons why the term seborrhea has held on so long is that "keratinization disorder" is quite a mouthful and not as familiar to most people as "seborrhea." Keratinization is the process of orderly turnover of the skin from the bottom of the epidermis to the top of the epidermis and its finally shedding as dead skin. In the normal dog, it takes about three weeks for skin cells to make their way from the bottom of the epidermis to the top; the dead cells may stay in place for another three weeks before eventually being shed. In the dog with a keratinization disorder, this process may dramatically speed up and the scaling occurs in a disorganized arrangement.

CLINICAL SIGNS

Dogs with keratinization disorders (seborrhea) have scaling on their skin surface and combined with surface microbes, often have infections, greasiness, smelly skin and dandruff. This "speeding up" of the keratinization process may be caused by a variety of problems, including allergies, hormonal problems, nutritional imbalances, immune problems or hereditary defects.

Certain breeds, such as the West Highland White Terrier and the Miniature Schnauzer, may have hereditary reasons for their scaling, which are often referred to as epidermal dysplasia and schnauzer comedo syndrome, respectively. Cocker Spaniels may be more susceptible to vitamin A-related imbalances and Siberian Huskies and Malamutes to zinc-related imbalances but the vast majority of seborrheic dogs have allergies. Many breeds are susceptible to hypothyroidism and seborrhea may be a manifestation of this as well. Immune-mediated diseases such

as pemphigus may be more common in Collies and Shetland Sheepdogs, and sebaceous adenitis is more common in Standard Poodles. Finally, dermatophytes (ringworm) and a variety of parasites can also cause seborrhea. All of these conditions may be impossible to distinguish simply by looking. Finally, some dogs may truly have seborrhea.

DIAGNOSIS

The diagnosis of keratinization disorders must therefore be an orderly process of carefully evaluating when and how the condition started, which breed is involved, how the condition has evolved and whether or not there are any other symptoms. Then, a variety of tests will be necessary which might include skin scrapings for parasites, fungal culture, biopsies to see what is going on in the skin, and a battery of routine and specific blood tests.

THERAPY

There is no specific treatment for seborrhea but hopefully, if the true cause is determined, successful therapy is possible. For animals in which a diagnosis can not be rendered, lifelong therapy with medicated shampoos and medications will likely be necessary. Some newer drugs, now available for the treatment of psoriasis in people (e.g., etretinate), have helped dogs with keratinization disorders of undetermined cause.

It is important to remember that

keratinization disorders may have an underlying cause such as allergies or hypothyroidism. The condition might therefore clear on its own if the underlying problem is addressed.

There has been much attention given to several specific conditions such as sebaceous adenitis and epidermal dysplasia. These appear to be strongly breed-related and may have an inherited nature. The biggest problem we have in making generalizations about their treatment is that they may not reflect the same condition in all breeds. Therefore, what works in treating sebaceous adenitis in Standard Poodles will not necessarily have the same effect in Vizslas. Successful treatments have ranged from essential fatty-acid supplements, to synthetic vitamin A derivatives (retinoids), to drugs that suppress the immune system (e.g., cyclosporine). Each patient should be managed as an individual and referral to a dermatologist familiar with the different breed tendencies is strongly advised.

EXTERNAL PARASITES

Fleas

Fleas are incredible products of evolutionary magic. Under ideal conditions they can complete their life cycle in three weeks and their pupal (cocoon) stage can survive for up to 20 months without feeding. Fleas can jump 300,000 times without stopping and can jump 150 times their length vertically or horizontally. This is equivalent to a man jumping the length of three football fields. Their acceleration at takeoff (140 G's) is 50 times that of a space shuttle after lift-off. Because most insecticides don't kill the immature forms which may be in the household, treating a dog only and not its environment is bound to end in failure.

There are many misconceptions about fleas that need to be addressed if control is to be effective. Fleas do not spend 90% of their time off the pet as is often reported in books and magazines. The cat flea (*Ctenocephalides felis*), which is the most common flea of both dogs and cats, starts feeding soon after it makes contact with a dog. It will then mate within the next two days. After that time, the flea is dependent on the dog for life support. A typical female flea will consume 15 times her body weight in blood during active reproduction. But, if a flea is removed from a dog after feeding, it will generally die within one to two days. Unfortunately, flea eggs are laid on the dog, but are not sticky, so fall off into the environment. These eggs provide a continual supply of fleas to plague house pets. A single female may deposit over 2,000 eggs during her lifetime, as many as 40 eggs per day.

Although most of the discussion needs to focus on the cat flea (*Ctenocephalides felis*), there are some other species of flea that also affect dogs. The dog flea (*Ctenocephalides canis*) is the most common flea of dogs in some parts

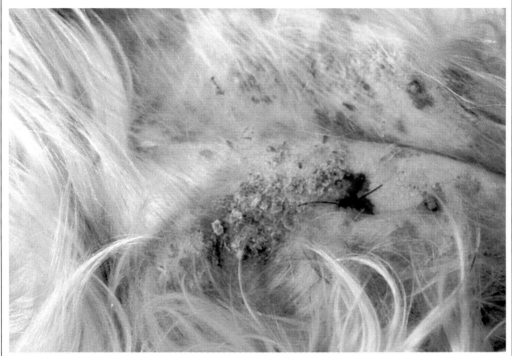

Scaling associated with a primary keratinization disorder in a Cocker Spaniel. A suture is present and marks the biopsy site used in diagnostic testing.

Scaling associated with a secondary keratinization disorder.

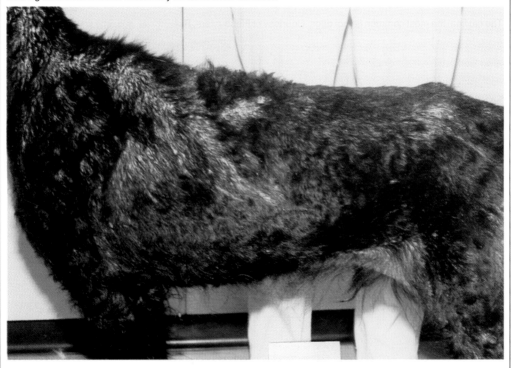

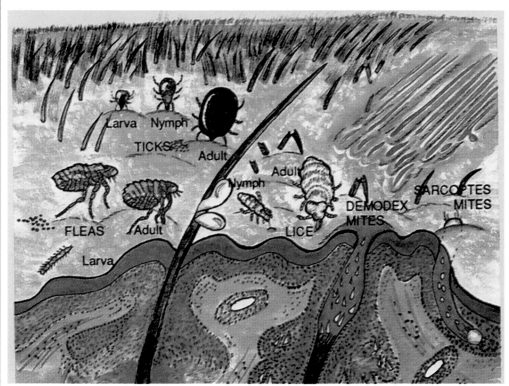

External parasites. Courtesy of Petcom, Inc.

The cat flea, the most common flea of dogs. Courtesy of Fleabusters, Rx for Fleas, Inc., Ft. Lauderdale, Florida.

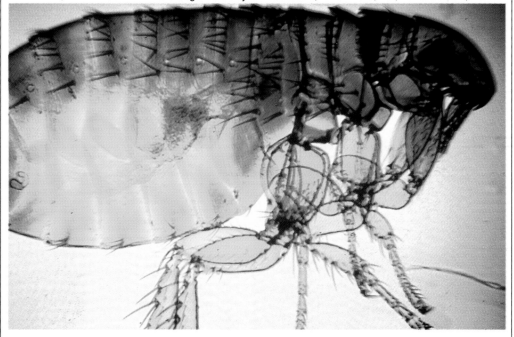

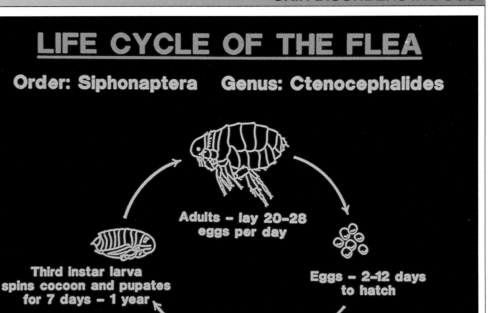

Life Cycle of the Flea. Courtesy of Fleabusters, Rx for Fleas, Inc., Ft. Lauderdale, Florida.

Normal Flea Population. Courtesy of Fleabusters, Rx for Fleas, Inc., Ft. Lauderdale, Florida.

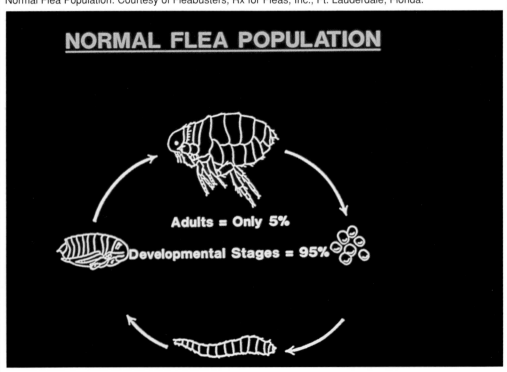

of Europe and in New Zealand. It is recovered in lesser numbers in North America. *Pulex irritans*, the human flea, and *Echidnophaga gallinacea*, the bird flea, can also account for infestations of dogs. Several other species of flea can temporarily reside on dogs. It is not unusual to find rabbit, rodent, or squirrel fleas on dogs that roam outdoors. These fleas often survive for only a short time on dogs and most likely do not remain reproductively active. They are therefore not a significant cause of infestation in dogs.

Where do most of the fleas come from? Fleas don't do well at high altitudes, low relative humidities, or when temperatures are very high (95°F) or very low (40°F). Developing larvae are relatively intolerant of cold and cannot survive freezing temperatures for more than a few days. But, they can do quite well indoors. Outside, the fleas normally reside on untreated dogs or cats, or on wild mammals such as raccoons and opossums. When these animals travel near homes in the spring, the eggs may fall off and develop in the environment. Newly emergent fleas are attracted by warmth, movement, and exhaled carbon dioxide from passing dogs and cats. And the cycle continues!

CLINICAL SIGNS

Not all dogs infested with fleas have problems. For others, however, the bite of only one flea is enough to make them scratch for five to seven days. The most common areas affected by fleas are the base of the tail, the back, the neck, and the belly. There is often evidence of itching and hair loss in the areas most commonly affected.

Fleas are large enough to be seen without magnification but they are unlikely to stay still when you're searching for them. They tend to scurry through the fur and so might be difficult to find. On dogs with flea infestation, however, the fleas are often quite numerous and not difficult to find.

DIAGNOSIS

A flea comb is a very handy device for recovering fleas from pets. Animals suspected of being infested should be combed for several minutes over their entire body, and the material collected should be examined with a hand lens. Fleas collected should be dropped into a container of alcohol, which quickly kills them before they can escape. Not finding evidence of fleas does not mean that they are not causing problems.

THERAPY

Flea control requires simultaneous treatment of all pets in the household, the indoor environment and possibly the outdoors. The less you allow your dog to contact other dogs and cats, the easier it will be to control the flea problem.

Flea collars, whether standard or electronic, will rarely get the job done when it comes to flea control. Also, flea shampoos will not do it— their effect is gone as soon as

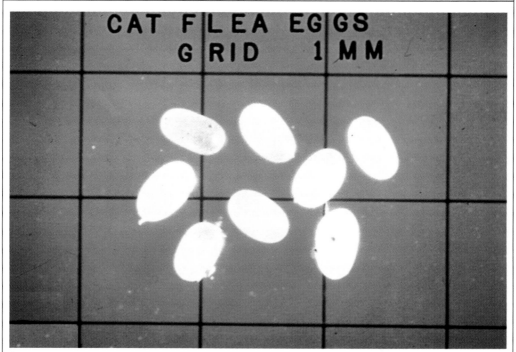

Cat flea eggs. Courtesy of Fleabusters, Rx for Fleas, Inc., Ft. Lauderdale, Florida.

Cat flea larvae. Eggs hatch in two to 14 days into tiny, whitish maggot-like larvae. Courtesy of Fermenta Animal Health, Kansas City, Missouri.

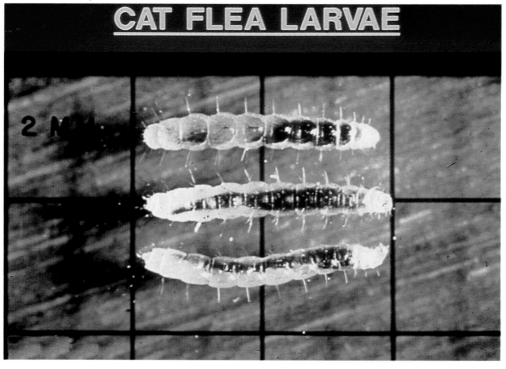

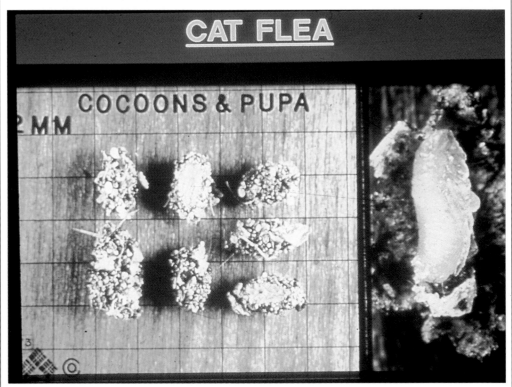

Cat flea cocoons and pupa. Larval fleas complete development in about three weeks and spin a cocoon which marks the pupal stage. Courtesy of Fermenta Animal Health, Kansas City, Missouri.

Dogs with fleas are often itchy even when they don't have hypersensitivity reactions. Courtesy of Fleabusters, Rx for Fleas, Inc., Ft. Lauderdale, Florida.

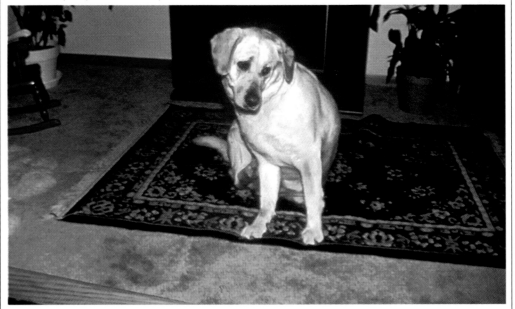

they're rinsed off. Any treatment that is going to work is going to have to involve treating the dog and its environment as well as repeating the treatment frequently enough to kill fleas that are hatching or being introduced from outdoors.

First, all animals in the household should be bathed with a cleansing shampoo to remove dirt and fleas and then a dip or the use of powders or sprays is needed to give some long-lasting effect. If you like natural products, consider adding sliced lemons to a pot of hot water and steeping the concoction for at least 12 hours, then sponging the solution on the pet on a daily basis as needed. The most useful and safe flea-control sprays contain both an insecticide (such as the safe pyrethrins and pyrethroids) together with an insect growth regulator, such as fenoxycarb or methoprene.

To clean up the household, vacuuming is a good first step but is not sufficient without some home treatment. Vacuuming stimulates flea pupae to emerge as adults, where they are easier to kill with insecticides. Also the vacuuming, if regular and thorough, will remove many eggs and pupae from the home environment. The vacuum bag should then be removed and discarded with each treatment.

Once vacuuming has been completed, the best approach is to use a safe insecticide to kill adult fleas in the house and then an insect growth regulator to stop the eggs and larvae in the environment.

Many veterinary-dispensed products combine the insecticide and insect growth regulator in a single product. The best way to apply these products is with a hand-pump sprayer or pressurized aerosol delivery system. Foggers can be used, but a sprayer is still useful to get at high-traffic areas and locations where the fogger aerosol may not penetrate (e.g., under tables, couches, etc.). When using foggers, it is best to use one for each room rather than relying on adequate dispersal throughout the entire home. In severe infestations, a second treatment with a safe insecticide should be performed in two to three weeks. The insect growth regulators (IGR's) are a marvelous new addition to our arsenal against fleas and are almost completely non-toxic.

In some new flea-control formulation, insect growth regulators are being given orally. They interfere with the development of chitin in the flea egg case and cuticle. Most affected flea eggs fail to hatch, and of those that do hatch, surviving larval stages fail to develop. One such product, lufenuron (Program: Ciba) is given orally, on a monthly basis, starting at least one month before the onset of flea season and continued throughout the entire flea season. Treatment is continued year 'round in areas where fleas are present throughout the year. Fleas are affected when they bite a dog and ingest the insect growth regulator. Since the products are not insecticides, the fleas don't die, but the eggs they produce do not give rise to more fleas. Since these products do not kill adult fleas, a safe insecticide (e.g., pyrethrins) should be periodically used.

Another option for home treatment is borax-containing preparations, which are currently being marketed across the country. These work best in home environments which are at least 40% carpeted. These products are safe and usually quite effective. However, at present, they are neither safer nor less expensive than the combination of insect growth regulators and pyrethrin-based insecticides.

When an insecticide is combined with an insect growth regulator, flea control is most likely to be successful. The insecticide kills the adult fleas and the insect growth regulator affects the eggs and larvae. However, insecticides kill less than 20% of flea cocoons (pupae). Because of this, new fleas may hatch in two to three weeks despite appropriate application of products. This is known as the "pupal window" and is one of the most common causes for ineffective flea control. To combat this effect, an insecticide should be applied to the home environment two to three weeks after the initial treatment.

If treatment of the outdoor environment is needed, most products need to be applied once or twice at ten-day intervals, then on a monthly basis for maintenance. A good strategy is to alternate products since resistance is becoming a more recognized problem in flea control. Another option is to add appropriate borax-containing products outside but be careful that they are not inadvertently eaten by pets. Some of the new insect growth regulators (e.g., fenoxycarb) are stable in sunlight so can be used outdoors in combination with an insecticide. It is not necessary to treat the entire property. Flea control should be directed predominantly at garden margins, porches, dog houses, garages, and in other pet lounging areas. Fleas don't do well with direct exposure to sunlight so generalized lawn treatment is not needed.

Recently, a very novel product was launched for outdoor flea control—worms! Biological flea control with specific nematodes (*Steinernema carpocapsae* in Interrupt:VLP) has been found to effectively control flea larvae in soil, turf, and sand. The nematodes work this way: in the soil they actively search for flea larvae or pupae, penetrate them and release bacteria that kill the flea forms. Preliminary studies indicate that, within a 24-hour period, there is 95% mortality of the immature flea. When all flea larvae and pupae have been killed, the nematodes die off and biodegrade. One application lasts up to four weeks. Since worms are normal members of the environment, there are no negative effects on soil, groundwater, crops, beneficial insects, or people. The product is too new to report on its ultimate impact on fleas, but it's always nice to see new approaches that don't rely on insecticides.

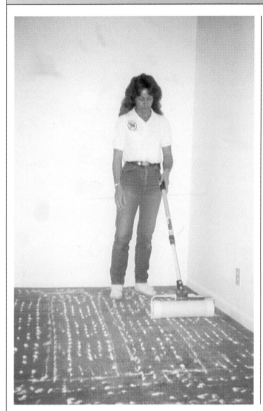

Insecticide Risks

Many people use a variety of insecticide products in the home and kennel environment but clearly relatively few are truly aware of the health concerns of handling such products. The most commonly used products are organophosphates, carbamates, pyrethrins, and pyrethroids, and all carry some risks.

Left: Applying polyborate (Borax) to the carpets for flea control. Courtesy of Fleabusters, Rx for Fleas, Inc., Ft. Lauderdale, Florida.
Below: *Steinernema carpocapsae*, the nemotode found in the new flea-control product Interrupt (VLP). Photo courtesy of Biosys.

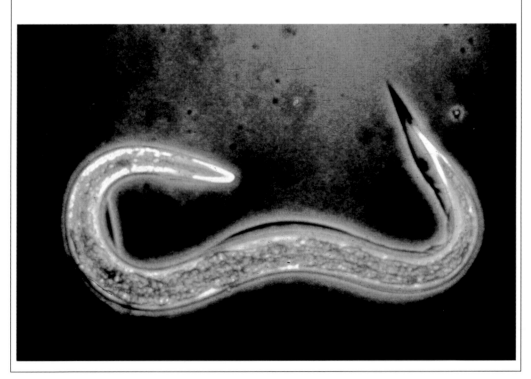

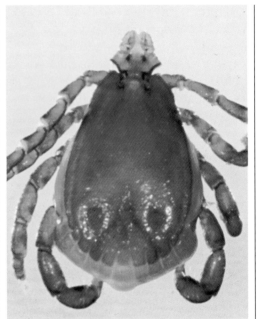

Rhipicephalus sanguineus, the Brown dog tick. Courtesy of Virbac Laboratories, Inc., Fort Worth, Texas.

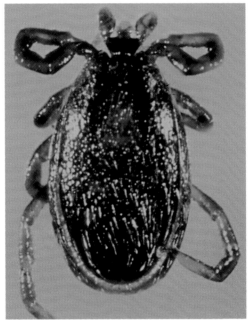

Ixodes scapularis, the deer tick. Courtesy of Virbac Laboratories, Inc., Fort Worth, Texas.

Dermacentor variabilis, the American dog tick. Courtesy of Virbac Laboratories, Inc., Fort Worth, Texas.

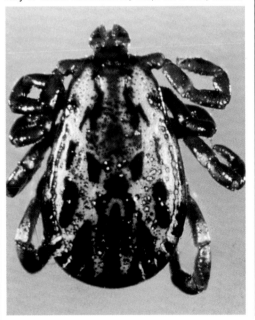

Dog skin parasitized by brown dog ticks. Courtesy of Dr. Thomas Lewis, Mesa Veterinary Hospital, Mesa, Arizona.

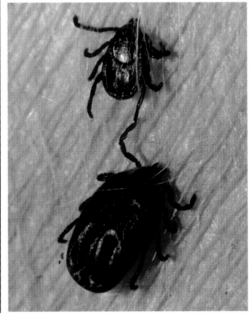

The organophosphates and carbamates have a higher incidence of acute toxicity in mammals (including people) than do other insecticides. Symptoms of intoxication might include: pinpoint pupils, blurred vision, tightness in the chest, wheezing, sweating, excessive tear production, salivation, nausea, vomiting, abdominal cramps, and diarrhea, as well as potentially more serious cardiovascular and neurological problems. These products should only be used in well-ventilated areas and extreme care should be used to avoid any skin contact. Do you exercise this degree of care when treating your pet? Possible long-term effects have not been completely studied, although effects on the immune system, the nervous system (decreased alertness, sleep disorders, memory loss, paranoia) and the reproductive system have been inferred. Many older preparations have not been adequately evaluated for cancer-causing risks as well. Some common organophosphates included in insecticides include malathion, chlorpyrifos, fenthion, dichlorvos, phosmet and chlorfenvinphos. Carbamates include carbaryl and propoxur. Are you exposed to any of these products?

Pyrethrins are derived from chrysanthemums and are considered to be relatively safe insecticides although acute toxicities are possible. Dermatitis is the most common adverse reaction to pyrethrin exposure in humans.

To protect yourself from the adverse effects of insecticides, endeavor to be aware. What is in that insecticide preparation you've been using? Learn about the active ingredients, expected duration of action, and toxicity. Do not apply insecticides more frequently or at higher concentrations than that recommended by label instructions. Be aware that concentrates (e.g., dips) carry a greater risk of accidental exposure than do diluted products. Therefore, choose dips that have a low order of toxicity, wear protective clothing, and apply them only in well-ventilated areas. If many animals need to be done, do not attempt to do them all yourself; share the duties and decrease the risk of exposure.

Your health is priceless and it pays to learn about the products you're handling and the potential risks you're taking. Either have a professional apply the insecticide for you or make sure you know how to use it safely.

Ticks

Ticks are found worldwide and can cause a variety of problems including blood loss, tick paralysis, Lyme disease, "tick fever," Rocky Mountain Spotted Fever, and babesiosis. All are important diseases which need to be prevented whenever possible. This is only possible by limiting the exposure of our pets to ticks. Although ticks are repulsive and suck blood, they are far more dangerous as carriers of microbes that cause serious diseases.

The life cycle of a tick runs about ten to 23 weeks, depending on climatic conditions and the availability of animal hosts. They don't jump or fly but they can crawl from 10–15 feet to reach an unsuspecting host. Each adult tick can lay between 4,000 and 5,000 eggs. Females die after laying all their eggs but males live to mate with several females.

For those species that dwell indoors, the eggs are laid mostly in cracks and on vertical surfaces in kennels and homes. Otherwise most other species are found outside in vegetation, such as grassy meadows, woods, brush, and weeds.

Ticks feed only on blood but they don't actually bite. They attach to an animal by sticking their harpoon-shaped mouthparts into the animal's skin and then sucking the blood. Some ticks can increase their size 20–50 times as they feed.

CLINICAL SIGNS

Ticks are large enough to be seen with the naked eye. Their oval bodies are usually seen sticking out perpendicular to the skin surface, the mouthparts sunk into the skin itself. Favorite places for them to locate are between the toes and in the ears, although they can appear anywhere on the skin surface.

Lyme disease, caused by *Borrelia burgdorferi* and spread by many ticks, can cause arthritis, inflammation of the heart muscle

(myocarditis), and kidney disease (glomerulonephritis). The characteristic rash that people get is very rarely reported in dogs. Most commonly dogs have anorexia, depression, joint pain, lameness, and fever. In later stages, they also have enlarged lymph nodes (lymphadenomegaly).

Ehrlichiosis in dogs typically causes depression, anorexia, fever, lymphadenomegaly, arthritis, and swelling of the scrotum and other body parts. After several weeks, some dogs will have bleeding episodes, especially nose bleeds and bruises, and consequently pale mucous membranes. This is caused by the effects of the organism on the platelets, the clotting cells of the blood. The severity of disease is influenced somewhat by the breed and the animal's own natural immune system. Human ehrlichiosis was first reported in 1986 and is caused by the same or closely related organisms to that affecting dogs. All evidence suggests that human ehrlichiosis is not transmitted directly from dogs to human beings but rather by ticks alone.

Tick paralysis is most commonly caused by female American dog ticks, although other species of ticks have also been reported to cause this condition. When the tick bites, it injects a toxin (poison) which will interfere with the stimulation of muscle by the nerves. The end result is paralysis, which usually starts in the back legs and spreads forward to the front legs. Complete recovery can

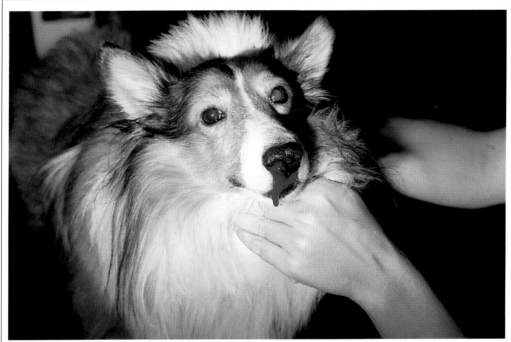

Dog with "tick fever" caused by ehrlichiosis with associated nose bleed. Courtesy of Dr. Jack Adkins, Brown Road Animal Clinic, Mesa, Arizona.

Dogs with ehrlichiosis often have bleeding tendencies because of the effect the organism has on the blood's clotting cells, the platelets. On the left are active, healthy platelets, looking like amoebae. On the right are the compromised platelets of a dog with ehrlichiosis. The platelets are rounded and incapable of performing normal clotting functions. Courtesy of Dr. Cynthia Holland, Protatek Reference Laboratory, Chandler, Arizona.

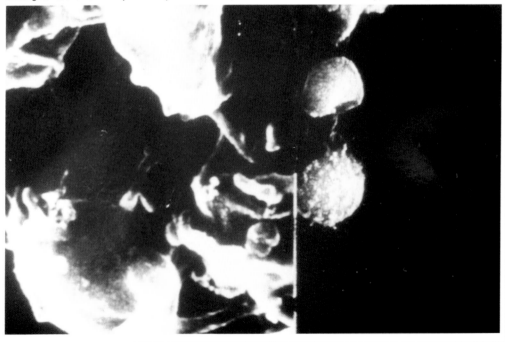

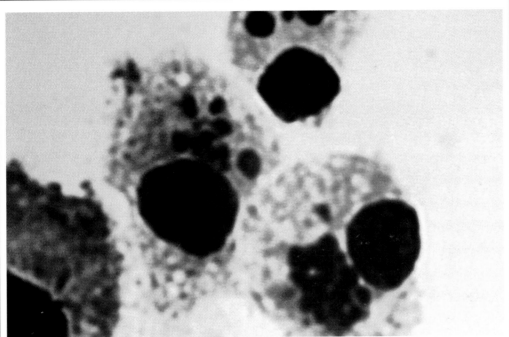

Inclusion bodies (morulae) of *Ehrlichia canis* within cultured canine white blood cells (monocytes). The organisms stain dark blue-purple while the nucleus of the cell is larger and stains reddish-purple. Courtesy of Dr. Cynthia Holland, Protatek Reference Laboratory, Chandler, Arizona.

Indirect Fluorescent Antibody (IFA) test for the diagnosis of canine ehrlichiosis. Inclusion bodies (morulae) with monocytes are made visible by a dye when patients have antibodies to this organism in their blood. Courtesy of Dr. Cynthia Holland, Protatek Reference Laboratory, Chandler, Arizona.

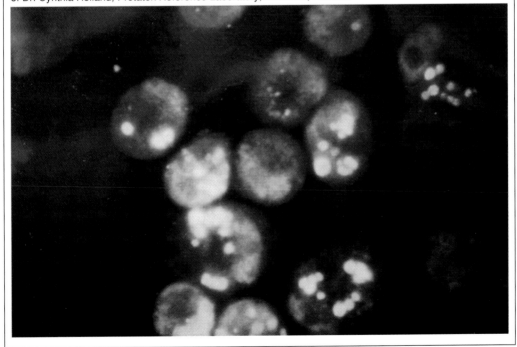

occur in two to three days after removal of the tick, but supportive care is vital.

Canine rickettsiosis, known as Rocky Mountain Spotted Fever in North America, is spread by several different ticks. The organism (*Rickettsia rickettsia* in North America and *Rickettsia conorii* in Europe) causes fever, depression, anorexia and pain during the first few days. Then, dogs may develop vomiting, diarrhea, enlarged lymph nodes, and swelling, especially of the scrotum. Bleeding episodes, neurological disease, and heart disease have also been reported. The North American syndrome tends to be more severe than that reported in Europe. Infection is carried principally by the American dog tick, but the Lone Star tick may also be an important carrier of infection.

Canine babesiosis is caused by *Babesia canis* and was first reported in the United States in 1934. Since that time it has become much more common, especially in the southern United States. The breed most commonly affected is the Greyhound, especially racing animals. In one survey of racing kennels in Florida, nearly 50% of the dogs were infected. This seems to mirror the incidences seen in other states that have dog racing. Clinical manifestations may include anemia, fever, loss of blood platelets, and jaundice. The disease is more common and more severe in young pups. Other animals may remain apparently healthy, despite infection. The organism that causes babesiosis in dogs is different from the one causing disease in people.

DIAGNOSIS

The diagnosis of tick infestation is not difficult if dogs are carefully inspected after walks through wooded areas. What is sometimes more difficult is diagnosing the diseases that ticks tend to carry. Not long ago Lyme disease (spread by ticks) was a novel diagnosis made by physicians and veterinarians alike. It wasn't until 1975 that the disease was recognized as a distinct form of arthritis in humans and the causative organism was not isolated and identified until 1982.

There is still much debate as to the accuracy of blood tests to predict actual Lyme disease versus exposure only. In addition, the development of antibodies to the bacteria (which is what is measured in the test) may take up to six months after the tick's transmission.

Ehrlichiosis, also known as "tick fever," is a tick-borne disease in which the organism (*Ehrlichia canis*) parasitizes blood cells, especially monocytes. The diagnosis can be made by finding the characteristic forms (morulae) of the parasite in blood smears or by using immunologic tests that detect circulating antibodies to the parasite.

Canine rickettsiosis is diagnosed with immunologic tests that detect antibody levels produced against the parasite. Since it is not unusual that early tests be negative, followup tests should be performed two weeks later to see if the antibody levels (titers) rise. A good ophthalmic examination can be very suggestive of the disease.

Canine babesiosis is diagnosed by an immunologic test that detects antibody levels produced against the parasite. Diagnosis can also be made by visualizing the tear-drop-shaped parasitic form (trophozoite) within infected red blood cells.

THERAPY

A good approach to prevent ticks is to remove underbrush and leaf litter, and to thin the trees in areas where dogs are allowed. This removes the cover and food sources for small mammals that serve as hosts for ticks. Ticks must have adequate cover that provides high levels of moisture and at the same time provides an opportunity of contact with animals. Keeping the lawn well maintained also makes ticks less likely to drop by and stay.

Because of the potential for ticks to transmit a variety of harmful diseases, dogs (and humans) should be carefully inspected after walks through wooded areas (where ticks may be found), and careful removal of all ticks can be very important in the prevention of disease. Insecticides and repellents should only be applied to pets following appropriate veterinary advice, since indiscriminate use can be dangerous.

If only a few ticks are present, they can be physically removed but it is important to remove the entire head and mouthparts, which may be deeply embedded in the skin. Removal is best accomplished with forceps designed especially for this purpose. Fingers can be used but should be protected with rubber gloves, plastic wrap, or at least a paper towel. The tick should be grasped as closely as possible to the skin and should be pulled upward with steady, even pressure. Care should be taken not to squeeze, crush, or puncture the body of the tick since exposure to body fluids of ticks may lead to the spread of any disease carried by that tick to the animal or to the person removing the tick. The tick should be disposed of in a container of alcohol or flushed down the toilet. If the site becomes infected, veterinary attention should be sought immediately.

Animals at risk of getting ticks should be regularly dipped. Flea/tick collars may have some effect and should be placed on animals in March, at the beginning of the tick season and changed regularly. Leaving the collar on when the insecticide level is waning invites the development of resistance, so change them as directed. Recently, a new tick collar has become available which contains amitraz (Preventic™: Allerderm/Virbac). This collar not only kills ticks but causes them to retract from the skin within two to three days. This greatly reduces the chances of ticks' transmitting a variety of diseases. A spray formulation has also recently been developed and marketed.

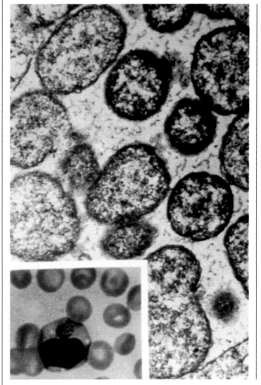

Left: Electron microscopic view of *Ehrlichia* inclusion body. Inset shows white blood cell (monocyte) with the morula. This is very rarely seen in blood films. Courtesy of Dr. Cynthia Holland, Protatek Reference Laboratory, Chandler, Arizona.

Below: Giemsa-stained blood smear of *Babesia canis* in red blood cells. Courtesy of Dr. Cynthia Holland, Protatek Reference Laboratory, Chandler, Arizona.

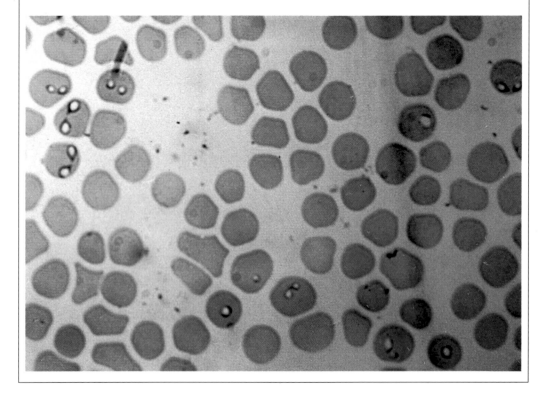

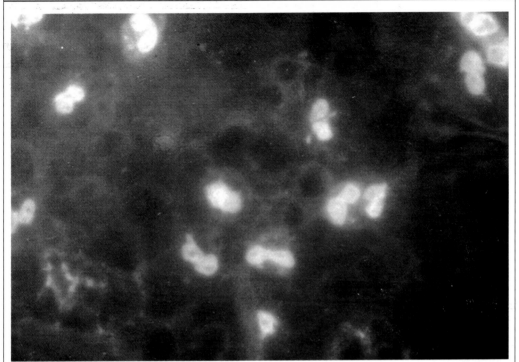

Indirect Fluorescent Antibody (IFA) test for *Babesia canis*. Courtesy of Dr. Cynthia Holland, Protatek Reference Laboratory, Chandler, Arizona.

Use proper instruments to remove ticks. Courtesy of EXTRACTIX tick extractor, Plaza Pet Clinic, Lebanon, Tennessee.

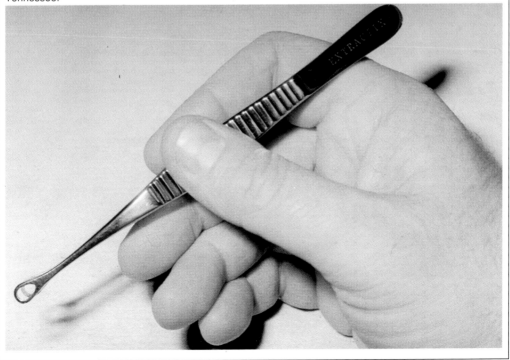

It might seem that there should be vaccines for all the diseases carried by ticks but only a Lyme disease *(Borrelia burgdorferi)* formulation is currently available. This bacterin appears to be effective in protecting vaccinated dogs but the situation is still being carefully evaluated. Most of the tick-borne diseases can be successfully treated with tetracyclines or their derivatives.

Mites

When mites cause problems in animals we call the condition mange. Some forms of mange are contagious to people but most aren't. Remember, mange itself is not a sufficient diagnosis. It is very important to learn the type of mite because risks and treatments often vary considerably.

DEMODICOSIS

Demodex mites are present on the skin of all animals but in some animals born with a defective immune system the numbers increase and begin to cause problems. Thus, many breeds appear predisposed to demodicosis, including Doberman Pinschers, Chinese Shar-Pei, Boxers, Great Danes, German Shepherd Dogs, Collies, Bull Terriers, English Bulldogs, Boston Terriers, Dalmatians, Old English Sheepdogs, Afghans, Dachshunds, Beagles and Staffordshire Terriers.

Most dogs acquire the mites while being nursed in the first two to three days of life. Mites can also be transmitted from one pup to another during this time, after which infestation is unlikely. It is thought that dogs only have problems with Demodex when they have some impairment of the immune system. All normal dogs carry the mites, so they are not considered contagious.

The extent of the immune deficit and its ability to be corrected determine the course of the disease. Localized disease (a few spots) tends to result in a spontaneous cure in 90% of cases by 18 months of age. Generalized demodicosis often requires significant therapeutic intervention and likely signifies more drastic impairment of the immune system. Though stress may trigger outbreaks in susceptible dogs, the mites themselves produce substances that further suppress the immune system. We can "cure" this secondary immune-system interference by treating the mites, but any underlying immune problems must also be addressed to achieve a real cure. Older animals that suddenly develop demodicosis should be very carefully screened for underlying reasons for the developing immune dysfunction.

Dogs with demodicosis may have a variety of skin problems depending on the degree of immunologic impairment. The skin disease itself is caused by the mites crowding out the hairs within the hair follicles, eventually destroying these follicles. Release of hair, bacteria and mites into the dermis causes infection, with associated

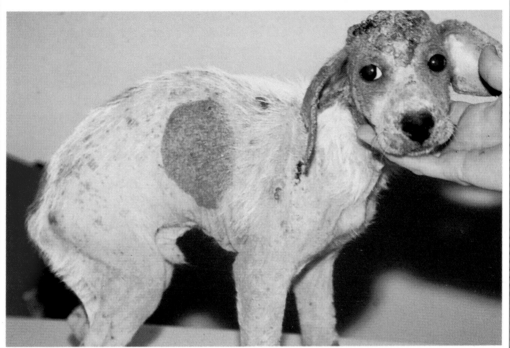

Demodicosis in a pup.

Skin scraping technique used in looking for mites.

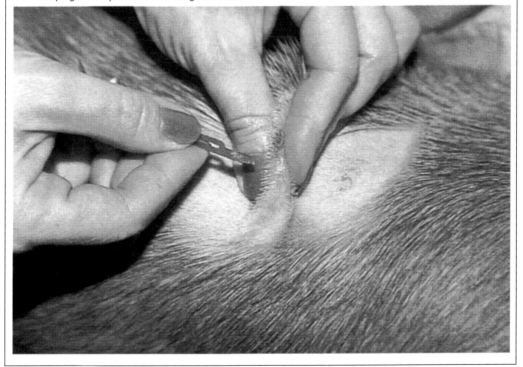

inflammation (redness) and hair loss. In fact, breeders used to refer to demodicosis as "red mange."

Demodicosis is not usually a difficult diagnosis to confirm. A veterinarian can squeeze the skin (to express the mites from the follicles) and scrape the skin surface with a scalpel blade until some blood is evident. The contents are then applied to a microscope slide and the Demodex mites look like little cigars with legs. In some breeds, such as the Chinese Shar-Pei, biopsies may be needed to get deep enough to locate the mites. Remember, the diagnostic process doesn't end here. It is also important to determine the immune system impairment that allowed the mite population explosion in the first place.

If the cause of the immune dysfunction can be cured, the mange will resolve on its own. If not, treatment involves killing the mites with special insecticides. Amitraz (Mitaban™) is the most common dip used, but experimentally, milbemycin oxime (Interceptor™) and ivermectin (Ivomec™) given daily has shown some promising results. It must be remembered that killing the mites will not restore the immune system to normalcy.

SARCOPTIC MANGE

Sarcoptic mange or "scabies" is probably the itchiest condition affecting dogs. The mite can also bite people and so is especially troublesome. Although it might bite people, the mite does not appear to be able to reproduce and lay eggs on people.

Trying to find this mite is a difficult task and so even if they are not found, treatment may be instituted if this problem is at all suspected. All animals in the household should be treated but humans do not usually require therapy. The treatment of scabies is often not difficult but there is some geographic evidence of resistance to a variety of different products. Routine insecticidal treatments must often be used on a weekly basis for six weeks to be curative. New products such as amitraz and ivermectin are often more effective and work in shorter periods of time but are currently not licensed for this use; they can often be used by veterinarians with owner consent.

CHEYLETIELLOSIS

Cheyletiellosis is caused by mites that have been affectionately nicknamed "walking dandruff." They are contagious to other animals as well as people. They are just large enough to be seen by a very keen eye, or with the use of a hand lens. These mites do not burrow but rather feed on the superficial debris present on the skin surface.

The clinical presentation is very variable and some animals may have no signs of problems, others have dandruff, and others are intensely itchy. The diagnosis is not as difficult as for sarcoptic mange, although the mites are not always easy to find. They can be collected by skin scrapings, acetate (transparent) tape impression, or even a modified vacuuming technique. The treatment options for cheyletiellosis are the same as for scabies and a cure is to be expected.

Ear Mites

Ear mites are probably the most common form of mange and are highly contagious among pets. Some animals may show no signs whatsoever, while others will have a dark black discharge in the ear canals that resemble coffee grounds. It is especially common in young puppies which have been housed closely with other animals.

The treatment of ear mites is more difficult than most owners expect. First, the mites are quite mobile, and merely squirting insecticide into the ears is rarely effective; the mites simply crawl out of the ears and as far away from the insecticide as possible (usually to around the tailhead) until it wears off and is safe for them to return.

Successful treatment requires treating all pets in the household with special ear drops once the ears have been cleaned out, as well as flea shampoos. If a whole-body flea shampoo is not done, the ear mites may just crawl out of the ears until the insecticide wears off, then crawl back in and start the problem all over again. Ivermectin is a very effective insecticide that has been used to treat ear mites, but it is currently not licensed for this purpose.

Chiggers

Chiggers latch on to dogs that might be roaming through forests or woods, causing a condition known as trombiculiasis. This problem is more prevalent in the late summer and fall. The bites of chigger mites are quite irritating and itchy, and most bites are on the head and feet.

The diagnosis may be suspected when pets roam through infested forests in late summer or fall, and can be confirmed by finding the mites. Occasionally the larvae may be seen as orange dots, but skin scrapings are often more helpful. Treatment is not difficult as the larvae are susceptible to many insecticides.

AUTOIMMUNE SKIN DISEASES

Everybody seems fascinated with autoimmune skin diseases. Perhaps it is because these diseases are relatively rare or because they are more common in some breeds than others. In any case, autoimmune skin diseases result from an overactivity of the immune system; the body itself produces abnormal antibodies that cause damage to the skin. Autoimmune diseases are sometimes described in simplified terms as an allergy to oneself but this does not accurately reflect what happens in these conditions. Whereas allergies may result in inflammation, autoimmune diseases cause actual destruction of tissues, which is clearly a quite different phenomenon.

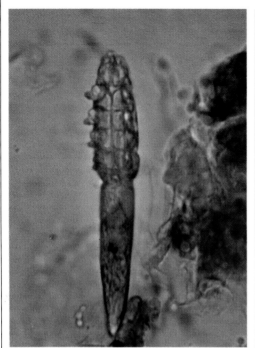

A Demodex mite.

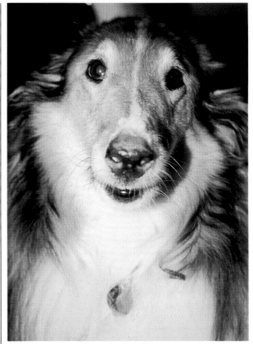

Cutaneous or discoid lupus erythematosus.

A Cheyletiella mite.

Pemphigus foliaceus produces a crusting skin condition that often first affects the face.

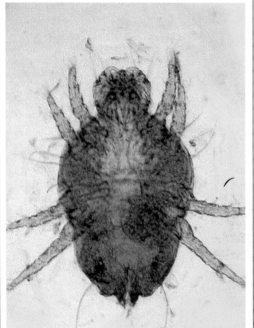

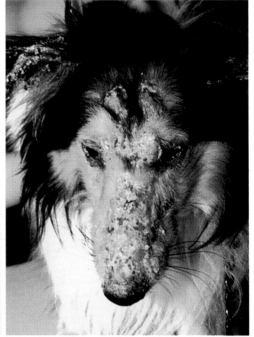

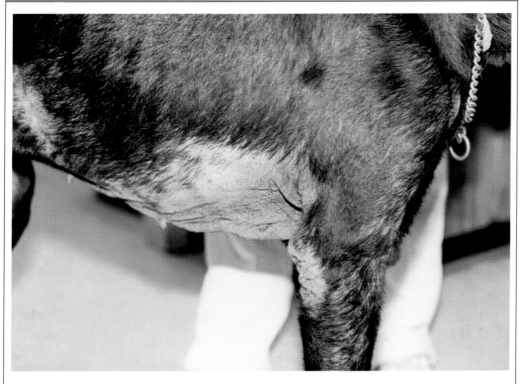

Above and below: Sarcoptic mange (scabies) is very itchy, and often results in hair loss and scabbing.

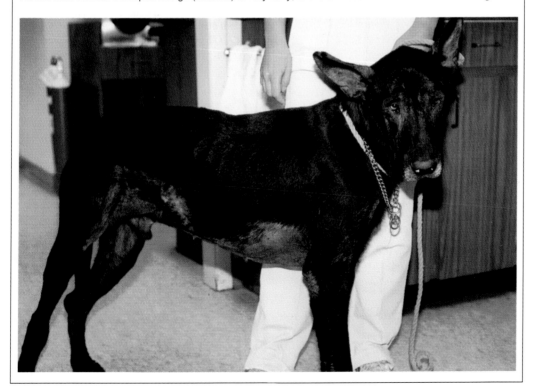

Lupus Erythematosus

Lupus erythematosus (LE) is a disorder that occurs in dogs as well as people. It is caused by abnormal antibodies that circulate in the blood and can cause quite widespread problems. One form of the disease affects many different organs (systemic lupus erythematosus or SLE) while the other (cutaneous or discoid lupus erythematosus) affects only the skin.

The most frequent clinical findings with SLE are fever which does not improve with antibiotics, arthritis, kidney disease, anemia, and skin problems, although many other disorders have been described. Collies, Shetland Sheepdogs and perhaps Doberman Pinschers are more commonly affected than are other breeds.

Cutaneous (discoid) lupus erythematosus often causes a facial rash. Collies, Shetland Sheepdogs and Alaskan Malamutes appear to be most commonly affected, and many of the cases of so-called "collie nose" are actually cutaneous lupus erythematosus. The important distinction between systemic and cutaneous lupus erythematosus is that cutaneous lupus does not involve other body systems and that the vast majority of cases of cutaneous lupus never evolve into systemic lupus erythematosus.

Specific diagnostic testing for SLE includes a variety of blood tests and biopsies; confirmation is not always a simple matter. Cases are often referred to dermatologists for appropriate diagnostic testing and treatment.

The therapy for SLE must be individualized but may be attempted with cortisone-like products (corticosteroids) and/or other medications that suppress the immune system and the production of abnormal antibodies. Unfortunately, all of these medications have potential side effects and monitoring blood and urine samples is an important part of the treatment regimen.

The therapy of CLE (DLE) differs from that of SLE in that heavy drug doses are usually not necessary. It is important that we be realistic in our treatment requirements and that we not "overtreat" patients with CLE. We should aim at limiting sun exposure (which worsens but doesn't cause the problem), use vitamin E to help lessen scarring, and use relatively lower doses of corticosteroids. This may not achieve 100% control but our primary goal is to lessen the impact of the disease and the medications, allowing the animal to optimize a quality lifespan.

Pemphigus and Pemphigoid

The term pemphigus (Greek for blister) is used to describe four related but different blistering diseases. Pemphigoid, which means pemphigus-like, has two variants of its own. Despite their names, blisters are rarely seen intact in cases of pemphigus and pemphigoid and the condition usually involves ulcers, marked scaling, and some-times "pimples." Appropriate diagnosis often requires biopsies and a referral to a specialist. Because these diseases are relatively rare, the ultimate cause may be missed and treatment commenced with antibiotics for infection.

Although any breed can be affected by pemphigus or pemphigoid, Collies, Shetland Sheepdogs, Doberman Pinschers and perhaps Akitas seem to have more than their share of problems with these conditions. No clear-cut genetic trend has been suggested, however.

The therapy of all forms of pemphigus and pemphigoid are similar but differ in degrees depending on the particular variant involved, the individual susceptibility, and the initial response to therapy. Prednisone (a corticosteroid) remains the initial treatment of choice because of its rapid onset of action, low cost, and ready availability. Unfortunately, corticosteroids alone are unsatisfactory in the majority of cases either because of side effects or inability to induce remission, but by combining them with other therapeutic agents such as azathioprine, cyclophosphamide, or gold, improved control and minimizing of side effects can be realized. Thus, corticosteroids coupled with either azathioprine or gold represents the best long-term choice in the treatment of pemphigus.

Uveodermatological (Vogt-Koyanagi-Harada-like) Syndrome

Uveodermatological syndrome, also known as Vogt-Koyanagi-Harada-like (VKH) syndrome is believed to be an autoimmune disease leveled against melanocytes, the cells responsible for producing pigment. The condition is characterized by a severe eye disorder which can result in blindness if not recognized and treated promptly. Skin changes include loss of pigment of the nose, lips, eyelids, and occasionally the entire body. The most affected individuals are in young adulthood, and the Akita appears to be the breed affected most often.

The diagnosis of VKH relies on appropriate biopsies. The mainstay of therapy is topical and/or systemic corticosteroids. Once blindness has occurred, the return of sight is unlikely, but early therapeutic intervention is usually successful.

MISCELLANEOUS SKIN PROBLEMS

Acral Lick Dermatitis (Lick Granuloma)

Few things are as frustrating to veterinarians as dealing with acral lick dermatitis, a problem caused by dogs' licking incessantly at a spot on their leg. Dogs start licking at a spot and before you know it they have removed layers of skin leaving a raw open area. The reason for this is still unknown.

Doberman Pinschers, Great Danes, German Shepherd Dogs, Labrador Retrievers and Irish Setters are affected most often, but a clear genetic trend has not been confirmed. Some recent research has even shown that there may be some nerve deficits in dogs that develop this condition. The old

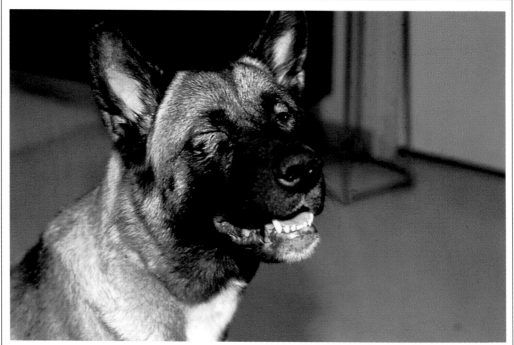

Uveodermatological (Vogt-Koyanagi-Harada) syndrome.

Self-inflicted damage done by a dog with acral lick dermatitis.

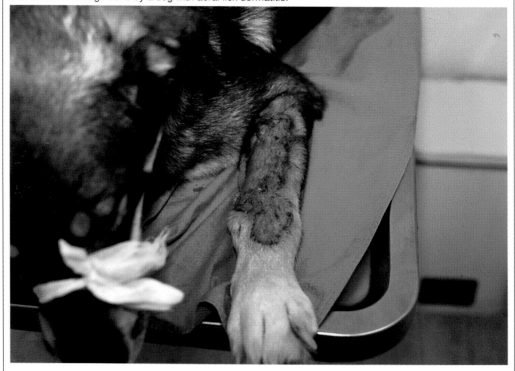

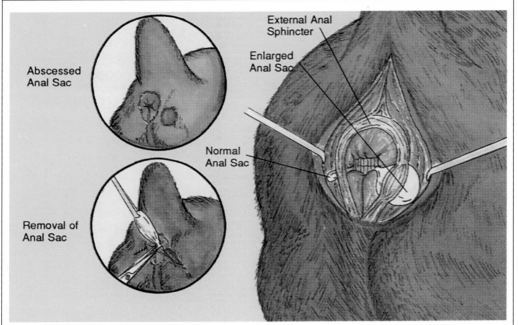

Location and anatomy of the anal sacs. Courtesy of Petcom, Inc.

reason to explain why this happened was to blame it on neurotic behavior—could be!

It is important to diagnose these cases carefully since some cases may actually be a result of another disease condition, which will need to be addressed. Therefore, often biopsies, microbial cultures and even radiographs are needed to help confirm a diagnosis.

Treatment is often frustrating because without knowing the cause, it is difficult to predict the chances of success. Most therapies use anti-inflammatory agents but a variety of other options exist, including tranquilizers, female sex hormones, anti-anxiety drugs and medications that reverse the effects of narcotics. More exotic treatments, such as injecting cobra antivenin into the site, radiation therapy and cryosurgery, have been used in the past but often have limited success.

Anal-sac Problems

Anal sacs are often incorrectly referred to as anal glands. These sacs are two pouches on either side of the rectum that act as reservoirs for secretions that may be associated with social recognition and territorial marking among dogs. All dogs have these sacs and most of the time they cause no problems at all. In normal conditions, when a dog is defecating, the expansion of the rectum compresses the sacs and the secretion is discharged with the stool. In some dogs, a problem exists, and they have difficulty emptying the sacs on their own. If the sacs fill with enough material they can become painful and even infected.

When there is a problem with the anal sacs, a dog may "scoot" its rear end across the ground or chew at the hind area to try to express the sacs. Most problems associated with the anal sacs are the result of impaction with material and then infection, so it is important to recognize the problem as soon as possible.

In uncomplicated cases, the anal sacs can be manually expressed by a veterinarian. If they have become infected, it may be necessary to flush the sacs with antiseptics, and antibiotics may be warranted. If the condition occurs frequently, another option is surgical removal of the sacs since they serve no critical function. The surgical approach to this area must be very careful because it is also the area where the nerves to the rectum are located.

Ear Problems

Ear problems in dogs are very common but there are many misconceptions about why they occur, how they are diagnosed and how they are best treated. Although some dogs do have hair in their ear canals that may cause obstructions, the vast majority of problems are not anatomic in nature. Similarly, although infections are commonly blamed on bacteria or yeasts, these microbes are rarely the cause of the problems. Then, what's going on?

Most ear problems are the result of allergies, hormonal problems, seborrhea, parasites or other matter in the ears, hereditary causes or immunologic disorders, not bacteria or yeasts. Sure, there are lots of microbes in the ear canal and you can find them on culture, but are they a cause of the problem or an effect? The fact is that there are supposed to be bacteria and yeasts in the ear canal—they belong there. They only cause a problem when the skin of the ear canal is inflamed, when the ear drum is ruptured or when there is a lot of debris in the ear canal for them to feed on.

If the pinnae, the flaps of the ears, are inflamed, you can be pretty sure that the primary cause is not an infection—why would an infection be extending up the flaps of the ears? Most of the time we must look past microbes and explore many of the possibilities listed above for an ultimate cause. This may involve microscopic examination of debris from the ears, careful inspection of the ear drums, blood tests and perhaps allergy tests. Bacterial cultures are occasionally necessary if oral antibiotics need to be prescribed, but remember that all cultures from the ear canal are likely to be positive for microbes—they belong there.

The treatment of ear problems will be most successful if an underlying cause can be determined. Repeated use of drops or ointments into the ears is often counterproductive, because resistance will become a problem, and many products contain cortisone-based products which cannot be administered long-term.

An accurate diagnosis will usually allow a safe and very effective form of therapy to be prescribed. As a last resort, surgeries of the ear canals can be done, but a success rate of perhaps 50% is all that can be realistically expected.

Finally, one other ear problem that should be discussed is aural hematoma. This results when a blood vessel bursts in the flap of the ear and blood collects between the cartilage and the skin. It is usually the result of severe head shaking, which may cause the hematoma to burst and bleed freely. Some recent research has shown that most dogs with a tendency to develop these hematomas have an immunologic problem. Treatment often involves draining the hematoma and "tacking down" the edges, but using medications to suppress the immune response may also be successful.

Superficial Necrolytic Dermatitis

Superficial necrolytic dermatitis (SND) is actually very rare in dogs, but it is included here because it is one of the most intensively studied skin disorders. It has been referred to by many different names in the literature, including glucagonoma syndrome, diabetic dermatopathy, metabolic dermatosis, hepatocutaneous syndrome, and necrolytic migratory erythema.

It appears that SND can result from several different underlying diseases, such as liver disease and pancreatic tumors (glucagonoma). Although at present the reason for the skin manifestations remain unknown, it appears that the underlying problems might result in nutritional imbalances, which then cause the skin lesions. Preliminary studies suggest that fatty acid and amino acid imbalances may be involved. This is supported by the fact that, in people, intravenous amino acid administration resulted in temporary resolution of the problem. It may be that the amino-acid deficiency in the skin is related to the liver impairment associated with the underlying disease. The research continues!

Dogs with superficial necrolytic dermatitis usually develop crusting and erosions on the muzzle, genitals, and feet. There may also be clinical signs associated with the underlying disease (e.g., liver disease, pancreatic cancer, etc.). Diagnostic testing should include blood counts, full biochemical profiles, and, if available, glucagon levels. Radiographs and ultrasound examinations of the abdomen may help confirm a suspected diagnosis.

If the underlying cause is not determined and corrected, most dogs eventually succumb. Although short-term remissions have been reported with prednisone, it should be remembered that corticosteroids can worsen many conditions, including liver disease and diabetes mellitus. Perhaps at this time, proper nutritional management in addition to addressing the underlying cause should be considered the treatment of choice. Surgery is recommended for cancers of the pancreas.

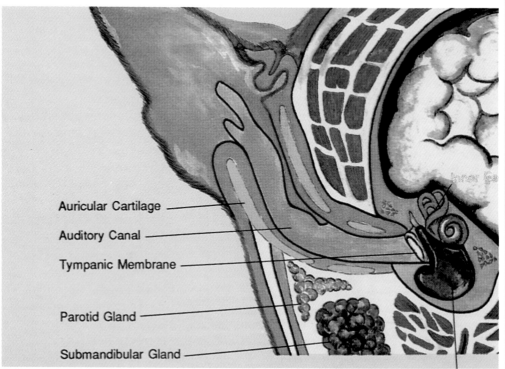

Auricular Cartilage

Auditory Canal

Tympanic Membrane

Parotid Gland

Submandibular Gland

Anatomy of the ear canal. Courtesy of Petcom, Inc.

Ceruminous (oily) otitis externa.

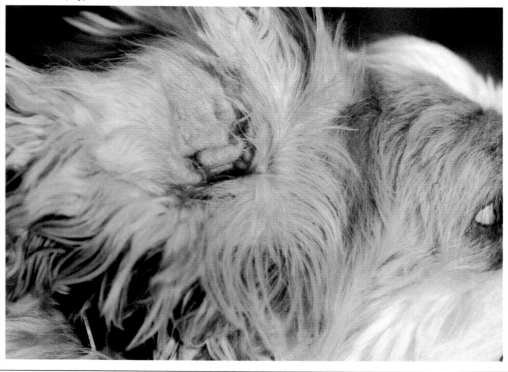

ADDITIONAL READING

Ackerman, L: *Guide to skin and haircoat problems in dogs.* Alpine Publications, 1993.

Ackerman, L: Inhalant allergies in dogs and cats. *Pet Focus,* 1990; 2(6): 91- 92.

Ackerman, L: Adverse reactions to foods and food additives. *Pet Focus,* 1990; 2(4): 67-70.

Ackerman, L: Dermatophytosis (Ringworm) in pets. *Pet Focus,* 1991; 3(3): 8-10.

Ackerman, L: Flea Control Update. *Pet Focus,* 1991; 3(2): 4-7.

Ackerman, L: Tick Control Update. *Pet Focus,* 1991; 3(4): 4-6.

Ackerman, L: Mange in dogs and cats- Part I. *Pet Focus,* 1991; 3(2): 20-22.

Ackerman, L: Mange in dogs and cats- Part II. *Pet Focus,* 1991; 3(3): 21-23.

Ackerman, L: Autoimmune Skin Diseases. *Pet Focus,* 1990; 2(5): 75-77.

Chu, H-J; Chavez, Jr., LG; Blumer, BM; et al: Immunogenicity and efficacy study of a commercial Borrelia burgdorferi bacterin. *Journal of the American Veterinary Medical Association,* 1992; 201(3): 403-411.

Codner, EC; Lessard, P: Comparison of intradermal allergy test and enzyme-linked immunosorbent assay in dogs with allergic skin disease. *Journal of the American Veterinary Medical Association,* 1993; 202(5): 739-743.

Dryden, MW: Biology of fleas of dogs and cats. *Compendium for Continuing Education of the Practicing Veterinarian,* 1993; 15(4): 569-578.

Duclos, DD; Jeffers, JG; Shanley, KJ: Prognosis for treatment of adult-onset demodicosis in dogs: 34 cases (1979-1990). *Journal of the Veterinary Medical Association,* 1994; 204(4): 616-619.

Hill, PB; Moriello, KA: Canine pyoderma. *Journal of the Veterinary Medical Association,* 1994; 204(3): 334-340.

Jeffers, JG; Shanley, KJ; Meyer, EK: Diagnostic testing of dogs for food hypersensitivity. *Journal of the American Veterinary Medical Association,* 1991; 198(2): 245-250.

Kasper, CS; McMurry, K: Necrolytic migratory erythema without glucagonoma versus canine superficial necrolytic dermatitis: Is hepatic impairment a clue to pathogenesis? *Journal of the American Academy of Dermatology,* 1991; 25: 534-541.

Mason, KV; Evans, AG: Dermatitis associated with Malassezia pachydermatis in 11 dogs. *Journal of the American*

Animal Hospital Association, 1991; 27(1): 13- 20.

Medleau, L; White-Weithers, NE: Treating and preventing the various forms of dermatophytosis. *Veterinary Medicine,* 1992; November: 1096-1100.

Plant, JD; Rosenkrantz, WS; Griffen, CE: Factors associated with and prevalence of high Malassezia pachydermatis numbers on dogs skin. *Journal of*

the Veterinary Medical Association, 1992; 201(6): 879-882.

Sosna, CB; Medleau, L: Treating parasitic skin conditions. *Veterinary Medicine,* 1992; June: 573-586.

Taboada, J; Harvey, JW; Levy, MG; Breitschwerdt, EB: Seroprevalence of babesiosis in Greyhounds in Florida. *Journal of the American Veterinary Medical Association,* 1992; 200(1): 47-50.

Disorders of the Bones, Joints, Muscles, and Nerves

The bones, joints, muscles, and nerves work in concert to allow animals to move normally. This collection of systems, the musculoskeletal system, the osteoarthrotic system, and the neuromuscular system, is discussed together because there is considerable overlap in their actions, and in the clinical syndromes that result when they are not functioning properly. Special attention is also given to those conditions with an inherited or congenital nature.

ORTHOPEDIC FOUNDATION FOR ANIMALS (OFA)

Many dogs are prone to developing inherited problems of their bones and joints. The most common of these are hip dysplasia and elbow dysplasia. Since these traits are often hereditary, an impartial registry was needed to record dogs that had no such problems so they could be used for breeding. The OFA is a nonprofit organization established in 1966 to collect and disseminate information concerning orthopedic diseases of animals and to establish control programs to lower the incidence of orthopedic diseases in animals.

Hip dysplasia is a common developmental disease in which the hip joints do not form correctly. The diagnosis is made by radiography and in order to standardize radiographic examination of dogs for dysplasia, a hip dysplasia registry was formed by the Orthopedic Foundation for Animals (OFA). The radiographs can be taken by your veterinarian but, if they are to be certified, they need to be sent to the OFA. Although puppy radiographs can be evaluated, a registry number can only be given to dogs older than two years of age. Each hip radiograph submitted to OFA is evaluated by veterinary radiologists and the hip joint conformation classified. Classifications of excellent, good and fair are considered within normal limits, and if the dog is two years of age or older, a breed registry number is assigned.

Elbow dysplasia is also a common orthopedic problem of dogs and may result from such strange-sounding causes as ununited anconeal process, fragmented medial coronoid process, osteochondritis of the medial humeral condyle or a combination of these. Like hip dysplasia, although problems may be evident earlier, certification can not be made until 24 months of age. Dogs with normal elbows on evaluation

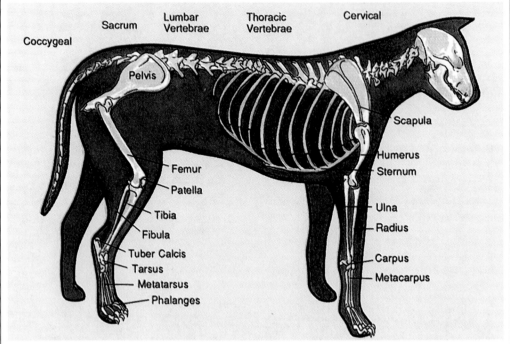

Coccygeal
Sacrum
Lumbar Vertebrae
Thoracic Vertebrae
Cervical
Pelvis
Scapula
Femur
Patella
Humerus
Sternum
Tibia
Fibula
Ulna
Radius
Tuber Calcis
Tarsus
Metatarsus
Phalanges
Carpus
Metacarpus

Normal canine skeleton. Courtesy of Petcom, Inc.

are given a breed registry number and are periodically reported to the parent breed club. Abnormal findings are reported only to the owner and submitting veterinarian.

The ultimate purpose of OFA certification is to provide information to dog owners to assist in the selection of good breeding animals; therefore, attempts to get a dysplastic dog certified will only hurt the breed by perpetuation of the disease.

For more information contact your veterinarian or the Orthopedic Foundation for Animals, 2300 Nifong Blvd., Columbia, MO 65201, (314)-442-0418.

GENETIC DISEASE CONTROL (GDC)

The Institute for Genetic Disease Control in Animals (GDC) is a nonprofit organization founded in 1990 which maintains an open registry for orthopedic problems, but does not compete with OFA. In an open registry like GDC, owners, breeders, veterinarians, and scientists can trace the genetic history of any particular dog once that dog and close relatives have been registered. The information about each dog automatically becomes linked in the open registry with relatives of that animal. An open registry delivers information on specific animals to breeders (for a fee) in order for the breeder to make knowledgeable selections of mates whose bloodlines indicate a reduced risk of producing genetic disease. Closed registries such as OFA tell only if an individual animal is free of clinical signs of the disease without providing information about parents, siblings, or half-siblings.

At the present time, the GDC operates open registries for the following orthopedic conditions: hip dysplasia, elbow dysplasia, and osteochondrosis. The diagnosis of all three are by radiographic evaluation. All films are read by at least two persons, a board-certified veterinary radiologist (Diplomate of the American College of Veterinary Radiology) and a board-certified surgeon (Diplomate of the American College of Veterinary Surgeons). In cases where there is question, an additional evaluation is made by a radiologist for a final consensus.

The GDC is currently developing guidelines for registries of: Legg-Calve-Perthes disease, craniomandibular osteopathy, and medial patellar luxation.

For more information, contact the Institute for Genetic Disease Control in Animals, P.O. Box 222, Davis, CA 95617, phone and FAX (916) 756-6773.

HIP DYSPLASIA

Hip dysplasia is a genetically transmitted disease that has been seen in most breeds of dogs. It was first diagnosed in the dog in 1935. Since that time, it has been diagnosed in most breeds of dogs, with the highest incidences in the larger breeds. Breeds with a particularly high prevalence of hip dysplasia include the St. Bernard, Boykin Spaniel, Bullmastiff, Newfoundland, Staffordshire

Positioning a dog for hip dyplasia radiographs. The only certain way to check for the presence of hip dysplasia is x-raying the dog. Courtesy of Dr. Jack Henry, Animal Emergency and Specialty Center,Woodland Hills, California.

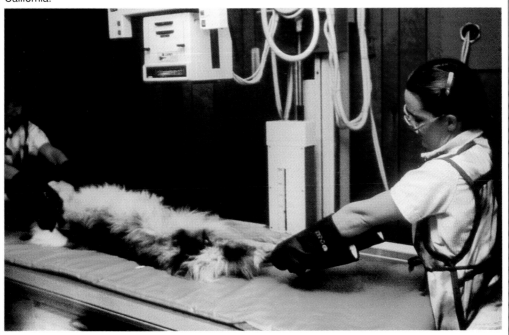

Terrier, Bloodhound, Field Spaniel, Bernese Mountain Dog, Kuvasz, Chesapeake Bay Retriever, Welsh Springer Spaniel, Golden Retriever, Norwegian Elkhound, Mastiff, Rottweiler, Gordon Setter, Chow Chow, Giant Schnauzer, English Setter, Old English Sheepdog, German Shepherd Dog, Portuguese Water Dog and Pembroke Welsh Corgi. Few diseases have attracted as much public and scientific interest and have generated as much knowledge and misconception as canine hip dysplasia. Why should that be? How can such a common condition create so much controversy?

Hip dysplasia is defined as an abnormal development of the hip (coxofemoral) joint. It is well known that hip dysplasia is an inherited disease but other factors are at least as important. The mode of inheritance is described as polygenic, meaning that the trait is influenced by several different genes. That means that it is impossible to predict with accuracy how pups will be affected when dysplastic parents are mated. However, in general, it is more likely that pups born to parents with normal joints will have normal hips themselves. Pups born to parents with hip dysplasia are at higher risk for developing hip dysplasia.

Part of the problem arises when we realize that the pups destined to be dysplastic will have normal hips at birth. In fact, a dog may be 24 months of age before hip dysplasia is diagnosed. Several secondary factors aside from inheritance influence the development of dysplasia. These include body size, body conformation, and growth patterns. It is well known that feeding a high-calorie diet to a dog at risk of developing hip dysplasia will increase the likelihood that dysplasia will, in fact, develop. This is because rapid weight gains are known to increase the incidence and severity of the disease. Likewise, feeding a lower caloric diet will decrease the incidence and severity of the disease.

It has also been shown that hind leg muscle mass is related to the prevalence of dysplasia. In German Shepherd Dogs, the greater the amount of musculature of the rear limbs, the lower the incidence of dysplasia. This points out that a well-balanced muscular support is necessary to maintain proper alignment and that generalized or specific weakness of the hip muscles can lead to adverse changes in the developing hip joint. Nutrition is also important in this regard. If the muscles of the hind limb fail to develop and reach functional maturity at the same time as the bones, joint instability may result. This eventually leads to degenerative osteoarthritis.

Clinical Signs

The primary abnormality in canine hip dysplasia is joint laxity, or a looseness of the hip joint. There just isn't a good fit. Because of this, there is play in the joint as the dog moves. This results in inflammation in the joint, which causes pain and lameness. However, there is a great deal of variability with individual dogs. Some dogs have severe dysplasia yet don't suffer much pain, while others with relatively mild changes may become severely lame. With chronic inflammatory changes, arthritis usually occurs in an attempt to stabilize the joint. Mild changes are usually evident in the first year of life. There may be hind-end lameness, changes in gait, difficulty in getting up, and associated pain.

Diagnosis

The diagnosis of hip dysplasia is confirmed by taking appropriate radiographs, which are registrable with OFA.

The Institute for Genetic Disease Control in Animals (GDC) recognizes that, with the USA as the exception, the world standard for screening for normal certification of hips is 12–18 months of age. Through the use of an open registry in Sweden and the evaluation at one year of age, the incidence of hip dysplasia has been reduced from 46% to 28% in five years in that country. In order to compensate for potential observer variations, the GDC requests re-evaluation of any borderline cases at two years of age and withholds certification until that time.

There are other methods of hip evaluation that deserve mention. Some veterinarians perform compression and distraction radiographic studies to provide a "laxity index." Some investigators feel that the laxity index at 16 weeks of age will accurately predict dysplasia, even when standard radiographs fail to detect a problem. There are other ways to judge laxity as well. Some veterinarians believe that careful manipulation of the joints in young (seven to 11 week old) pups (Bardens-Hardwick technique) provides a reasonably accurate picture of their risk for developing dysplasia. Another manipulative diagnostic technique (Ortolani) can be performed in older dogs. An excellent time to have early studies done is when the non-breeding animal is anesthetized for ovariohysterectomy (spay) or orchiectomy (neuter).

The University of Pennsylvania has developed a new method for predicting the development of canine hip dysplasia and has initiated a nationwide collaborative effort named PennHIP. This program uses a new stress-radiographic technique for evaluating hip laxity. Hip laxity or looseness can be detected 2.5 times more reliably with this new technique. Laxity is graded on a scale 0 to 1 and dogs with laxity greater than 0.3 are considered susceptible to developing hip dysplasia. PennHIP collaborators are required to send all radiographs, of good or bad hips, to PennHIP for evaluation. The data will then be included in the study, providing the base to determine specific breed laxity indexes. The grading will be refined as more cases are evaluated by collaborators.

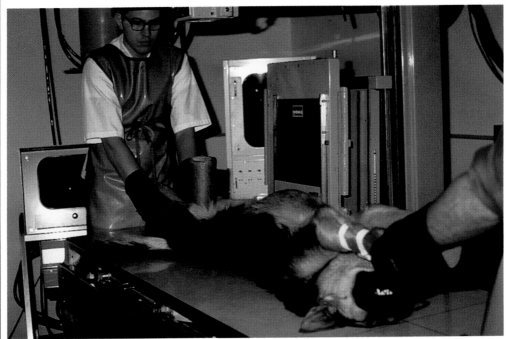

Hip dysplasia may not be diagnosed until a dog reaches 24 months of age. Only radiographs can reliably determine its presence.

Pictorial representation of the flattened femoral head that occurs with hip dysplasia. Courtesy of Toronto Academy of Veterinary Medicine, Toronto, Canada.

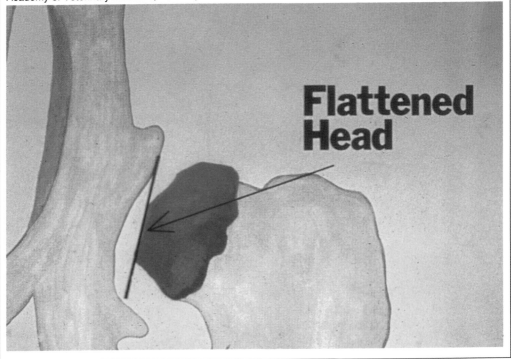

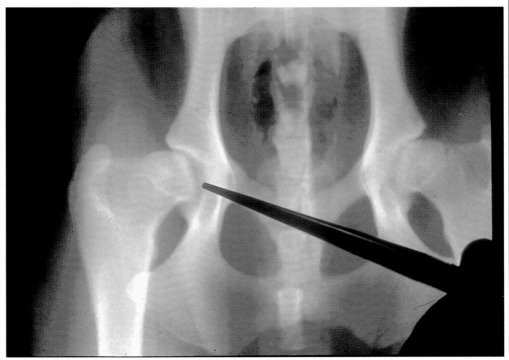

Radiograph of a dog with hip dysplasia. Note the flattened femoral head at the marker. Courtesy of Toronto Academy of Veterinary Medicine, Toronto, Canada.

Pictorial representation of the joint luxation that occurs as a consequence of hip dysplasia. Courtesy of Toronto Academy of Veterinary Medicine, Toronto, Canada.

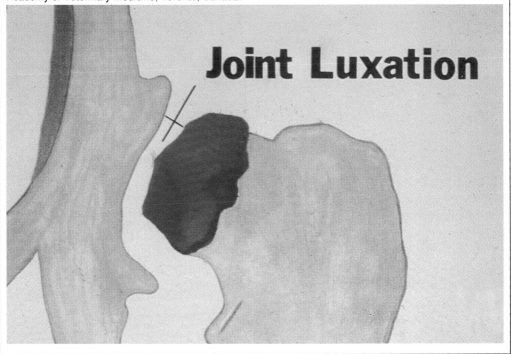

Treatment

A diagnosis of hip dysplasia is not necessarily a sentence of life in pain for a dog. There are both medical and surgical options for management. Although Orthopedic Foundation for Animals (OFA) certification radiographs are not taken until two years of age, evaluation for possible treatment may be necessary by six months of age.

One of the simplest treatment

The more a dog runs and exercises over this critical period, the more stress is put on the hip joint and the greater the likelihood of laxity developing. It seems likely that if laxity does not develop by two years of age, then the risk of developing dysplasia after this time is greatly reduced.

Medical therapy is used for dogs that have pain and discomfort associated with their dysplasia. It is not always easy to determine when

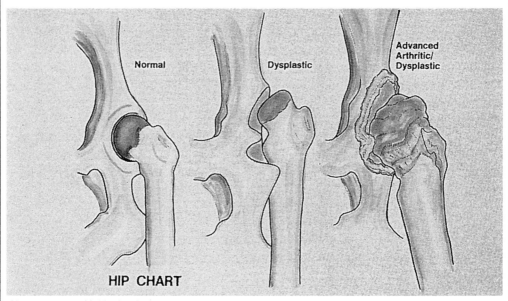

Normal   Dysplastic   Advanced Arthritic/ Dysplastic

HIP CHART

Changes seen with hip dysplasia. Courtesy of Petcom, Inc.

measures is to enforce exercise restriction for the first 18 months of life in animals at risk of developing hip dysplasia. This is the critical time for joint development. Recent studies performed in England showed that over 70% of immature dogs diagnosed with hip dysplasia achieve good pet-quality function over a ten-year study period without medications or surgery.

our pets are in pain, but we view their discomfort with sympathy and try in earnest to spare them any pain, whenever possible. Together with pain relief, dysplastic dogs are put on a diet so that they are bearing the least amount of weight possible on the damaged joints.

Pain relievers used in the dog include ASA (aspirin), indomethacin, naproxen, ibuprofen, flunixin meglumine, phenylbutazone, and piroxicam. Aspirin-like products were first introduced in the late 19th century and are still important anti-inflammatory agents today. They likely represent the first line of pain relief for animals, although dosing is important and ulceration in the digestive tract is a possible complication, as it is in people. Dogs appear to be more sensitive to ibuprofen than do people, and stomach ulcers may result; since ibuprofen offers no advantages over aspirin and causes more side effects, its use in animals is not recommended. The use of naproxen is usually limited to cases of bone- and joint-related pain in dogs that are poorly responsive to aspirin. Most animals that develop ulceration while on therapy benefit from immediately discontinuing the medication but some require blood transfusions, administration of antacids, administration of cimetidine, and surgical repair.

Aspirin-related compounds are the oldest and still the best medical options for the control of pain in pets. Side effects are possible, and dosing is important but risks are less with these products than with the more potent nonsteroidal anti-inflammatory agents. It is important to remember that aspirin and other anti-inflammatory agents provide pain relief but do nothing to reverse or impede the progression of degenerative joint disease (osteoarthritis).

A new medical approach to the treatment of early or advanced degenerative osteoarthritis secondary to hip dysplasia involves the use of a product called polysulfated glycosaminoglycan or PSGAG. PSGAGs are naturally occurring components of the joint cartilage and when purified and injected into a muscle, they increase the rate of repair of damaged cartilage and joint fluid production. Although results are preliminary and no controlled studies in dogs have been performed, there have been several reported successes with this compound in selected cases.

When should a patient receive conservative management as opposed to specific surgical treatment? This depends on the age of the dog, the intended use of the dog, the degree of osteoarthritis, the severity of the lameness and the financial capability of the owner. There appears to be a 50-60% chance that a given patient may respond conservatively over a long period of time. Surgical treatment would be reserved for the remaining 40-50% of patients. Unfortunately, there is no way to predict into which category any one particular dog will fall. Surgery should be considered before too much muscle atrophy occurs. The worse the state of the surrounding muscles, the harder it is to have a good surgical outcome.

There are several different surgical approaches used to manage dogs with hip dysplasia. If there is little or no arthritis present, a stabilizing reconstruction of the hip joint is recommended. When significant arthritis is present, a BOP

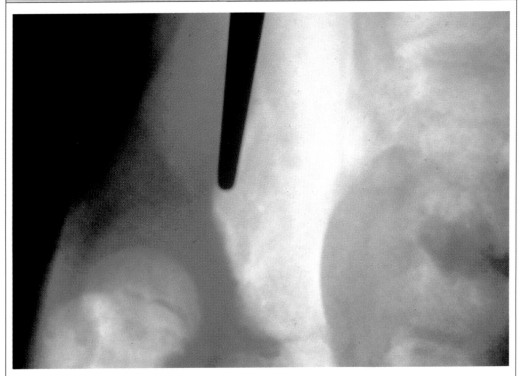

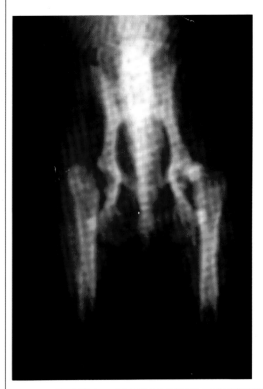

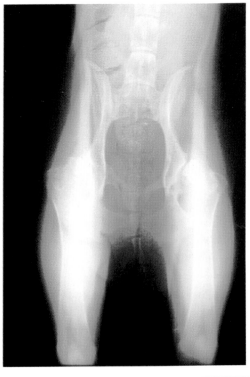

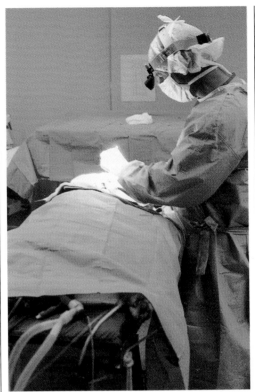

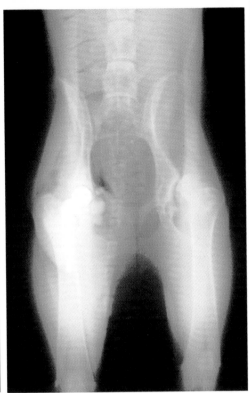

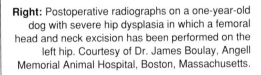

Hip replacement surgery being performed by Dr. Jack Henry, as above.

Dog following total hip replacement surgery by Dr. Jack Henry, as above.

Right: Postoperative radiographs on a one-year-old dog with severe hip dysplasia in which a femoral head and neck excision has been performed on the left hip. Courtesy of Dr. James Boulay, Angell Memorial Animal Hospital, Boston, Massachusetts.

Opposite, top: Radiograph of a dog with hip dysplasia. Note the joint luxation at the marker. Courtesy of Toronto Academy of Veterinary Medicine, Toronto, Canada.
Opposite, bottom left: Standard radiograph from a five-year-old Curly-Coated retriever with one-sided (unilateral) hip dysplasia. Note normal hip joint on the right (left side of photo) with femoral head (a), acetabulum (b), and area of round ligament attachment (arrow). There is severe arthritis present in the other hip. Note thickening of the femoral head (c) and the new bone production around the joint (fuzziness). Courtesy of Dr. James Boulay, Angell Memorial Animal Hospital, Boston, Massachusetts.
Opposite, bottom right: Severe hip dysplasia with subluxation of hip joint.

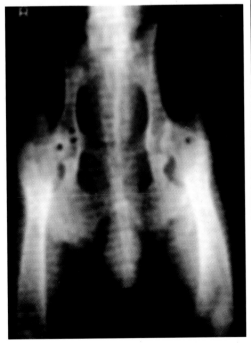

(biocompatible osteoconductive polymer) shelf arthroplasty, or a total hip replacement technique is used.

One of the more aggressive techniques used to stabilize the hip joint is the pelvic osteotomy. In this procedure, the pelvis is surgically "cut" and tilted to obtain better coverage of the head of the femur. The goal is to try to create a normal hip joint. This procedure is not suitable if there is considerable arthritis present in and around the joint.

Since its introduction in 1976, the total hip replacement has become the only method available that can replace normal hip joint function once advanced osteoarthritis is present. In this technique, the femoral head and neck are replaced with a stainless steel component and the acetabulum is replaced with a plastic cup prosthesis. A five-year followup study of 221 total hip replacements revealed an overall success rate of 91%. Total hip replacement can be done on both hips, although many dogs do very well with one replacement. The major disadvantages of this surgery are that the expertise required to perform this type of surgery, and the costs involved, limit its availability. For dogs under 50 pounds and those with one-sided dysplasia, the surgical removal of the femoral head and neck (excision arthroplasty, femoral head ostectomy, FHO) may provide satisfactory results if a total hip replacement is not possible.

The BOP shelf arthroplasty is a useful technique but not without controversy. Fibers and blocks of a product called biocompatible osteoconductive polymer are implanted to help form a shelf that improves the coverage of the head of the femur. It has been used in Europe on people but has not been used long-term in the United States. There are questions related to short-term outcome, long-term outcome, and potential complications in dogs. It seems clear that pain relief is achieved after the surgery but the other claims being made are harder to substantiate.

Prevention

The best way to avoid hip dysplasia is to only buy or breed dogs that have disease-free joints based on appropriate radiographs. This method of breeding is called mass selection. This will lower the incidence of hip dysplasia but not remove it entirely. The incidence can be further reduced by selecting dogs for breeding based on family performance and progeny testing. Ideally, there should be no history of hip dysplasia for three generations back in any dog or bitch intended for breeding.

The control of hip dysplasia is best achieved through selective breeding programs since it is an inherited disease. The following breeding criteria have been demonstrated to more rapidly reduce the frequency of dysplasia in a population of dogs: breed only normal dogs; the normal dogs should come from normal parents and grandparents; the normal dogs should have greater than 75% normal litter-mates; the sire should have a record of producing normal pups that exceed the breed average; and replacement bitches should have better hip conformation than their parents and grandparents.

Nutritional intervention may also lessen the incidence of hip dysplasia in some breeds. It has now been well established that overfeeding pups contributes to hip dysplasia. Dogs with weight gain above the standard weight curve of the breed have a higher incidence of hip dysplasia, as well as more severe diseases than dogs with weight gain below the standard curve. Calcium supplementation of puppies at risk also poses dangers for an increased susceptibility to both hip dysplasia and osteochondrosis in susceptible animals.

Ascorbate (vitamin C supplementation) has been advocated for the prevention of hip dysplasia since it is a necessary cofactor in collagen manufacture. It is reasoned that ascorbate deficiency might thus contribute to joint laxity. Although this has never been scientifically proven, many breeders supplement pups with ascorbic acid in an attempt to lower their risk of developing hip dysplasia.

Recently it has been proposed that dietary electrolytes may play a role in canine hip dysplasia. Electrolytes are minerals dissolved in the tissues, including potassium, sodium, and chloride. Recent investigations have suggested that controlling the balance of dietary electrolytes in breeds with a high incidence of hip dysplasia can reduce the severity of hip-joint laxity in these dogs. A dietary electrolyte balance (DEB) can be calculated by subtracting the amount of negatively charged electrolytes (chloride) from the positively charged ones (potassium and sodium). Hip-joint laxity is minimized if the difference (DEB) can be kept to less than 20 meq/100 g, preferably less than 10 meq/100 g in a nutritionally balanced dog food.

In conclusion, hip dysplasia is a genetic disease best controlled through early detection and selective breeding. In dogs with the potential for dysplasia, early clinical and radiographic examination by your veterinarian may be able to provide early detection of the disease. For those dogs with early signs of dysplasia, a reconstruction of the joint should be strongly considered, and for those dogs with advanced arthritis, careful consideration should be given to medical and surgical treatments currently available.

OSTEOCHONDROSIS

We have known about osteochondrosis since the late 1950s and yet it receives considerably less press than hip dysplasia. Osteochondrosis is a degenerative condition of cartilage, seen in young dogs, in which the cartilage cells fail to develop properly into mature bone. This results in localized areas of thickened cartilage that are very prone to injury since they are not well attached to the underlying bone. Therefore, although the condition is called osteochondrosis, which means a degenerative condition of bone and cartilage, this is essentially a disorder affecting cartilage, not bone.

In time, when osteochondrosis causes flaps of cartilage to be exposed in the joint, inflammation results. At this time, it is referred to as osteochondritis dissecans (OCD), describing the inflammatory component and the fact that cartilage has become "dissected" and exposed. If the flap becomes dislodged, it may be referred to as a "joint mouse." In dogs, the condition affects the front legs preferentially (shoulder, elbow) but can also affect the back legs (hip, stifle) and even the vertebrae in the neck. Related conditions include ununited anconeal process and fragmented coronoid process.

The factors that cause osteochondrosis are many, but trauma, poor nutrition, and hereditary abnormalities have all been explored. The most likely associations made to date suggest that feeding diets high in calories, calcium and protein promotes the development of osteochondrosis in susceptible dogs. Also, animals that are allowed to exercise in an unregulated fashion are at increased risk, since they are more likely to sustain cartilage injuries. The fact that OCD occurs mainly in large-breed dogs suggests that the increased weight-bearing needs of the cartilage may make it prone to damage. There is also some evidence that a variety of hormones (such as calcitonin, somatotropin, thyrotropin, and sex hormones) may influence the development of osteochondrosis.

Osteochondrosis of the canine shoulder. A radiograph of the elbow (left) is also included. Courtesy of Dr. Jack Henry.

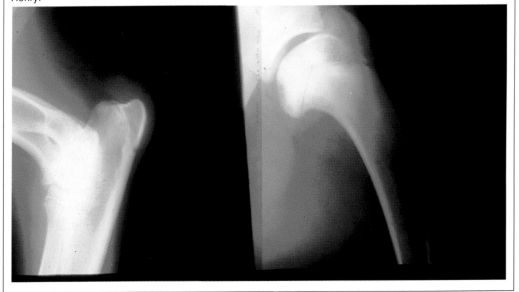

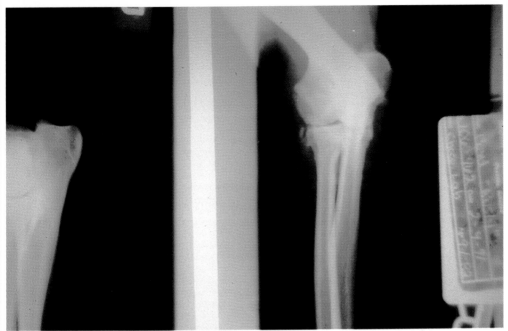

Fragmented coronoid process of the elbow, a manifestation of elbow dysplasia. Courtesy of Dr. Jack Henry.

Clinical Signs

Osteochondrosis is a disorder of young dogs, with problems usually starting between four and seven months of age. Large-breed dogs are most likely to be affected. It is found in many of the same breeds that are prone to hip dysplasia, especially the Akita, Bouvier des Flandres, Bloodhound, Bernese Mountain Dog, Bullmastiff, Bulldog, Chinese Shar-Pei, Chow Chow, Doberman Pinscher, English Springer Spaniel, Fila Brasileiro, German Shepherd Dog, Golden Retriever, Irish Wolfhound, Leonberger, Labrador Retriever, Mastiff, Newfoundland, Otterhound and Rottweiler. Other breeds may also be affected, but less often. In the early stages of osteochondrosis, there are usually no clinical signs (symptoms). Only when a cleft forms in the cartilage and inflammation ensues is the condition clinically evident. The usual manifestation is a sudden onset of lameness. In time, the continued inflammation results in arthritis in those affected joints.

OCD of the head of the humerus (shoulder) is probably the most common manifestation of this condition in dogs. Although large breeds such as the Rottweiler, Newfoundland, Golden Retriever, and Labrador Retriever are commonly affected, smaller breeds such as the Chihuahua, Whippet, Miniature Poodle, and Greyhound can also be affected. Most cases are seen in pups less than seven months of age, but one-third of all cases are not detected until a year of age. The classic picture is one of lameness, and usually only one leg is involved initially. Affected dogs can't support their weight on the leg and so walk with a shortened stride, often raising their heads as the weight is placed on the bad leg. Both front legs eventually become involved in about 50% of cases. In time, if the problem is not addressed, the joint eventually becomes incapacitated with arthritis.

In some studies, osteochondrosis of the elbow is reported even more frequently than disease of the humerus. This area is anatomically complex because it involves the intimate association of the bones of the forearm (radius and ulna) with the upper arm (humerus). Three conditions are usually lumped under the category of osteochondrosis of the elbow. They are ununited anconeal process, fragmented coronoid process, and OCD of the medial humeral condyle. This triad of disorders is usually referred to by breeders collectively as elbow dysplasia.

The most common of the three is fragmented coronoid process (FCP), in which part of the elbow joint breaks away from its bony anchor. It occurs in large breeds of dogs, especially Labrador Retrievers, Rottweilers, Golden Retrievers, German Shepherd Dogs, and Newfoundlands. A genetic trend is thought to be important, but this has only been truly documented in Rottweilers. In about 60% of cases, there is also a problem with OCD of the medial humeral condyle. Apparently, not all cases of FCP are due to osteochondrosis; some are

due to mechanical stresses.

OCD of the medial humeral condyle is very similar to the disorder seen in the shoulder. It just involves the lower end of the humerus rather than the upper part. The inner (medial) aspect of the lower humerus (condyle) retains thicker cartilage longer than the outer (lateral) aspect, and therefore, this site is more prone to osteochondrosis. When cracks and fissures form in the cartilage, it is prone to the classic changes of OCD.

Ununited anconeal process (UAP) occurs when the bone-growth center in the anconeal process of the elbow fails to unite with the ulna of the foreleg. This union normally occurs in medium- and large-breed dogs at four or five months of age. If it has not fused by five months of age, there will be joint instability and the pain and inflammation associated with OCD.

Osteochondrosis of the hind legs is much less common than OCD of the shoulder or elbow. In addition, some cases heal spontaneously, which may explain in part why it is more rarely reported. Affected dogs have lameness of one or both back legs and a shortened stride on the affected leg. Also, the joint capsule may be swollen on the affected leg. This condition (OCD of the hock or stifle) is most commonly seen in large-breed dogs (especially the Rottweiler, Labrador Retriever, and Golden Retriever) although it is reported in many other breeds as well. Although OCD of the knees (stifle joints) is commonly seen in people, it is a rare cause of problems in dogs. There appears to be a breed tendency in the German Shepherd Dog and Great Dane.

Diagnosis

The diagnosis of OCD is often strongly suspected when a young dog of a breed at risk suddenly becomes painfully lame. This lameness may worsen in wet or cold weather or when the leg is extended. Careful manipulation by a veterinarian can usually pinpoint the site of the problem. It is imperative that the manipulation be exact so as not to confuse elbow problems with those in the shoulder, or hip problems with those in the stifle. The opposite limb should also be carefully evaluated, even if there are no problems evident.

Radiographic studies of the joints are very useful for establishing a diagnosis. Unfortunately, cartilage material does not show up well on radiographs. Heavy sedation or anesthesia is usually necessary so that the painful limb can be stretched and properly positioned. If finances allow, it is worthwhile to take radiographs of both limbs for comparison purposes. Radiographs should also be taken of other joints on the same limb (e.g., elbow, shoulder) to evaluate for other potential sites of involvement. Early cases may show minimal decrease in bone density; moderate cases may have a flattened contour; and advanced cases are often associated with a concave defect

and considerable arthritis.

It is very difficult to actually see a fragmented coronoid process on radiographs because this area is often obstructed by other bones. However, there are tell-tale signs that accompany the condition, such as bony deposits (osteophytes) found on the rim of the anconeal process. The coronoid process can be visualized with sophisticated linear tomography, but this is available from relatively few referral centers. When dogs younger than seven months of age have lameness suggestive of FCP but no radiographic changes, they should be re-evaluated in four to six weeks to see if there is evidence of degenerative changes to support the diagnosis. Sometimes, however, surgery is necessary to confirm, as well as treat, the condition.

The elbow registry of the Orthopedic Foundation for Animals (OFA) serves to provide a standardized evaluation of the elbow joints for canine elbow dysplasia, regardless of specific cause. Abnormal elbows are graded by radiologists from I to III depending on the extent of joint damage, with Grade III being the worst. Normal elbows on individuals 24 months or older are assigned a breed registry number and are periodically reported to parent breed clubs.

The Institute for Genetic Disease Control in Animals (GDC) provides evaluation of elbows for degrees of arthrosis as recommended by the International Elbow Working Group, as determined at the 1992 meeting, and also for joint incongruity, ununited anconeal process, fragmented medial coronoid process, and evidence of osteochondrosis.

Radiographs are necessary to diagnose OCD of the hind legs. Flap lesions of the hock (tarsocrural) joint are most common in the Rottweiler, but difficult to visualize in this breed because other anatomic structures are usually in the way. OCD flaps in this joint often contain bone, in contrast to OCD flaps in other joints which usually contain cartilage. Other changes in and around the joint may provide important clues to diagnosis. OCD of the stifle results in flattened and irregular contours and loss of bone density, typical of the condition. If facilities allow, arthroscopic surgery can be used to diagnose and treat OCD of the hind legs.

Treatment

The management of dogs with OCD is a matter of much debate and controversy. Some recommend surgery before permanent damage is done. Others recommend conservative therapy of rest and pain-killers. Each side has proponents. What seems clear is that some dogs will respond to conservative therapies, while others need surgery.

The conservative approach utilizes non-steroidal anti-inflammatory drugs such as aspirin and polysulfated

Ununited anconeal process, another manifestation of elbow dysplasia. Courtesy of Dr. Jack Henry, Mesa Veterinary Hospital, Mesa, Arizona.

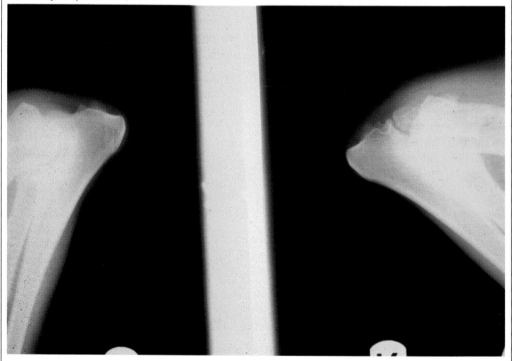

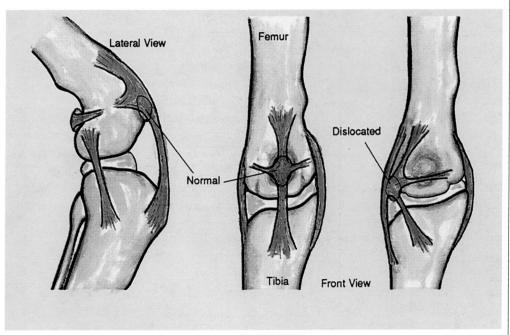

Graphic representation of medial patellar luxation. Courtesy of Petcom, Inc.

glycosaminoglycan (Adequan®-Luitpold). Aspirin reduces pain and lameness but doesn't promote healing. Most veterinarians agree that the use of cortisone-like compounds (corticosteroids) creates more problems than it treats in this condition. Polysulfated glycosaminoglycan (abbreviated PSGSG) is a natural product with claims of protecting and repairing cartilage. It is being used experimentally in dogs and is not yet licensed for use in this species. Usually it is given as an intramuscular injection every four days for six doses, and then every four to six weeks as needed.

Surgery is often helpful if performed before there is significant joint damage. The edges of the cartilage defect are trimmed with a bone curette or scalpel back to healthy bone. The central portion of the defect is completely removed. The defect then fills with fibrous cartilage. The result is usually excellent if the surgery was performed before arthritis sets in. Those dogs that have recurrent problems after surgery likely have retained loose cartilage fragments within the joint.

For OCD of the elbow, surgery is usually needed as soon as the diagnosis is made. Conservative medical therapy is not likely to be as helpful as with OCD of the shoulder. For ununited anconeal process (UAP), the process is surgically removed or fixed in place with a lag screw. This is an effective remedy for the painful joint condition but does not fully stabilize the joint. Degenerative joint disease continues, but at a much slower rate.

Dogs with fragmented coronoid process (FCP) may benefit from enforced rest and polysulfated glycosaminoglycan, but other anti-inflammatory drugs tend to delay cartilage healing. In addition, anti-inflammatory agents decrease pain and encourage dogs to use the leg. This is not desirable for this condition since it puts further stress on the joint. There are several different surgical techniques described for managing this condition. Surgery is the treatment of choice for OCD of the medial humeral condyle.

Dogs with hind-leg OCD do not respond well to conservative therapy. If arthritic changes have not yet set in, surgery is the treatment of choice.

Prevention

There is strong evidence to support the contention that OCD of the elbow is an inherited disease. Therefore, breeding stock should be selected from those animals without a history of osteochondrosis, preferably for several generations.

LEGG-CALVE-PERTHES DISEASE

Legg-Calve-Perthes disease is a disorder of the hip joint seen in young, small-breed dogs. It is also known as aseptic necrosis of the femoral head. The Yorkshire Terrier appears to be particularly prone. It is most commonly seen in dogs between four and 12 months of age. The exact cause is unknown but only one leg is involved in the

majority (85%) of cases. A genetic trend (autosomal recessive with incomplete penetrance) has been suggested.

Clinical Signs

Affected dogs are usually lame and often experience pain when the leg is moved or manipulated. There is often substantial atrophy of muscle in the affected area. Once again, this tends to be a disease of young dogs, most being under a year of age when the problem is first detected.

Diagnosis

The diagnosis can be strongly suspected on the basis of radiographic studies, and is confirmed by surgical biopsies. For some unknown reason, the bone of the femoral head just dies (avascular necrosis) and collapses in upon itself. The Institute for Genetic Disease Control in Animals (GDC) plans to provide a registry for this condition in the near future.

Treatment

The time-honored treatment for this condition is surgical removal of the femoral head (femoral head ostectomy). This is because there is little chance that the problem will resolve itself.

PATELLAR LUXATION

The patella is the kneecap and patellar luxation refers to the condition when the kneecap slips out of its usual resting place and lodges on the inside (medial aspect) of the knee. It is a congenital problem of dogs but the degree of patellar displacement may increase with time as the tissues stretch and the bones continue to deform. The condition is seen primarily in toy and slightly larger breeds of dogs.

Clinical Signs

Medial patellar luxation may be graded by veterinarians as to how much laxity there is in the patella. For example, a Grade 1 luxation may not even be noticed by owners. However, a veterinarian can manually move the patella over its bony ridge but it spontaneously returns to a normal position once released. A Grade 2 luxation is characterized by a kneecap that may skip off its bony ridge occasionally, resulting in lameness. It does eventually return to its normal position. A Grade 3 luxation varies from an occasional lameness to a more persistent weight-bearing lameness. The kneecap tends to spontaneously luxate out of its normal position when the leg is manipulated. Grade 4 luxation is characterized by persistent lameness and the patellas no longer remain in their normal positions.

Diagnosis

The diagnosis can be made by manipulating the knee joint to see if the kneecap luxates towards the inner (medial) aspect of the leg. There is usually little or no pain associated with this process. Radiography can be used to document persistent luxation and to evaluate for other abnormalities, such as arthritic changes.

Therapy

Conservative therapy can be attempted in animals over one year of age and consists of enforced rest, weight reduction, and controlled exercise. Anti-inflammatory agents can be used if pain is evident but, when animals are feeling better, they should not be allowed uncontrolled exercise or they may further damage the joint.

In younger dogs and those with persistent lameness, surgery should be used to correct the problem. There are several successful surgical techniques for this condition. After surgery, dogs should have enforced rest for six weeks while healing, and leash activity only. The results are excellent in most cases.

DEGENERATIVE JOINT DISEASE (DJD)

Degenerative joint disease (DJD) is a disorder in which there is degeneration of joint cartilage and the formation of new bone at the joint surface. The common name for the condition is osteoarthritis, but this is an inaccurate term because the cause is not inflammatory. In many parts of the world, the condition is called arthrosis or osteoarthrosis, which correctly describes the condition as degenerative rather than inflammatory.

Degenerative joint disease (DJD) can be a primary or secondary event. In most cases, there is a problem in the joint and the degeneration occurs as a secondary event, usually associated with abnormal stress on the joint. Primary degenerative joint disease becomes more common with age, especially in dogs over ten years of age. It is considered a "normal" part of aging, reflecting the wear and tear of life on old joints.

Clinical Signs

The clinical signs (symptoms) of DJD in dogs should come as no surprise. Affected dogs have more difficulty getting up and getting around and may have lameness and pain. DJD may be seen in young dogs as a consequence of osteochondrosis or other joint disorders, or in older dogs associated with aging. As the degeneration becomes more severe, the joint becomes stiffer, more painful, and more likely to cause lameness. DJD that occurs secondary to inherited or acquired joint diseases is almost always more severe than the primary degenerative changes of aging.

Diagnosis

Degenerative joint disease (DJD) can usually be suspected on the basis of a thorough veterinary evaluation, but radiographs are important in determining the severity and extent of the damage. The more drastic changes include scarring of the cartilage, bony deposits (osteophytes), bone remodeling, and changes in the contour of the joint surfaces. In most cases, both limbs are

Medial patellar luxation in which the knee caps are resting on the inside of the knee joint. Courtesy of Dr. Jack Henry.

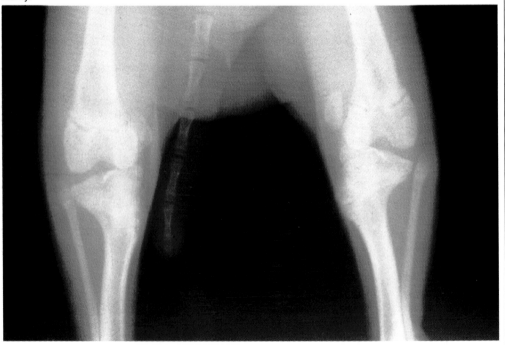

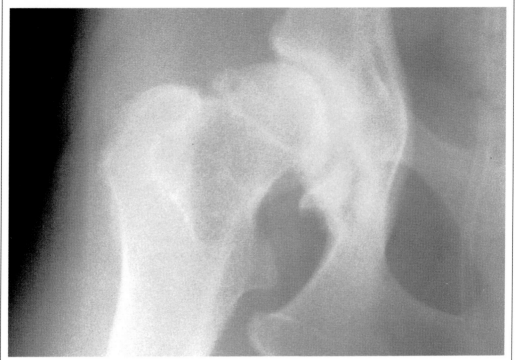

Degenerative joint disease (arthritis) seen in the hip joints of this dog with hip dysplasia.

involved, although there may be considerable variability in the amount of involvement in each. Unlike primary DJD, in which the basic anatomy of the joint remains intact, secondary DJD often has structural, anatomical, and functional abnormalities associated with the underlying cause of the problem.

Treatment

There is no cure for DJD in people or in animals. The best that can be hoped for is to minimize pain and discomfort and to increase mobility. For most cases, conservative therapy is all that is needed. This might include the use of anti-inflammatory agents, weight reduction, adequate periods of rest, and regular but limited exercise.

The anti-inflammatory agent of choice is usually buffered aspirin. More potent anti-inflammatory agents are often prescribed for people with DJD but these often have a high rate of side effects in dogs.

A final option for dogs with severe, crippling DJD is surgery. This is only warranted in certain instances since, in some cases, it can actually complicate joint function.

OSTEOMYELITIS

Osteomyelitis is an inflammatory and often infectious disorder of bone and bone marrow. It most commonly results from bacterial infections (e.g., *Staphylococcus, E. coli,* and mixed infections) but occasionally results from fungal or viral infection. It can also result as a foreign body reaction, most often to surgical implants. The presence of bacteria alone is not enough to cause osteomyelitis. Usually there must also be some interference with normal immune function, such as occurs when the blood supply to the bone is compromised in some fashion.

Clinical Signs

Osteomyelitis usually occurs within the first few weeks of a surgery, such as fracture repair. In some geographic areas, fungal infections (e.g., coccidioidomycosis) are common and will result in osteomyelitis. Brucellosis can also cause osteomyelitis. Regardless of the cause, the result is pain and swelling in the affected leg and the dog is often depressed, anorexic and feverish.

In time, pus production ensues and the area may drain like a wound. It can also remain localized as an abscess. Chronic osteomyelitis results when the process is not completely controlled. Lameness, pain, and draining are common manifestations.

Diagnosis

The diagnosis may be suspected based on clinical findings, and radiographs (x-rays) usually show swelling and bony changes. However, the changes in the bone may not be evident for several weeks into the course of the condition. Ultrasound examination may be useful in locating abscess compartments beneath the skin surface.

Radiographs may show suspicious changes but don't confirm the diagnosis or isolate the cause. This can be accomplished with bone biopsies. Sophisticated diagnostic techniques such as technetium phosphate bone scans and magnetic resonance imaging can detect osteomyelitis very early in its course but are not routinely available for animals.

Most routine blood profiles do not help further in narrowing the diagnostic possibilities. However, examining cultures of blood for microbes and performing immunologic tests for fungi may help uncover the presence of systemic (body-wide) infections.

Therapy

Ideally therapy should be directed at the underlying cause. This can be predicted based on bacterial and fungal cultures taken by various bone biopsy techniques and tests on blood for microbes. Since staphylococci are the most common cause of osteomyelitis, treatment is usually commenced with antibiotics effective against these organisms, such as the cephalosporins (e.g., cephalexin). The treatment can then be altered when the specific microbes involved have been identified.

Surgery is often needed if an abscess is present or if antibiotics fail to improve the situation within 72 hours. The surgical procedure is used to remove dead or decaying tissue, encourage normal drainage, and to directly sample material for culture. Antibiotics then need to be given for one to two months and progress should be followed by radiographs every two weeks.

For chronic osteomyelitis, treatment needs to be more intensive (and heroic) since there has probably been some bone death. This weakens the bone and makes any infection there less susceptible to antibiotic therapy. Any defects need to be completely removed so that healing can occur and drainage and antibiotic therapy can be effective. Many high-tech treatments have also been evaluated, such as antibiotic-impregnated bone cement or plaster of Paris, hyperbaric oxygen, and even electrically generated silver ions.

PANOSTEITIS

Panosteitis is an inflammatory condition that affects the leg bones of large and giant-breed dogs, especially German Shepherd Dogs. The cause is currently unknown but a genetic nature has been proposed. The condition affects males more frequently than females and is often recurrent or periodic in nature. Most dogs are less than a year of age, but occasionally they may be as old as six years of age when first affected.

Clinical Signs

Dogs typically have a sudden shifting-leg lameness, often accompanied by lethargy, anorexia, and fever. The front legs are affected first. There is typically no evidence of trauma to make one think that an injury may have taken place. When pressure is applied to the affected area, pain is often evident.

Diagnosis

Panosteitis is diagnosed by radiography. In early cases, the only noticeable change is a decreased density of bone in the area where the nutrient blood supply enters the bone. The decreased density is believed to result from removal of fat cells from the inner cavity of the bone (bone marrow). Later, the area becomes coarse or granular on radiographs which may arise from bony proliferation in the area. There is no relation between the severity of radiographic findings, the degree of lameness, and the amount of pain experienced. Blood counts and biochemical profiles usually display no abnormalities.

Therapy

There is no specific treatment for panosteitis but the condition tends to be self-limiting. In the interim, anti-inflammatory therapy (e.g., aspirin) is given to manage lameness and any pain experienced.

HYPERTROPHIC OSTEODYSTROPHY

Hypertrophic osteodystrophy is a disease of young, primarily large-breed dogs that affects the leg bones. The most common breeds affected are the Irish Setter, German Shepherd Dog, and Great

Dane. They are typically affected at a young age, often at three to four months of age. The condition is associated with inflammation of affected bones and a derangement of normal bone development.

The cause of hypertrophic osteodystrophy is the subject of much debate. It is thought that an infectious process is most likely, but no organisms have been consistently isolated. Other theories suggest that it may be involved with a relative imbalance of vitamin C or result from excessive supplementation with other vitamins and minerals. Yet others suggest that it is a genetically conditioned defect of bone growth.

Clinical Signs

Affected dogs experience lameness, often in the wrist areas (distal radius and ulna) of the front legs. The upper leg bones may be swollen, warm, and painful. Affected dogs may experience anorexia, fever, depression, and even weight loss. These signs may come and go in an intermittent pattern.

Diagnosis

The diagnosis is confirmed by radiography. A light line is often seen parallel to the growth plate of the affected bone and there is associated swelling of the tissues around the growth plate. This is often accompanied by a cuff of new bone growth. In severe cases, the process will result in bone deformity. Blood panels may have increased serum alkaline phosphatase levels but calcium and phosphorus levels are usually normal. This helps differentiate this condition from panosteitis.

Panosteitis, an inflammatory condition of the long bones. Courtesy of Dr. Jack Henry.

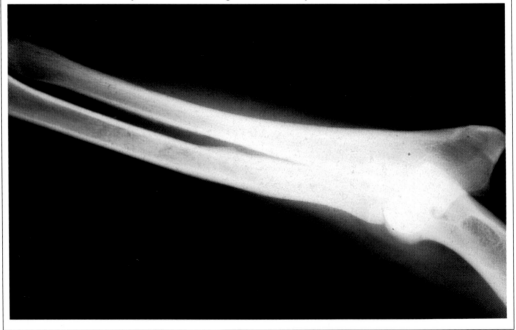

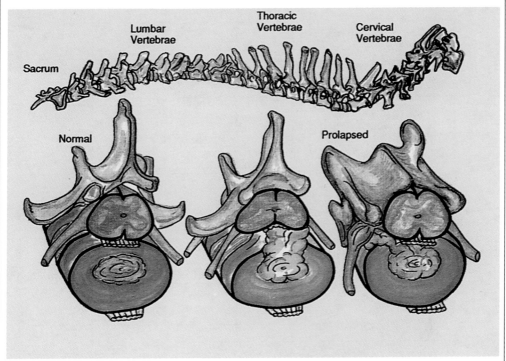

Graphic representation of intervertebral disk disease. Courtesy of Petcom, Inc.

Therapy

Because the cause of this condition is not known, there are no specific treatments. Episodes often last a week and complete, spontaneous remissions have been reported. Affected dogs are placed on a balanced diet and often treated with anti-inflammatory agents (e.g., aspirin) and cage rest. Although it might seem reasonable, vitamin C is not given to these animals because it might accelerate abnormal bone growth and remodeling. Antibiotics may be given on the grounds that some type of infection is presumed, even if not proven. Surgery is sometimes needed to correct severe bone deformities.

CRANIOMANDIBULAR OSTEOPATHY

Craniomandibular osteopathy is a proliferative bone disease that typically affects the lower jawbone (mandible), the tympanic bullae of the inner ear, and, occasionally, other bones of the head. The cause is unknown but clearly the condition is not cancerous or inflammatory, although it certainly appears that way.

Clinical Signs

Affected animals are less than one year of age and the breeds most commonly affected are Scottish Terriers, West Highland White Terriers, and Cairn Terriers. It is seen less frequently in the Boxer, Labrador Retriever, Great Dane and Doberman Pinscher.

The condition does not cause

clinical problems in all cases. However, affected animals often have difficulty chewing and swallowing and may experience some pain when opening their mouths. They may experience atrophy of those muscles used for chewing and have visible thickening of the jawbone. This may or may not be painful, and there may be fever intermittently.

Diagnosis

The diagnosis is usually suspected when a young dog of a breed at risk experiences the clinical signs listed above. The diagnosis is confirmed by radiography, in which selected bones of the head show thickening associated with proliferation of bone. The teeth are normal. Radiographs should be repeated every three months to monitor progression or regression of the condition.

Blood profiles of affected dogs may demonstrate increased serum calcium levels and some enzymes, such as serum alkaline phosphatase. Bone biopsies can also be used to confirm the diagnosis, since they show removal of normal bone and replacement with coarse bone that expands beyond the normal boundaries of the bone itself.

Therapy

There are no effective therapies available, but luckily the condition is often self-limiting. The abnormal bone growth slows, often stops, and may even recede by about a year of age. In the interim, symptomatic therapy consists of anti-inflammatory therapy (e.g., aspirin), feeding soft foods, and perhaps tube feeding if opening the mouth is painful.

Surgeries may be performed if the mouth can't be opened, but should be considered a heroic effort and are rarely completely successful. Sometimes euthanasia is necessary if animals can't eat and are in much pain.

INTERVERTEBRAL DISK DISEASE

Everyone has heard of a slipped disk, but some may be surprised to learn that this is a common problem in the dog. The Dachshund is the most common breed affected, and by some estimates, this breed may account for up to half of all cases reported. Other breeds at risk are the Pekingese, Basset Hound, and French Bulldog. Approximately 85% of herniated disks occur in the lower back, and 15% in the neck region.

The intervertebral disk is like a jelly donut with a tough fibrous outer layer and a jelly-like inner layer. In some instances, the jelly-like inner layer protrudes or "herniates" through the fibrous layer and puts pressure on the spinal cord. This causes intense pain and limited use of the limbs controlled by those obstructed nerves.

There can be different reasons why the disk material herniates and causes such damage. In breeds with stunted legs (chondrodystrophoid breeds) such as the Dachshund, 75-100% of all disks may be degenerated by one year of age. In other breeds, degeneration of the disks occurs with old age. Therefore, intervertebral disk (IVD) disease is most often seen in young chondrodystrophoid breeds and in older dogs of other breeds. The Doberman Pinscher is the only large, nonchondrodystrophoid breed that is commonly affected with cervical intervertebral disk disease.

Clinical Signs

The cardinal sign of IVD disease is intense pain. Other signs (symptoms) depend on where the herniation occurred. When a disk ruptures in the neck (cervical disk disease), pain is usually the only problem noted. That's because the spinal cord space is relatively wide there and so there is less chance that the cord itself will become compressed. These dogs will often cry out in pain, and not want their head or neck to be manipulated or moved.

When a disk ruptures in the lower back (thoracolumbar disk disease) the presentation can be much more severe. Often there is paralysis of the hind legs and pressure is applied by the herniated material onto the disk. In a very short period of time, the pain subsides as the spinal cord damage interferes with the ability to recognize pain. These cases are surgical emergencies.

Diagnosis

Many times, the clinical presentation of IVD syndrome is so specific that diagnosis is not difficult. However, in relatively mild cases, other conditions need to be considered. Radiographs and some special radiographic studies may be needed to confirm the diagnosis and location of the herniation.

When IVD syndrome is suspected, radiographs are usually taken of both the neck and back areas, even when the clinical picture suggests where the problem is likely to be. This is because other areas of potential herniation will need to be evaluated. Radiographs may demonstrate a narrowing or wedging of the disk space but the disk material itself does not show up on the films. In time, the disk material will mineralize and then it will be evident on standard radiographs. Occasionally it will be necessary to inject dye into the spinal canal (myelography) to identify the exact location of the problem.

Treatment

Intervertebral disk disease can be managed medically or surgically but there are definite guidelines to suggest which is more appropriate. Medical therapy may be adequate when there is mild-to-moderate pain but no evidence of spinal cord damage (e.g., paralysis). Strict cage rest must be enforced and a variety of anti-inflammatory drugs are used to reduce the swelling in the spinal cord. The drug regimen often includes corticosteroids ("cortisone") which works very fast at reducing inflammation in this region. Muscle relaxants may also be prescribed. This form of therapy is most appropriate for dogs with cervical disk disease.

For dogs with thoracolumbar disk disease, paralysis, and loss of deep pain sensation, surgery should be immediate. If the pressure on the spinal cord is not reduced within about 24 hours, permanent nerve damage is likely. Many different surgical techniques are available to decompress the spinal canal and remove the herniated disk material. At the time of surgery, the surgeon may elect to fenestrate other disks in the area that are at risk of future rupture. Since IVD syndrome in chondrodystrophoid breeds is likely to involve more than one disk

eventually, this is considered a preventive measure against the need for future surgeries.

Medical therapy can be attempted for thoracolumbar disk disease as long as there is still pain sensation and incomplete paralysis. This suggests that the damage to the spinal cord is more superficial, and less likely to be permanent. Unfortunately, dogs successfully managed with medical therapy have a 40% chance of recurrence. For dogs that have had deep pain loss for over 24 hours, the chances for complete recovery are slim, so conservative therapy would be just as effective as surgery in these cases. With perseverance and a dedicated owner, even these animals might regain some function in weeks or months.

A group of Dachshunds that all have had back surgery for intervertebral disk disease. Courtesy of Dr. Don Levesque, Veterinary Neurological Center, Phoenix, Arizona.

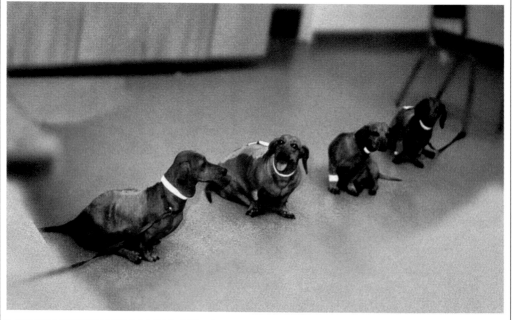

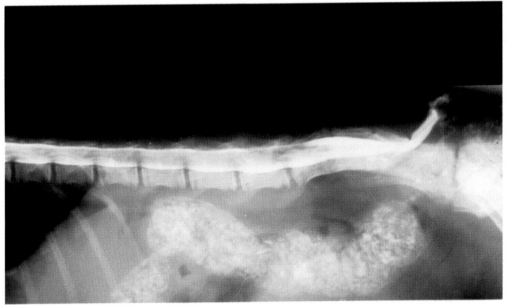

Example of a myelogram, in which contrast media has been injected into the spinal canal. Courtesy of Dr. Don Levesque, Veterinary Neurological Center, Phoenix, Arizona.

CERVICAL VERTEBRAL INSTABILITY (WOBBLER SYNDROME)

This condition is caused by an instability of the disks in the neck. Sometimes it is referred to as cervical spondylopathy. It is most common in the Doberman Pinscher and Great Dane, but can be seen in any large or giant breed of dog. Why the condition occurs is a matter of controversy, but the effects are well known. Affected dogs develop clinical signs (symptoms) associated with a narrowing of the spinal canal and compression of the spinal cord. Preliminary research suggests that excess dietary calcium, genetic factors, and overfeeding may all be involved.

Clinical Signs

When the spinal canal is narrowed, there is increased compression of the spinal cord which results in neck pain, and sometimes a difficulty or inability to walk. Most Great Danes with problems start between three to 18 months of age, while Dobermans usually develop clinical signs at four to ten years of age. By contrast, affected Basset Hounds usually have clinical problems before six months of age.

Even though the underlying problem is a bony instability of the spine, the effects are neurologic, and due to compression of nerves of the spinal cord itself in this area. Although the clinical signs may appear suddenly, they usually are progressive, getting worse over time. Most of the weakness is seen in the hind legs and hips even though the problem is centered in the neck region. Doberman Pinschers may also have rigidity of their front legs. This is uncommonly seen in other breeds. Although there may be resistance to moving the neck, neck pain itself is usually not a major part of the syndrome.

Diagnosis

The diagnosis may be suspected based on characteristic clinical signs, but radiographs are needed for confirmation. Plain radiographs typically show narrowing (stenosis) of the spinal canal in the neck and associated degenerative changes in the affected joint and intervertebral discs. Injecting dyes to outline the defect (myelography) is important, especially if surgery is to be performed. This serves to highlight the defect and show the extent of the compression.

Therapy

Conservative therapy is typically prescribed initially, even if surgery is to be performed later. This involves restricted activity and the administration of corticosteroids (cortisone-like compounds) to reduce the inflammation in the spinal canal. This conservative therapy will often improve the clinical signs (symptoms) but cannot be expected to correct the underlying spinal defect. Some dogs can be maintained on long-term cortisone therapy with adequate control, but most others eventually develop progressive problems.

Surgical decompression and stabilization is the treatment of choice for this condition but it is not universally successful. This is probably not a suitable alternative if permanent spinal-cord damage has already occurred, or if multiple spinal defects are present. The procedure can be accomplished by several different surgical techniques.

CRUCIATE LIGAMENT RUPTURE

The cruciate ligaments crisscross within the knee joint and serve an anchoring function. Rupture of the anterior cruciate ligament is very common in dogs and is the leading cause of knee subluxation in this species. It is often seen in middle-aged and older house pets and results from mild trauma, such as jumping off a couch. It can also be seen in younger dogs secondary to moderate or severe trauma, such as sudden hyperextension of the knee joint. With trauma to the cruciate ligaments, problems may also occur in the collateral ligaments and the medial meniscus.

Clinical Signs

The lameness that results from cruciate ligament rupture is not always painful. Affected dogs may carry the leg for a while, then eventually start putting more weight on the leg. Unfortunately, although they may start using the leg, more damage is likely to occur in the knee as the body attempts to stabilize the joint.

In time, if the ligament damage is not corrected, degenerative joint disease will set in and cause permanent damage to the joint.

This might also include damage to the medial collateral ligament, and the medial meniscus.

Diagnosis

Anesthesia is often necessary to completely evaluate the range of motion of the knee (stifle) joint. When the animal is suitably relaxed, the lower aspect of the leg can be advanced further than it should. This is known as a "drawer" sign, because the lower leg moves forward like the opening of a dresser drawer. This reaction is hard to elicit in most dogs that are awake because they may tense the muscles of the hind leg, making adequate manipulation difficult.

Diagnostic arthroscopy has been used to diagnose cruciate ligament rupture. This is performed by introducing a viewing device into the stifle joint. Although it is considered a less invasive diagnostic tool than surgery, this technique requires advanced instruments and extensive experience to correctly localize and identify the ruptured ligament. Removing fluid from the joint for analysis (arthrocentesis) may also confirm the presence of a degenerative joint disorder.

Therapy

The treatment of choice for rupture of the anterior cruciate ligament is surgery. However, in very small dogs, enforced rest for 12–16 weeks may allow adequate healing to occur. If this doesn't work, surgery should be performed as early as possible to diminish the risk of permanent joint damage. In dogs more than 30 pounds (15 kg), less than 20% can be expected to improve without surgery. Conservative therapy may be considered when permanent joint damage has occurred and stabilization through surgery is not possible or likely.

There are many different surgical techniques used to repair the ruptured ligament, as well as removing debris and damaged tissue and tightening the joint capsule. Static transfer techniques use tendons or prosthetic materials to reconstruct the torn ligament. Dynamic transfer techniques use existing functioning muscles to replace the damaged ligament. These surgeries will not absolutely prevent further degenerative joint disease, but usually slow its progression and lessen its severity. Most veterinarians recommend bandage or cast support for two to six weeks after surgery, to help support the joint while it heals. When the bandage or cast is finally removed, limited activity (e.g., leash walking) and physical therapy (e.g., swimming) are encouraged.

OSTEOSARCOMA (MALIGNANT BONE CANCER)

Osteosarcoma is the most common bone tumor in the dog. This is an important cancer because it is difficult to treat and because it preferentially affects certain breeds. German Shepherd Dogs, Great Danes, Saint Bernards, Boxers, Irish Setters, Labrador Retrievers, Doberman Pinschers, and Collies are at increased risk.

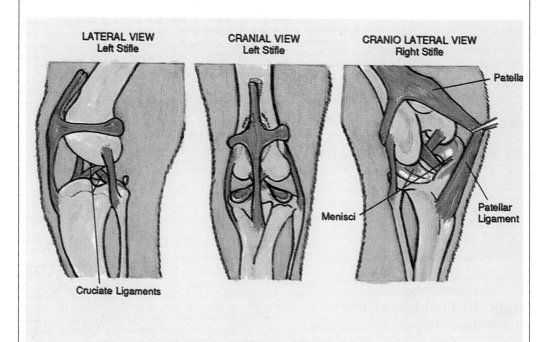

Graphic representation of the knee (stifle) joint. Courtesy of Petcom, Inc.

Clinical Signs

Most osteosarcomas originate in the long bones of the legs. Less than 25% start out in the flat bones. The usual picture is one of sudden lameness over a two to five day period. There may be associated swelling, but this is not a consistent finding. If the tumor has eaten through the supportive matrix of the bone, the affected leg might sustain a spontaneous fracture. Osteosarcoma is invariably fatal and the cancer spreads to the lungs in 80% of cases.

Diagnosis

The diagnosis of osteosarcoma may be suspected when an older dog of a breed at risk has sudden lameness. Radiographs of the affected leg are often suggestive since there may be typical changes seen in the bone tissue. However, it is usually not possible unequivocally to make the diagnosis based on radiographs alone. Biopsies, surgical samples of the tissue, provide absolute confirmation once evaluated by a trained pathologist.

Treatment

The treatment of osteosarcoma is somewhat controversial because it is one of those cancers that has proven most difficult to manage. Amputation of the affected leg is an option but it is imperative to check other areas of the body first for evidence of tumor spread. There are also

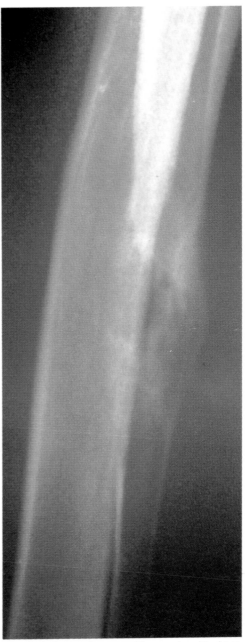

"Fuzziness" appearing around the margins of the bone in a dog with osteosarcoma.

many studies that seem to show that amputation is no assurance of increased survival. In most cases, the cancer has spread prior to the surgery.

Osteosarcoma does not respond to many anti-cancer drugs, but some headway is being made with cisplatin, a platinum-based drug. Current studies suggest that cisplatin therapy may increase survival times to about 11 months following diagnosis. Otherwise, it is rare to see dogs with osteosarcoma survive longer than nine months, regardless of the form of treatment.

DISORDERS OF THE NERVOUS SYSTEM

SEIZURE DISORDERS

A seizure is a sign of an abnormality in the brain. It results from a sudden uncontrolled activity of nerve cells (neurons), for a variety of reasons. There are different types of seizures, representing different degrees of involvement of the brain. These are classified as either generalized or partial seizures. Generalized seizures involve the entire body with loss of consciousness. Partial seizures, or focal seizures, involve only a portion of the brain and usually only a portion of the body.

Not all seizure disorders can be classified as epilepsy. Idiopathic epilepsy does not result from underlying brain diseases. It reflects a trait of the neurons to start seizures on their own.

There are many causes of seizures other than epilepsy.

Hypoglycemia (low blood sugar) may be seen in young puppies, or in diabetic dogs receiving too much insulin. Similarly if calcium levels get too low, such as in the lactating bitch (puerperal tetany), seizures can result. Dogs with liver disease may have high blood levels of ammonia because the liver can't fulfill its detoxifying role—the result could be seizures. Exposure to heavy metals (e.g., lead poisoning), insecticides (especially organophosphates), or rodent poisons (e.g., cholecalciferol) can also result in seizures. Finally, trauma, heatstroke, viral (e.g., distemper, rabies), fungal (cryptococcal meningitis), parasitic (e.g., toxoplasma), congenital (e.g., lysosomal storage diseases) and immunologic (e.g., granulomatous meningoencephalitis) disorders can all result in seizure activity.

Clinical Signs

Idiopathic epilepsy is usually first seen in dogs between one and three years of age. The animals are normal between seizures. The seizures often cluster, with three or four seizures occurring over a one-to-two-day period. They also tend to be cyclic, with the clusters recurring regularly over an interval of several weeks to several months. The length of the cycle is often constant in an individual. These seizures may occur while the animal is resting.

Idiopathic epilepsy may be an inherited disorder, at least in some breeds. Breeding studies have shown a genetic basis for the disorder in German Shepherd Dogs, Belgian Tervurens, Keeshonden, Beagles, and Dachshunds. The disorder is also quite common in some other breeds, including Poodles, Saint Bernards, Irish Setters, Siberian Huskies, Cocker Spaniels, Wire Fox Terriers, and Labrador and Golden Retrievers.

The generalized seizure usually involves certain phases. The aura is the first phase. In this phase the animal may appear restless, fearful, abnormally affectionate or show other behavioral changes. The ictus phase, the actual seizure phase, follows the aura. Here the animal usually loses consciousness and the limbs become stiff. This is followed by paddling movements of the limbs. Crying, urination, defecation and salivation may also occur. This phase may last from seconds to minutes. The final phase is post-ictus. During this phase one may see confusion, circling, blindness or sleepiness. It may last from several minutes to a few days. There is no apparent correlation between the length of the post-ictus phase and the length or severity of the ictus phase.

Status epilepticus is a condition of prolonged seizure activity lasting longer than five to ten minutes. It may also occur as repeated shorter seizures without recovery between attacks. While this is not common, it can result in severe brain damage and even death. Immediate veterinary care is necessary.

Diagnosis

A presumptive diagnosis of idiopathic epilepsy may be made clinically in a young dog that has seizured only once and has no physical abnormalities. However, if the dog has seizured more than once or has any other detectable abnormalities, a more complete workup is required.

A general approach to diagnosing the seizuring pet is to look for other body systems that might be involved in the process. For example, low blood sugar, liver disease, poisons, and trauma can all cause seizuring. Therefore, generalized tests such as blood counts, blood chemistries and urine profiles are often the first requested.

More involved evaluation might include examining the cerebrospinal fluid, the liquid that bathes the brain and spinal cord. By examining this fluid we are often able to detect signs of disease processes involving the brain. This is particularly helpful when brain infections or immunological diseases are suspected.

Electroencephalography (EEG) monitors the electrical activity of the brain just as electrocardiograms measure electrical conduction of the heart. This equipment is not available at most veterinary hospitals and referral to a veterinary neurologist is usually required. While many seizuring animals will have normal EEGs between seizures, this specialized test is sometimes helpful when a disease process

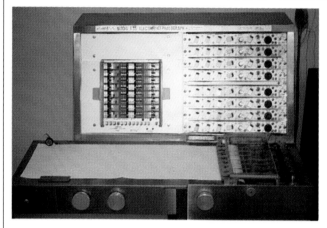

Electroencephalography (EEG) machine used to measure electrical currents through the brain. Courtesy of Dr. Don Levesque, Veterinary Neurological Center, Phoenix, Arizona.

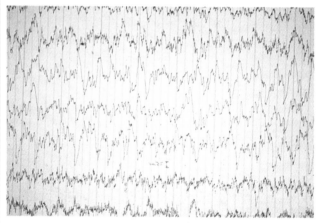

An electroencephalograph in which each line represents the electrical activity in different areas of the brain. Courtesy of Dr. Don Levesque, Veterinary Neurological Center, Phoenix, Arizona.

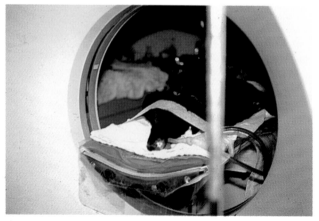

Positioning a dog for a CT (CAT) scan. Courtesy of Dr. Don Levesque, Veterinary Neurological Center, Phoenix, Arizona.

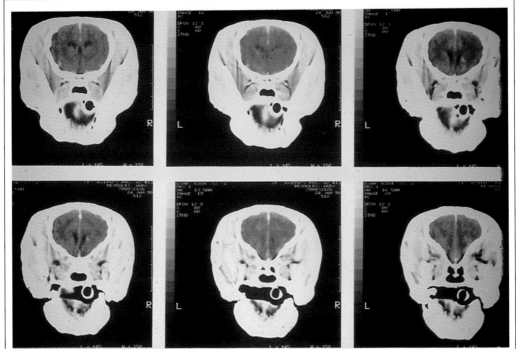

Example of CAT scans from a dog. Courtesy of Dr. Don Levesque, Veterinary Neurological Center, Phoenix, Arizona.

Example of MRI scans from a dog. Courtesy of Dr. Don Levesque, Veterinary Neurological Center, Phoenix, Arizona.

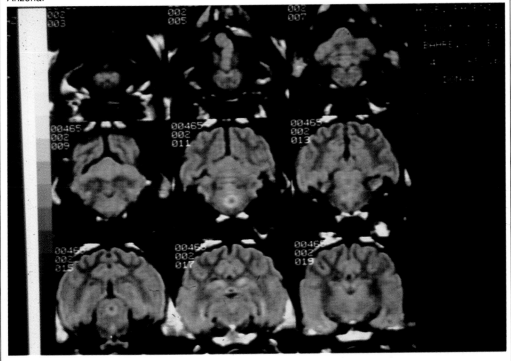

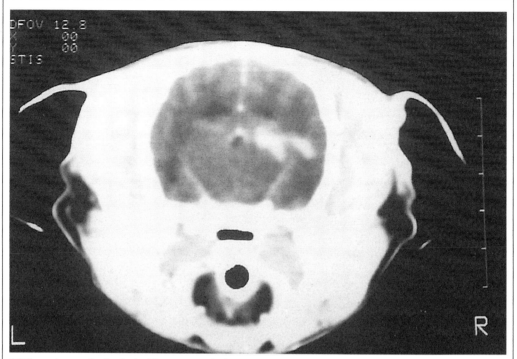

CAT scan image of a dog brain. The gray area in the central region represents the brain, and the white area within the brain is a granuloma that caused seizures in this animal. Courtesy of Dr. Michael J. Knoeckel, University of California, Davis.

such as a tumor or infection is affecting the brain.

Radiographs of the skull are helpful if a fracture or malformation is suspected, but the brain itself cannot be seen well with this test. CT (computed tomography) scans, which are also referred to as CAT scans (computed axial tomography) consist of a series of radiographs run through a computer, resulting in a picture of the brain itself. Another method of visualizing the brain is by magnetic resonance imaging (MRI). Unfortunately, neither CAT scans nor MRIs are readily available in veterinary medicine. They often require referral to a veterinary teaching hospital or a specialty practice.

Therapy

Treatment of seizures will vary with the cause. If there are metabolic problems (hypoglycemia) or organ problems (liver failure), it is most important to correct the underlying problem. The seizures will usually then stop on their own. With infectious processes (viruses, bacteria, fungi) the effort should be to clear the infectious agent from the brain and decrease inflammation. Tumors in the brain can occasionally be surgically removed and others may be better treated with radiation.

By far the most common cause of seizures in dogs is idiopathic epilepsy, and many drugs are useful in treatment. Unfortunately, many of the anti-seizure medications used in human medicine don't work particularly well in animals.

The most common anti-seizure drug used in veterinary medicine is phenobarbital. It is very good at preventing seizures and has few side effects. The animal may have an increase in appetite and thirst and, occasionally, temporary weakness while becoming accustomed to the drug.

It is important to periodically check the level of phenobarbitol in the blood. This is done by taking a blood sample immediately before giving the anticonvulsant medication so the concentration of drug is measured when lowest. This blood level shows if the amount of drug given needs to be increased, decreased or kept the same.

If the seizures cannot be controlled with phenobarbital, other drugs may be added to the phenobarbital as combination therapy. Primidone is probably the second most commonly prescribed seizure medication in dogs and cats; other products which have been used in people but with less successful results in pets include diphenylhydantoin, valproic acid, and carbamazepine. In recent years, potassium bromide has been used successfully in canine epileptics resistant to phenobarbital and primidone.

Successful control of seizures doesn't always mean they stop completely. Often we must be satisfied with reducing the frequency and intensity of the seizures to a level acceptable to pet and owner. For instance, if we reduce an animal's seizures from one per month to one every six or seven months, this may be the best control possible. Each case should be evaluated on an individual basis with both the animal's well-being and the owner's acceptance in mind.

Although complete elimination of seizure activity may not be achieved, it is still important to reduce the seizures in both intensity and frequency as much as possible. While a few short seizures are not a medical emergency, repeated seizures can lead to an increase in both the frequency and severity of the seizures.

DEAFNESS

Deafness refers to a loss of hearing, and it can be complete or partial. There are many reasons for a pet to become deaf. Some are congenital and there are a number of breeds in which degeneration of the inner ear from birth have been reported. Most cases seen in the young are inherited, but a small percentage may be acquired. The genetic transmission is usually dominant, but autosomal recessive and sex-linked inheritance has also been reported. The deafness in many canine breeds has been shown to be hereditary.

Although the incidence of congenital deafness is presumed rare, the occurrence of deafness may reach 30% in selected breeds. Some of the breeds affected include: Dalmatian, Australian

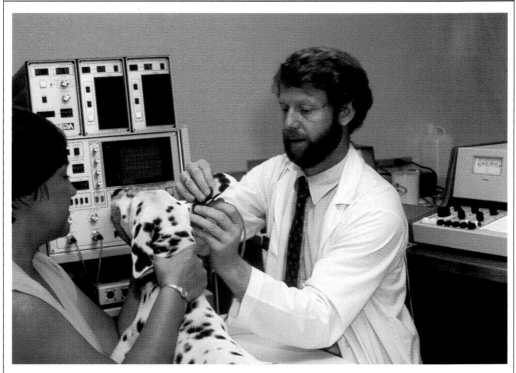

Above: Dr. Don Levesque of the Veterinary Neurological Center, Phoenix, Arizona, performs BAER testing of a Dalmatian.

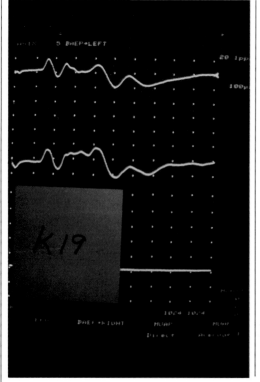

Left: Example of a normal BAER test. Courtesy of Dr. Don Levesque, Veterinary Neurological Center, Phoenix, Arizona.

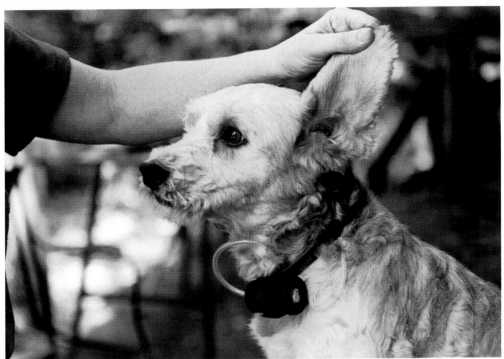

A hearing aid made especially for dogs. Courtesy of Dr. A. Edward Marshall, Auburn University, College of Veterinary Medicine, Auburn, Alabama.

Expansion of the skull sometimes occurs in young dogs with hydrocephalus. Courtesy of Dr. Don Levesque, Veterinary Neurological Center, Phoenix, Arizona.

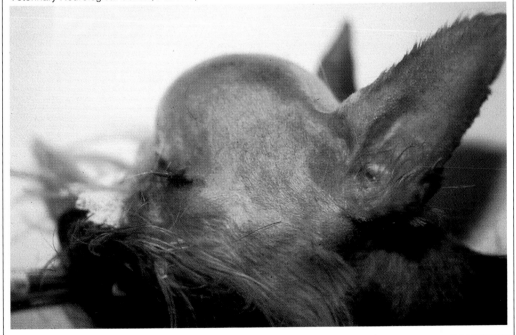

Heeler, English Setter, Australian Shepherd, Boston Terrier, Old English Sheepdog, Bulldog, Bull Terrier, Sealyham Terrier, dapple Dachshund, merle-colored Collie, Shetland Sheepdog, Norwegian Dunker, Foxhound, merle-colored and harlequin Great Dane, Scottish Terrier, Border Collie, Fox Terrier, Samoyed, Great Pyrenees, Greyhound, Beagle, West Highland White Terrier, Rhodesian Ridgeback, Beagle, and Doberman Pinscher. As you might guess from reviewing this breed list, there is an increased incidence with merle (Collie, Shetland Sheepdog, harlequin Great Dane, dappled Dachshund, American Foxhound, Norwegian Dunker) or piebald (Bull Terrier, Samoyed, Great Pyrenees, Sealyham Terrier, Greyhound, Bulldog, Dalmatian, Beagle) genes, and excessive white coat coloration.

Deafness may involve one (unilateral) or both (bilateral) ears and unilateral deafness may not be noticed by owners. The incidence for Dalmatians has been shown to be 8% bilateral deafness and 22% unilateral deafness for a total of 30% of all Dalmatians. Unilateral and/or bilateral deafness affects 75% of all-white Norwegian Dunkers but the incidence in normally colored dogs is not known.

There are other causes of deafness that are not genetic. Older dogs lose hearing progressively (presbycusis) as a consequence of aging. Certain drugs can also cause deafness because they have a toxic effect on the inner ear (ototoxicity).

This is most common with the aminoglycosides (aminocyclitol antibiotics), which include gentamicin, streptomycin, neomycin, and kanamycin. Gentamicin and neomycin are common ingredients in ear medications and can cause much damage if inserted into an ear in which the eardrum has ruptured. Deafness can also result from a bad infection in the outer or middle ear.

Clinical Signs

Owners of a deaf dog or cat may not become suspicious of the deficit until the pet reaches one year of age or older, attributing strange behaviors to stubbornness or stupidity rather than deafness. When ear infections precede deafness, there is a clear association between ear-canal disease and then the onset of deafness as a consequence.

Diagnosis

The evaluation of hearing in pets can be done with several specialized procedures, including impedance audiometry and brain stem auditory evoked responses (BAER). The impedance audiometry refers to measurement of changes in the eardrum as pressure in the external canal is changed. This is useful when the deafness is a result of ear-canal disease or damage to the eardrum.

BAER measures the electrical potentials generated in the inner ear and brain stem. The test is performed by delivering audible clicks to one ear and recording a series of brain-stem wave forms via electrodes. It is a specialized procedure which is only available from specialty practices and veterinary medical teaching hospitals. This test does not require the pet's cooperation, is painless, and can usually be performed without the need for tranquilization. It is normally performed in animals at least six weeks of age, and is an excellent screening test for breeds at increased risk of congenital deafness.

Therapy

It is often difficult to raise completely deaf dogs because they may bite when startled and do not respond to voice commands. The only way that such a dog might become a good pet is if his owners are willing to take considerable time in training, including use of hand signals. Also, the dog must never be outside alone because he will not hear other animals or vehicles approaching him. Pets with unilateral deafness can make good pets, but should not be bred since they might be carriers of the gene which could cause deafness in future generations.

There are some measures that can be taken for the deaf dog. Hearing aids are available for partially deaf, older dogs, but are not inexpensive and take considerable time getting the pet conditioned to the device. The single most important consideration in selecting candidates for the hearing device is the willingness of the owner to spend time conditioning the dog to accept the device. To use the device, dogs must have a healthy ear canal and no history of ear infections. Since the device is only an amplifier, the dog must have at least some degree of hearing to begin with.

HYDROCEPHALUS

Hydrocephalus is a condition in which the brain swells from the accumulation of cerebrospinal fluid (CSF). The cause can either be congenital or secondary to some obstructive process to the outflow of CSF. It is thought that congenital hydrocephalus might result from infections, toxins, or nutritional disorders while pups are still in the womb.

Clinical Signs

Primary hydrocephalus occurs most commonly in small breeds of dogs such as Chihuahuas, Pomeranians, and Boston Terriers. It causes seizures, problems with vision, and behavioral abnormalities. In young dogs, the skull may expand as the cerebrospinal fluid accumulates and forces the skull outward. Even with treatment, affected animals may have permanent learning deficits.

Diagnosis

Confirmation of the diagnosis often requires specialized tests such as electroencephalography (EEG), ultrasonography (ultrasound examination through fontanelles), or computed tomography (CT scans). Neurological examinations, radiographs of the skull and pressure measurements of the cerebrospinal fluid are often highly suggestive but not confirmatory in all cases.

Therapy

Treatment for hydrocephalus is directed at lowering the volume of cerebrospinal fluid and encouraging proper drainage. Corticosteroids such as prednisone are thought to decease the production of CSF, but there are dangers to using them long-term. Diuretics (water pills) such as furosemide (Lasix) may also be helpful in this regard.

For animals with severe disease, surgical drainage may be contemplated, but this is a sophisticated procedure in which a permanent drainage tube (ventriculovenous shunt) is placed in the brain. When seizures result, they must be treated with appropriate medications, such as phenobarbital.

MYASTHENIA GRAVIS (MG)

Myasthenia gravis (MG) is a disease affecting the interaction of nerves and muscles and both congenital and acquired forms occur in the dog. Congenital MG most likely results from an inherited (suspected autosomal recessive) defect in the receptors for acetylcholine, an important neurotransmitter. The most common breeds affected are the Jack Russell Terrier, Smooth Fox Terrier, English Springer Spaniel, and Samoyed. The acquired form is an immune-mediated disease in which antibodies are produced against those receptors. Large breeds are more frequently affected, especially the German Shepherd Dog.

Clinical Signs

The clinical picture of myasthenia gravis is one of muscle weakness. With the congenital form, weakness is noted by six to eight weeks of age when the pups are just learning to walk. In Smooth Fox Terriers, the condition has been seen in association with an enlarged esophagus (megaesophagus) as well.

In the acquired form, most dogs are older than two years of age when first affected. There is a noted association between this condition and a benign tumor of the thymus gland (thymoma). In older dogs, the clinical picture is more variable and the weakness is usually first evident as tiring easily after exercise. When walking, the stride may be seen to be shorter than usual, but there is typically recovery after a short rest. With fatigue, there may be drooping of the face and animals may even have difficulty holding up their heads. Chewing and swallowing may become difficult and an enlarged esophagus (megaesophagus) is frequently seen with acquired MG. This can result in pneumonia caused when ingested foods are retched up and then enter the respiratory passages (aspiration pneumonia).

Diagnosis

The most used diagnostic test for MG is the Edrophonium chloride (Tensilon) response test, but it should be administered by experienced individuals since side effects may be noted. Dogs with MG tend to improve within 30 seconds of the injection, then revert back to fatigue within five minutes. A modification of this test can also be performed with neostigmine methylsulfate (Prostigmin). In animals with MG, radiographs of the chest are taken to see if there is evidence of thymus tumors or enlarged esophagus.

The diagnosis can also be made with nerve conduction studies, antibody titers, and indirect immunologic tests. The antibody titers (to acetylcholine receptors) are only useful for cases of acquired MG and those with severe manifestations; thymus tumors tend to have the highest titers. The indirect tests incubate blood serum with normal dog muscle to determine if immune complexes form at the junctional area where nerves meet muscle. This test is useful in animals suspected of having MG but without significant titers.

Therapy

There is little that can be done for pups with congenital myasthenia gravis. The acquired condition is much more amenable to therapeutic management. In these older dogs, treatment can consist of using anticholinesterase drugs, reducing abnormal antibody production, and surgically removing the thymus if a tumor is present.

Pyridostigmine bromide (Mestinon) is currently considered the drug of choice for acquired MG in dogs. It doesn't repair the defect but it does delay the destruction of acetylcholine, giving it the maximum opportunity to interact with the nerve muscle junction. Neostigmine (Prostigmin) has also been used for this purpose. When using these anticholinesterase agents, it is important that caution be exercised in selecting any other drug to be used in the affected dog. That is because several other drugs, including some antibiotics, heart medications, and anticonvulsants, may interfere, and actually potentiate the signs of myasthenia gravis.

The principle of lowering antibody levels is only useful in cases of acquired myasthenia gravis. Corticosteroids such as prednisone, and chemotherapies such as cyclophosphamide and azathioprine, have been used to push down antibody levels. Patients receiving these medications must be monitored closely for side effects. Successful use of these products often allows reduction in the amount of anticholinesterase that needs to be administered.

Surgical removal of the thymus is only considered in those animals that don't respond well to the medical forms of therapy. Obviously, this surgery is only indicated if there is actually a tumor present on the thymus. Even after the surgery, pyridiostigmine and prednisone still need to be administered.

POLYRADICULONEURITIS

Acute polyradiculoneuritis, also known as coonhound paralysis, was originally reported as a form of paralysis that resulted seven to ten days after an encounter with a raccoon. It is now known that raccoon exposure is not the critical aspect of the clinical condition; only certain dogs are susceptible. The cause is not known, but is thought to be an immune-mediated syndrome similar to Landry-Guillain-Barre syndrome in people.

Clinical Signs

For those hunting dogs with exposure to raccoons, the onset of clinical signs is usually seven to 14 days after exposure. There is a sudden onset of hind-leg weakness and within 48 hours the front legs are involved as well. The muscles also become weak and begin to atrophy, and tests of spinal reflexes reflect the nerve damage that has occurred. Despite the lack of reflex action, these animals are usually exquisitely sensitive to pain, and even a light touch may seem painful to these individuals. Occasionally the paralysis affects the breathing centers and can result in death if not treated promptly.

Diagnosis

The diagnosis is usually suspected based on the clinical presentation and is confirmed by electromyographic (EMG) studies of affected muscle. The EMG findings are consistent five to seven days after the onset of clinical signs. Cerebrospinal fluid (CSF) analysis may reveal increased protein levels, but otherwise is not diagnostic for the condition.

Therapy

There is no specific treatment for polyradiculoneuritis, but fortunately the situation tends to improve spontaneously three to six weeks from the onset of signs. Recovery occurs in the reverse order of appearance, so the front legs are often the first to recover strength and movement.

The important aspects of therapy are supportive care, such as insuring comfortable bedding, physical therapy, and making sure animals are turned and bathed regularly. Most severely affected animals will also need to be given food and water by hand. Oxygen supplementation will be needed in animals experiencing respiratory paralysis. Corticosteroid use is controversial, but probably should only be used within the first three days. After that, they increase the risk of urinary tract infections and pneumonia.

MENINGITIS

Meningitis is an inflammatory disease of the covering of the brain and intervening cerebrospinal fluid.

When the brain itself is also involved, it is referred to as meningoencephalitis, and meningomyelitis when the spinal cord is involved.

The most common cause of meningitis is infection, usually with bacteria or fungi. An inflammatory reaction of blood vessels (vasculitis) is causative in some cases, and yet others have unknown (idiopathic) causes.

Clinical Signs

Meningitis can occur in any breed and any age but the idiopathic varieties are usually reported in dogs less than 18 months of age. These conditions are thought to result from some abnormal immunologic response. Vasculitis as a cause of meningitis has been reported in several breeds, including the Beagle, Bernese Mountain Dog, and German Shorthaired Pointer.

Meningitis can cause weakness, seizures, dementia, neck pain, head tilt and many other clinical signs. Since meningitis is often associated with systemic illnesses, it is not surprising that there might also be respiratory disease, eye disease, fever or other manifestations.

Diagnosis

Meningitis is typically diagnosed by examining the cerebrospinal fluid. This fluid tends to have increased white blood-cell counts, increased protein, and elevated pressures. The fluid can also be used to culture microbes or to use in immunologic tests for viruses and fungi.

Therapy

The treatment of choice for dogs with infectious meningitis is antibiotics selected on the basis of bacterial and fungal cultures. Then appropriate therapy can be instituted and needs to be continued for at least three to four weeks. The culture information needs to be combined with the knowledge that only certain antibiotics penetrate the brain to reach concentrations sufficient to kill microbes.

For dogs with idiopathic meningitis, presumed to be immune-mediated in origin, and for those with vasculitis, corticosteroids are often given. This treatment is given in fairly large doses for the first few weeks, then gradually tapered. It often needs to be continued for several months. It is important that an appropriate diagnosis be made because corticosteroids should not be given to dogs with infectious meningitis.

ADDITIONAL READING

Boulay, JP: Canine hip dysplasia. *Pet Focus*, 1990; 2(1): 7-10.

Corley, EA; Hogan, PM: Trends in hip dysplasia control: Analysis of radiographs submitted to the Orthopedic Foundation for Animals, 1974 to 1984. *Journal of the American Veterinary Medical Association*, 1985; 187(8): 805-809.

Dupuis, J; Harari, J: Cruciate ligament and meniscal injuries in dogs. *Compendium for Continuing Education of the Practicing Veterinarian,* 1993; 15(2): 215-232.

Fox, S; Walker, A: Symposium on osteochondrosis in dogs. *Veterinary Medicine,* 1993; 88(2): 116-153.

Jones, RD; Baynes, RE; Nimitz, CT: Nonsteroidal anti-inflammatory drug toxicosis in dogs and cats: 240 cases (1989-1990). *Journal of the American Veterinary Medical Association,* 1992; 201(3): 475-477.

Knoeckel, MJ: Seizure disorders in the dog and cat. 1990; 2(3): 30-32.

Lewis, DD; McCarthy, RJ; Pechman, RD: Diagnosis of common developmental orthopedic conditions in canine pediatric patients. *Compendium for Continuing Education of the Practicing Veterinarian,* 1992; 14(3): 287-301.

Lust, G; Rendano, VT; Summers, BA: Canine hip dysplasia: Concepts and diagnosis. *Journal of the American Veterinary Medical Association,* 1985; 187(6): 638-640.

Richardson, DC: The role of nutrition in canine hip dysplasia. *Veterinary Clinics of North America, Small Animal Practice,* 1992; 22(3): 529-540.

Roperto, F; Papparella, S; Crovace, A: Legg-Calve-Perthes Disease in dogs: Histological and ultrastructural investigations. *Journal of the American Animal Hospital Association,* 1992; 28(2): 156-162.

Sackman, JE: Pain. Part II. Control of Pain in Animals. *Compendium for Continuing Education of the Practicing Veterinarian,* 1991; 13(2): 181-192.

Slater, MR; Scarlett, JM; Donoghue, S; et al: Diet and exercise as potential risk factors for osteochondritis dissecans in dogs. *American Journal of Veterinary Research,* 1992; 53(11): 2119-2124.

Strain, GM: Congenital deafness in dogs and cats. *Compendium for Continuing Education of the Practicing Veterinarian,* 1991; 13(2): 245-252.

Toombs, JP: Cervical Intervertebral Disk Disease in Dogs. *Compendium for Continuing Education of the Practicing Veterinarian,* 1992; 14(11): 1477-1487.

Wallace, MS; et al: Gastric ulceration in the dog secondary to the use of nonsteroidal anti-inflammatory drugs. *Journal of the American Animal Hospital Association,* 1990; 26(5): 467-472.

Eye Problems

The eye is a masterpiece of specialized function. It allows us and our pets to have a fuller appreciation of the world around us. Do you still believe that dogs are color-blind? Not so, but they don't see colors exactly the same as people do. Vision is controlled by the impact of light on the rods and cones present in the retina at the back of the eye. Do animals have cones, those cells necessary to distinguish color? The answer is yes, and therefore we shouldn't be surprised that animals should be able to distinguish colors. Do they see the same colors we do? In all likelihood, they see blues and violets just as we do, but, since dogs lack green cones, their perception of green, yellow and orange is likely poor.

This should translate to mean that dogs can distinguish red from blue but would find it difficult to distinguish green from yellow or orange from red. And, as was mentioned earlier, colors in the blue-green zone would appear white. Although dogs have developed exceptional senses of smell and touch, it is still reassuring that they don't spend their lives in shades of gray.

CANINE EYE REGISTRATION FOUNDATION (CERF)

The Canine Eye Registration Foundation (CERF) is an international organization devoted to eliminating hereditary eye diseases from purebred dogs. This organization is similar to the Orthopedic Foundation for Animals (OFA).

CERF is a nonprofit organization that screens and certifies purebred dogs' eyes as free of heritable eye diseases. All information gained through this program is confidential; only the dog owner and the veterinary ophthalmologist have access to the records.

CERF is a cooperative program involving board-certified veterinary ophthalmologists, breed clubs, breeders, and dog owners. Dogs are evaluated by veterinary eye specialists and the findings are submitted to CERF for documentation. The information is compiled by a computer and is used to evaluate and predict trends in heritable eye diseases in different breeds of dogs. The goal is to identify purebreds without heritable eye problems so they can be used for breeding. Some of the problems the eye specialists screen for include progressive retinal atrophy, cataracts, and eyelid disorders.

Dogs certified free of ocular disease can be used in breeding programs. However, if they are known to carry genetic defects, they should not be used for breeding even if they are currently free of eye disease.

It is recommended that dogs considered for breeding programs be screened and certified by CERF on a minimum of a yearly basis. People interested in acquiring puppies should request that the parents be evaluated to reduce the likelihood of heritable eye conditions.

For more information on CERF, contact: Canine Eye Registration Foundation, SCC-A Purdue University West Lafayette, IN 47907, 317-494-8179.

GENETIC DISEASE CONTROL (GDC)

The Institute for Genetic Disease Control in Animals (GDC) is a nonprofit organization founded in 1990 and maintains an open registry for several hereditary conditions. In an open registry like GDC, owners, breeders, veterinarians, and scientists can trace the genetic history of any particular dog once that dog and close relatives have been registered. The information about each dog automatically becomes linked in the open registry with relatives of that animal. An open registry delivers information on specific animals to breeders (for a fee) in order for the breeder to make knowledgeable selection of mates whose bloodlines indicate a reduced risk of producing genetic disease. Closed registries such as OFA and CERF tell only if an individual animal is free of clinical signs of the disease without providing information about parents, siblings, or half-siblings.

The Poodle Club of America (PCA) at their October 1992

Basic anatomy of the eye. Courtesy of Petcom, Inc.

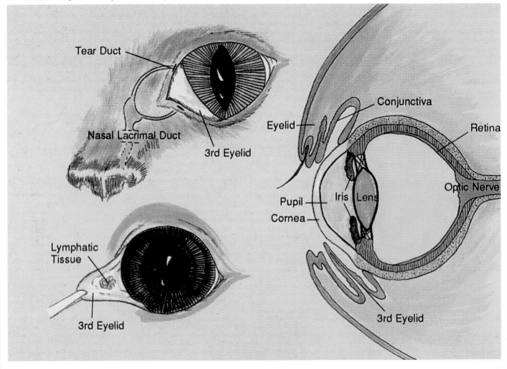

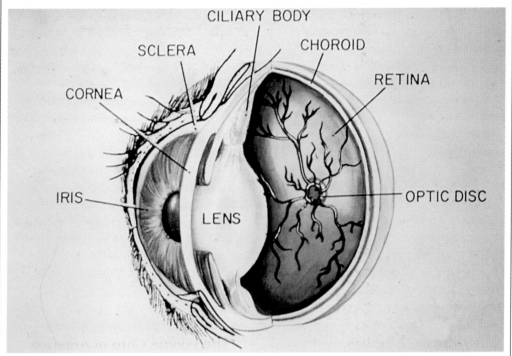

CILIARY BODY

SCLERA

CHOROID

RETINA

CORNEA

IRIS

LENS

OPTIC DISC

Internal anatomy of the eye.

meeting had endorsed the formation of an open registry for genetic diseases of the eye to be established and administered by the GDC. This organization also started research data bases for a variety of different inherited diseases. The GDC represents the first open registry of hereditary diseases in North America that aids in genetic selection of breeding stock and supports research for the control of genetic diseases of dogs. GDC also offers professional genetic evaluations and scientific support services.

For more information, contact the Institute for Genetic Disease Control in Animals, P.O. Box 222, Davis, CA 95617, phone and FAX (916) 756-6773.

ANATOMY AND PHYSIOLOGY OF THE EYE

The eyes are complicated units that translate light waves into images in the brain. There are many steps necessary to perform this miraculous function, and many different components to the system. Some of these components are located outside the eye, while others are inside. Because of their visual-processing functions, the eyes are often compared to cameras and some of these comparisons are valid. To understand some of the problems that affect the eyes, it is therefore important to have at least some familiarity with the components of the eye and how they function.

The eyes are protected from the environment by upper and lower eyelids. These eyelids serve several important functions, including controlling the amount of light entering the eye, protecting the eye, and distributing the tear film over the eye surface. Eyelashes are found only on the upper eyelids of dogs.

The third eyelid, or nictitating membrane, serves the same functions as the external eyelids. This membrane originates at the inner (medial) margin of the eye and covers the eye diagonally. It is supplied with its own tear (lacrimal) glands which contribute significantly to the tear film. The secretions of these glands are used to lubricate the eye and prevent it from drying out.

The cornea is the clear covering of the front of the eye. It is richly supplied with nerves, and corneal damage is extremely painful. The unique transparent nature of the cornea allows 99% of the light to pass without scatter.

The iris is the colored portion of the eye. The various colors depend on the amount of pigment in the iris. The iris actually acts as a diaphragm within the eye, opening and closing depending on the amount of light available. A dilated iris, or large pupil, is needed to capture more light in poor illumination. A constricted iris, or small pupil, shields the eye from excessive light and glare in bright areas. The iris also plays a role in focus and accommodation.

The ciliary body produces clear aqueous humor (translation from Latin: "watery fluid") which is formed from blood components. The eye needs clear fluid because blood and blood vessels would obscure vision. The aqueous fluid passes through the pupillary opening and is then drained at the filtration angle. This works like the plumbing in a house. Drainage is essential or the fluid "backs up" and causes problems. An increase in pressure from blockage of the drainage system is called glaucoma. The ciliary body must produce aqueous humor but it is equally important that it be properly drained or the consequences can be severe. The ciliary body is not as well developed in dogs as it is in people.

The lens is proportionately larger and more spherical in domestic animals than in man. Suspensory ligaments (lens zonules) hold the lens to the ciliary body. The muscle of the ciliary body contracts and relaxes to change the shape of the lens, thus focusing images on the retina for vision at different distances; this is called accommodation. Gradual hardening of the lens is called lenticular sclerosis and is a normal consequence of aging in dogs. This should not be confused with cataracts. A cataract is an opacity or cloudiness on or within the lens.

The retina is the "film" in the eye's video unit, the structure which records the image. There are two basic light-perceiving cells: rods, which are sensitive to dim light, and cones, which are sensitive to bright light. Colors are perceived by the cones, which vary in their sensitivity to different wavelengths of light.

Nocturnal animals such as dogs and cats have a "tapetum lucidum" (Latin for "shining carpet") located in the upper half of the retina. Plate-like cells, without much pigment, optimize reflection of incoming light—like the reflectors on our bikes and cars—for good twilight and night vision. This causes their eyes to appear luminous or have an "eye sheen" when light is directed on them in the dark. All of the nerve fibers of the retina gather at the optic disk where they come together to form the optic nerve. The optic nerve exits the eye and becomes the optic tract, which courses to the brain.

In summary, the eye focuses light rays through the cornea and lens onto the retina resulting in a small inverted image. The light-perceiving cells of the retina (rods/cones) convert the light stimuli to chemical reactions which are, in turn, converted to nerve impulses which travel to the brain.

EYELID DISORDERS

There are several disorders that affect the upper and lower eyelids of dogs, as well as the nictitating membrane (also known as the third eyelid). The most common are ectropion, entroprion, distichiasis, and prolapsed gland of the nictitans. The majority are breed related and a genetic basis is suspected.

Ectropion refers to eyelids that are "turned out" and often have the appearance of drooping. It is most commonly seen in the lower lids. Breeds observed with ectropion include the Bloodhound, Cocker Spaniel, Springer Spaniel, Mastiff, and some retrievers.

Entropion occurs when the eyelids "turn in" toward the eye, often resulting in abrasive damage to the cornea. The lower lids are the ones most commonly involved. Breeds commonly observed with entropion include the Chinese Shar-Pei, Chow Chow, Golden Retriever and Rottweiler.

Distichiasis refers to lashes that may project towards the surface of the eye from abnormal locations, such as the openings of specialized (Meibomian) glands in the eyelids. Breeds with a high incidence of distichiasis include American and English Cocker Spaniels, Shih Tzu, Poodles, Bulldogs, St. Bernards, Pekingese, and Golden Retrievers. The condition is suspected of being a genetic disorder.

Prolapsed gland of the nictitans (frequently referred to as a cherry eye by breeders) refers to an enlarged gland at the base of the nictitating membrane that is displaced from its normal position. It is seen as a red mass above the margin of the nictitating membrane. It is most commonly seen in Cocker Spaniels, Bulldogs, Boston Terriers, Shih Tzu, and other breeds.

Clinical Signs

Ectropion is the sagging of the lower eye lid so that the conjunctival lining of the eye can be easily seen. It is a breed characteristic in Cocker and English Springer Spaniels,

Bloodhounds, Newfoundlands, and many other breeds. Because the lids don't conform to the eyeball, these dogs may be prone to inflammatory reactions of those lining membranes. This is known as conjunctivitis and there are many other causes as well.

Entropion is an inward-rolling of the lids. In the Chinese Shar-Pei, this may be noted as soon as the eyes are open, soon after birth, or in the adult. Anatomic entropion is seen in sporting breeds, Chow Chows, and Chinese Shar-Pei.

Distichiasis may not be problematic because the hairs may be soft and fine, and may float on the tear film of the eye. If the hairs are coarse and stiff, or if the eyes become dry, problems can develop. Corneal ulceration, scarring or pain can result from the hairs contacting the surface of the eye.

Pain may be evidenced when dogs blink repeatedly (blepharospasm) or have weepy, runny eyes.

Prolapse of the gland of the nictitans is easy to see as a red ball of tissue protruding from beneath the nictitating membrane. Most dogs are quite young when this develops, and it is not rare that both eyes be simultaneously affected.

Diagnosis

Diagnosis is rather straightforward for these disorders as they can all be detected by thorough visual examination. Magnification will be needed to detect the aberrant hairs of distichiasis.

Therapy

All of the eyelid disorders are best managed by surgery. These

Ectropion. Notice the drooping lower lid. Courtesy of Dr. Dan Lavach, Eye Clinic for Animals, Garden Grove, California.

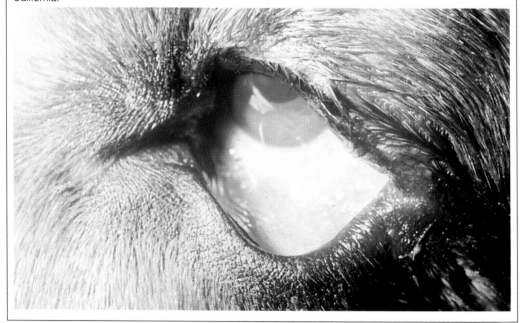

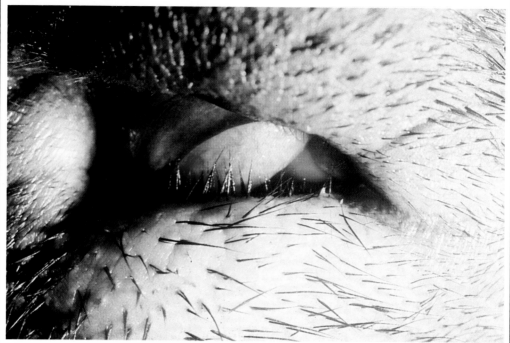

Entropion. The lid folds inward. Courtesy of Dr. Dan Lavach, Eye Clinic for Animals, Garden Grove, California.

Prolapsed gland of the nictitans ("cherry eye"). Courtesy of Dr. Dan Lavach, Eye Clinic for Animals, Garden Grove, California.

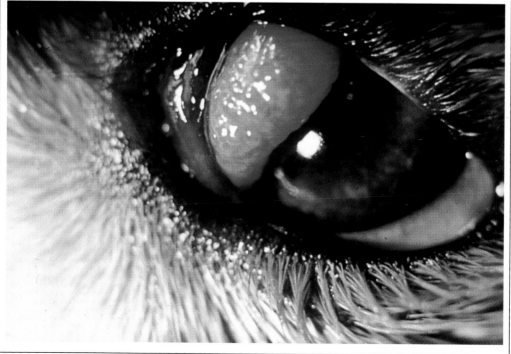

surgeries are performed to provide relief to affected dogs. They are not meant to alter conformation in dogs used for show purposes.

The surgical treatment for ectropion often involves removing a wedge of tissue from the lid margin. This is used only if the ectropion is resulting in conjunctival or corneal diseases. Additional "tightening" procedures may be used for best cosmetic results.

Entropion involves more complicated techniques to properly reposition the lids. In the Chinese Shar-Pei, temporary sutures are often needed to revert the lids. This is often done at three to four weeks of age. The final surgery is not performed until five to seven months of age when the adult dimensions of the eye are achieved. The most common procedure is to remove an ellipse of tissue parallel to the lid margin so that the lid then returns to a more normal location.

Distichiasis can be treated by a number of options. The abnormal hairs can be plucked periodically to provide temporary relief. Unfortunately, they often regrow. More sophisticated techniques such as electrocautery or electroepilation can be used. Surgery or cryosurgery can be used in stubborn cases. There is still the possibility of recurrence or scarring with any of these procedures.

The old treatment for prolapsed gland of the nictitans was to surgically remove it. However, it is now known that this gland produces a significant amount of tear film, so it should be preserved whenever possible. Most surgeries today conserve the gland and "tack it down" into its normal location. The problem can recur with any of the surgical techniques, at which time the surgery will need to be repeated.

CONJUNCTIVITIS

The conjunctiva is the lining membrane of the eyelids and sclera. When it gets red and inflamed, the condition is referred to as conjunctivitis. In dogs, the most common causes for conjunctivitis are allergies and bacterial infections. True bacterial conjunctivitis is rare in dogs but bacterial infections are common complications of already inflamed tissues. Sometimes conjunctivitis is subdivided into infectious and non-infectious causes.

Clinical Signs

There is quite a bit of variability when it comes to the clinical presentation of conjunctivitis. However, all cases of conjunctivitis are inflamed. Dogs with inhalant allergies might have runny eyes (epiphora) or rub them with their paws or on carpets or furniture. If the cause of the allergy is seasonal (e.g., ragweed), the conjunctivitis will be seasonal as well.

Bacterial conjunctivitis is usually associated with some degree of pus or mucus accumulation in the eyes. It is usually secondary to other ocular conditions, such as ectropion or keratoconjunctivitis sicca (dry eye).

Diagnosis

The cause for the conjunctivitis should always be investigated. Careful examination of the eye and lids may provide interesting clues. If there is mucus or pus present, samples may be taken for microscopic evaluation and for culture. A Schirmer tear test should also be performed to make sure that the dog is producing adequate amounts of tears.

For dogs with suspected allergic conjunctivitis, intradermal allergy testing can be performed. This is a modified version of the human test, in which different pollens, molds, and environmentals are injected into the skin and the response evaluated.

Therapy

To be successful, the underlying cause for the conjunctivitis must be addressed. Dogs with allergies might be treated with immunotherapy (allergy shots), antihistamines, fatty acids, and corticosteroids. Mild corticosteroid eye drops also help relieve inflammation. However, neither topical nor oral corticosteroids are desirable for long-term use.

Bacterial conjunctivitis is treated with antibiotic eye drops, often given at least four times a day. It is imperative that any underlying problems be dealt with, or the condition is likely to recur once the antibiotics have been discontinued. This is critical because it must be remembered that bacteria frequently complicate conjunctivitis but rarely ever cause it.

KERATOCONJUNCTIVITIS SICCA (KCS)

Keratoconjunctivitis sicca (KCS), or "dry eye," is a common condition seen in dogs. Breeds that appear to be especially prone to the disease include the Cocker Spaniel, Miniature Dachshund, Bulldog, Lhasa Apso, Miniature Schnauzer, Pug, Chinese Shar-Pei, Shih Tzu, West Highland White Terrier, Bloodhound, Pekingese, and Yorkshire Terrier.

KCS results from reduction in the amount of watery tears produced by the lacrimal glands. The underlying reasons for this condition are numerous. Some are congenital (present at birth), some are due to toxins (including drugs), some due to infection (e.g., chronic conjunctivitis), some due to hypothyroidism, and some due to abnormal immunologic reactions. Most cases are immune-mediated, meaning there is an abnormal immune response targeting the lacrimal glands. Regardless of cause, it is important that the condition be recognized early and appropriately treated while it can still be corrected.

In keratoconjunctivitis sicca, the lack of corneal tear film results in patchy, dry areas on the corneal surface. The dried cornea, deprived of oxygen and nutrients from the tear film, rapidly undergoes destructive changes. This can result in brown pigmentation, scarring, ulceration, and blood vessel growth on the surface of the eye.

Clinical Signs

It is impossible to visually determine if there is adequate tear film being produced. What is apparent is that a lack of tear film causes mucus to accumulate in the eyes. The eyes may then become painful and inflamed. At no time is it necessarily obvious that the eyes are "dry." With long-term tear loss, vision is progressively lost due to "clouding" or opacification of the inside the lower eyelid for one minute. It absorbs tears which can then be measured to determine whether or not tear production is normal.

Two of the most common causes for KCS are immune-mediated disorders and drug reactions. Sulfa drugs are the most common cause of drug-induced KCS. However, overall, immune-mediated disorders are probably the most

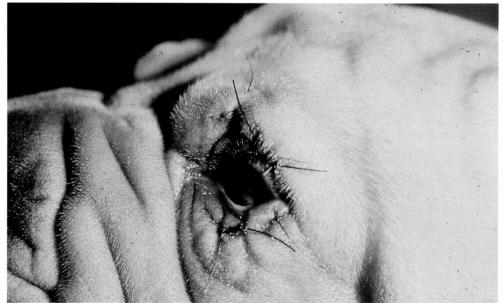

Entropion surgery in a young Chinese Shar-Pei. Courtesy of Dr. Dan Lavach, Eye Clinic for Animals, Garden Grove, California.

cornea, and the eyes may be permanently damaged.

Diagnosis

The diagnosis of KCS is relatively straightforward but finding the underlying cause can be more difficult. The amount of tear film being produced can be measured with a special paper strip. This is known as the Schirmer tear test. The thin strip of paper is placed common cause. Therefore, additional blood tests such as antinuclear antibody (ANA) and rheumatoid factor (RF) tests are typically run in a patient with KCS and no history of drug administration. The ANA and RF tests may be positive in 25-30% of cases.

Therapy

The goal of therapy is to restore

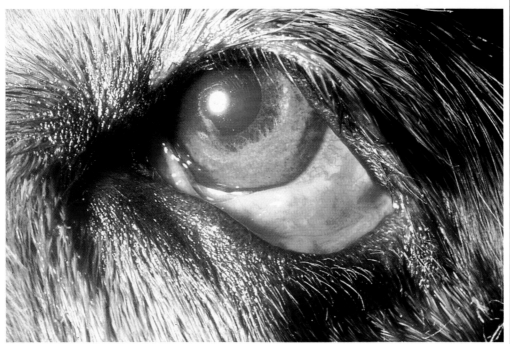

Conjunctivitis of unknown cause. Courtesy of Dr. Dan Lavach, Eye Clinic for Animals, Garden Grove, California.

Keratoconjunctivitis sicca ("dry eye"). Note the accumulation of mucus and debris. Courtesy of Dr. Dan Lavach, Eye Clinic for Animals, Garden Grove, California.

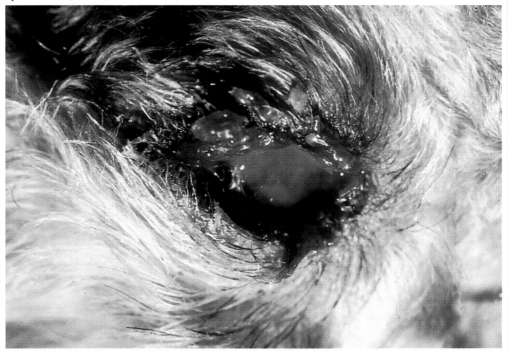

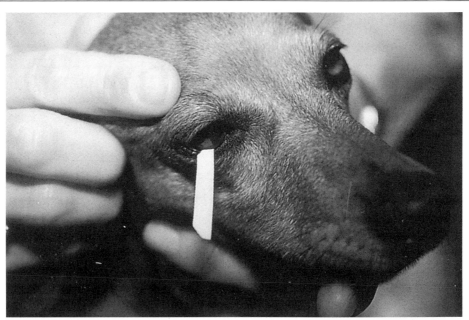

The Schirmer tear test measures the volume of tear production. Courtesy of Dr. Karen McWhirter, Roadrunner Mobile Veterinary Clinic, Tucson, Arizona.

or supplement tear production. This may be as basic as discontinuing a particular drug, or as sophisticated as using drugs to restore normal tear production. There are also some surgical options which can re-route salivary ducts to provide saliva as a tear substitute. Antibiotics are also often necessary because the dry-eye syndrome tends to promote the overgrowth of microbes on and around the eyes and in the mucus that accumulates.

A new drug, cyclosporine A, has been extremely useful in stimulating tear production in dogs with immune-mediated KCS. Although it is expensive, it is currently the best treatment. Cyclosporine is prepared in a purified oil base and administered topically, twice daily, to the affected eyes. The best responses are seen in dogs that have only mild or moderate tear loss. There is considerable breed variation when it comes to responding to cyclosporine therapy. Cyclosporine should be used for at least three weeks before the long-term benefits are evaluated. Artificial tears may need to be applied to the eyes until tear production approaches normal levels. Artificial tears can be purchased as over-the-counter products at most pharmacies. These solutions should be applied as frequently as possible.

Pilocarpine, a drug used to treat glaucoma, is sometimes used in the management of KCS. It can be applied to the food to be given orally, or administered topically. Neither route seems to be consistently successful, and side effects may be observed if too much drug is given.

For those animals that do not respond to medical therapy, there is a surgical option called parotid duct transposition. It involves surgically re-routing one of the salivary ducts to the eye underneath the skin. In this way, saliva replaces tears in lubricating the eyes. Dogs which have had this procedure generally require very little medication afterward. However, for those dogs with immune KCS associated with salivary deficiency as well (known as Sjogren's Syndrome in people), this option is not satisfactory.

PANNUS

Pannus, also known as chronic superficial keratitis, refers to a condition where pigment and blood vessels grow across the cornea, appearing like a dark film. The most common breed affected with pannus is the German Shepherd Dog.

The cause of the condition is still a matter of much debate. It is believed that genetics may play some role but studies have not shown the condition to be passed from generation to generation. The role of ultraviolet light and immune reactivity are also being considered. Dogs living at high altitudes and low latitudes often are more commonly affected.

Clinical Signs

Although the presentation of pannus may be quite variable, there are some generalizations that can be made. In most cases, pigment infiltrates the clear cornea, usually starting at the outer edge and moving inward. The outer lower corner of the eye is usually the site at which the process starts.

In time, blood vessels grow into the cornea where none existed previously. Finally, connective tissue grows in causing a brown stain on the corneal surface and associated scarring. The disease may cause discomfort when progressing but, in general, this is not a painful eye disease.

Diagnosis

The diagnosis is often suspected based on the clinical signs, especially if a German Shepherd Dog is involved. If necessary, a referral to a veterinary ophthalmologist can confirm the diagnosis.

Therapy

Currently, there are no cures for pannus. Treatment is directed at halting the process before further damage is done. Once scarring and pigment have been lodged in the cornea, the condition is considered irreversible.

The usual treatment of choice to slow the progression of the disorder is corticosteroids. These are administered by injection under the lining of the eye and by eye drops. Treatment is usually lifelong. Of course, there are side effects to corticosteroid use. They will delay the rate of healing and this can prove troublesome if the cornea is wounded in any way. Any evidence of eye pain while on corticosteroids merits immediate veterinary evaluation.

There are some other options in managing pannus. Beta-irradiation can be used when medication alone proves insufficient. Also, surgery can be performed to remove the pigmented and damaged portion of the cornea. This surgical procedure is known as superficial keratectomy. Surgery appears to be a temporary method of control leading to loss of vision in dogs. Ulcerative keratitis is not a diagnosis, only a description of what happens when other processes cause an ulcer on the corneal surface. Ulcers can result from trauma, infections, or secondary to other problems such as eyelid defects or keratoconjunctivitis sicca.

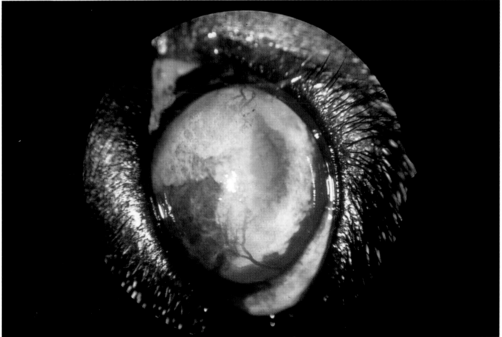

Pannus. Note the pigment and blood vessels on the surface of the cornea. Courtesy of Dr. Dan Lavach, Eye Clinic for Animals, Garden Grove, California.

because the chances of relapse are high. Cyclosporine has also been used experimentally in the management of pannus, with some success.

ULCERATIVE KERATITIS

Ulceration of the cornea, also known as ulcerative keratitis, is an epithelial erosive disease and one of the most common ocular diseases

When the cornea is injured, it takes time to heal. Because of its relatively poor blood supply, the cornea tends to heal more slowly than other tissues. This healing can become protracted if the underlying problem is not corrected, or if the wound becomes infected.

Refractory epithelial ulcers are those that don't heal as antici-

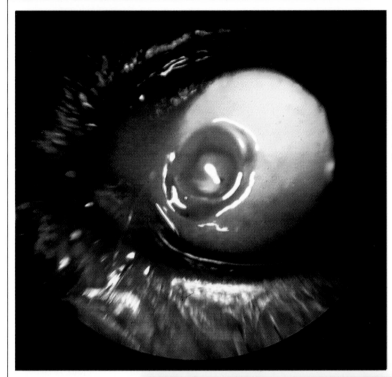

A deep corneal ulcer (desmetocoele) on a six-month-old Shih Tzu. Courtesy of Dr. Dan Lavach, Eye Clinic for Animals, Garden Grove, California.

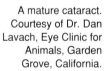

A mature cataract. Courtesy of Dr. Dan Lavach, Eye Clinic for Animals, Garden Grove, California.

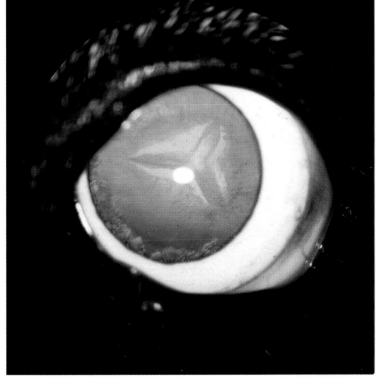

pated, even in the absence of trauma and infection. Some may be due to an inherited epithelial dysplasia such as that seen in Boxers, while others result from substantial damage having been done to the lower layers of the cornea, prohibiting complete healing.

Clinical Signs

Most corneal ulcers result from trauma. Affected dogs often squint (blepharospasm) and have a watery eye (epiphora). In most cases, only one eye will be affected. Because of the pain involved, it is difficult to thoroughly examine the eye.

For ulcers that are healing on their own in an uncomplicated fashion, there might be some white haziness evident on the cornea.

Diagnosis

The diagnosis of corneal ulcers takes more than just noticing an ulcer on the corneal surface. It is important to search for the underlying cause. The eyelids and eyelashes must be examined for abnormalities that could traumatize the cornea. For example, if the eyelids roll inward (entropion) or there is an aberrant lash (trichiasis), there may be an anatomical reason for the ulcer.

The cornea is typically evaluated with magnification to detect changes in contour and the extent of damage. Corneal swelling (edema) occurs whenever significant areas of corneal epithelium are absent. The presence and pattern of blood vessels infiltrating the cornea help determine severity

and duration of the ulcer. Since blood vessels can only invade the cornea at a rate of 1mm/day, extensive blood-vessel networks indicate that the condition has gone on for some time.

Stains such as fluorescein are used to confirm the presence of an ulceration. A small fluorescein strip is applied to the eyeball and will stain an ulcer temporarily green. Rose bengal stain is also used for this purpose by some veterinarians.

Other diagnostic tests are also of value. With proper instrumentation, examination of the anterior chamber of the eye can provide useful information. This examination may help detect corneal perforation, in which the ulcer extends all the way through the layers of the cornea.

Ideally, samples can be collected for bacterial culture and then the eye can be anesthetized topically and additional samples collected for microscopic examination. This should allow proper selection of antibiotics, which will be needed during therapy.

Therapy

There is no single treatment that is effective in all cases of ulcerative keratitis, but most dogs do well if they receive immediate veterinary attention. Topical antibiotics are important since infections will delay the healing of corneal ulcers. Ideally, the selection of antibiotics will be based on microscopic examination and cultures. Fortunately, many corneal ulcers are not associated with infection. In uncomplicated cases, the antibiotic drops need to be instilled in the eyes every six hours. For eyes that are already infected, it may be necessary to instill drops every one to four hours. For rapidly progressing ulcers, a daily injection of antibiotics may be given under the lining of the eye. This does not replace eye drops but it might reduce the frequency at which they must be given. In experimental circumstances, recombinant epithelial growth factor has been given to animals with epithelial erosive disease. These patients have faster corneal healing times than when the product is not used.

Since corneal ulcers are painful, analgesics are often administered to help relieve pain. Also, since trauma is frequently the cause, lubricants may also be used to help protect the eye from further damage. After the infection has been successfully treated and the cornea is healing uneventfully, corticosteroids may be used (judiciously) to help prevent scarring. Since corticosteroids delay healing, they must always be used cautiously. Therapeutic contact lenses have been used in some locations to protect the cornea, relieve pain, and facilitate healing but, because of the variation in size and curvature of canine corneas, it is often difficult to get a good "fit." Collagen corneal bandage lenses help reduce discomfort by covering nerves, and protecting and lubricating growing corneal cells.

Surgery may be required to manage corneal ulcers. If the corneal ulcer is not too deep and not infected, the dog's third eyelid (nictitating membrane) can be pulled across the eye and sutured in place as a protective covering. This does protect the eye but is not suitable in all cases, because it doesn't allow eye drops to be used and there might still be some friction possible between the eye and the lid. Conjunctival flaps provide excellent protection as well as tissue support. This allows the body's immune system to help in the healing process and in getting rid of infections. Reconstructive surgeries are needed in more extensive cases.

For refractory epithelial ulcers, recognition is the most important part. These will typically heal with conservative therapy but progress is slow. The best treatment is to trim away the damaged cornea and apply antibiotics and analgesics as necessary. The eye is re-examined weekly, and more of the damaged tissue is trimmed away each time. This can all be done with just a topical anesthetic. If the ulcer fails to respond, surgery is indicated.

CATARACTS

Cataracts are relatively common in dogs. However, most of the time, the term is used incorrectly. As dogs age, they may develop a haziness on their eyes. This is not a cataract. This is a normal consequence of aging, known as lenticular or nuclear sclerosis.

Most cataracts in dogs are

hereditary and are seen in young and middle-aged individuals more commonly than older dogs. In fact, the majority of canine cataracts are seen in animals under five years of age. Breeds with a high incidence of hereditary cataracts include: Afghan Hound, Cocker Spaniel, Beagle, Boston Terrier, Chesapeake Bay Retriever, German Shepherd Dog, Chow Chow, Golden Retriever, Irish Setter, Labrador Retriever, Miniature and Toy Poodles, Miniature Schnauzer, Old English Sheepdog, Siberian Husky, Staffordshire Bull Terrier, Standard Poodle and West Highland White Terrier.

Although most cataracts seen in dogs have a hereditary basis, other causes such as ocular inflammation, diabetes, injuries or inherited retinal diseases do occur.

Clinical Signs

There are different types of cataracts but these cannot be recognized by owners. With cataract progression, what is noticed over time is that there is a gradual loss of vision. Pets are very good at adapting to this gradual vision loss so blindness may seem sudden to owners, even though it was a long time developing. Of course, not all cataracts lead to blindness. Incomplete cataracts may impair vision but not enough to seriously affect a dog's visual ability.

Diagnosis

Cataracts are diagnosed by an ophthalmoscopic examination of the eye. Often, these cases are referred to ophthalmologists so that the type of cataract can be determined and the heritability predicted. Ophthalmologists can

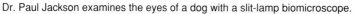

Dr. Paul Jackson examines the eyes of a dog with a slit-lamp biomicroscope.

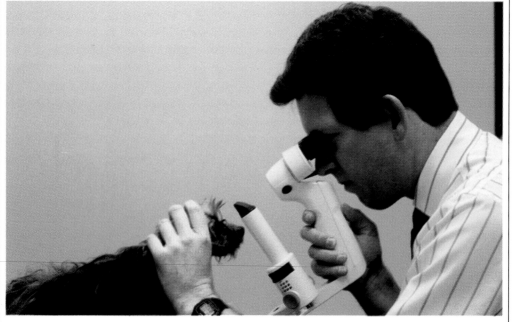

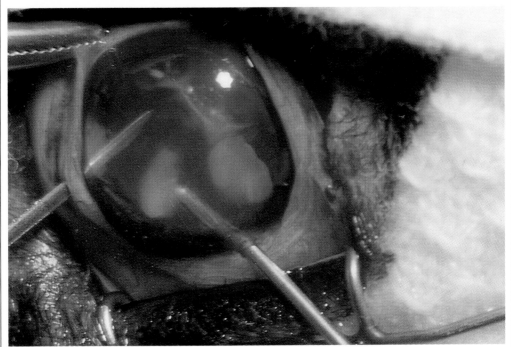

Cataract surgery using phacoemulsification technique. The small instruments inside the eye remove the cataract by a "vacuuming" method. Courtesy of Dr. Dan Lorimer, Michigan Veterinary Specialists, Southfield, Michigan.

Chronic glaucoma. Note the painful eye and the extension of blood vessels. Courtesy of Dr. Dan Lavach, Eye Clinic for Animals, Garden Grove, California.

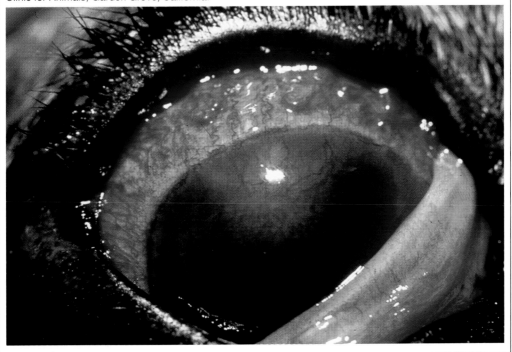

perform a detailed slit-lamp (biomicroscope) examination of the eye, which is much more precise than the standard ophthalmoscopes used in general practice. This is especially important if breeding is being considered or if surgery is being contemplated.

Therapy

There are no medicines that are effective in treating cataracts. Therefore, surgery is the only option if the cataracts seriously impair vision. Animals usually do quite well after surgery.

There are a number of options when it comes to cataract surgery. Most involve surgically removing the defective lens; lens implants are not routinely done in animals.

One method of removing cataracts surgically is called phacoemulsification. It is less invasive and may provide a better outcome for some animals. It involves placing a small ultrasonic instrument in the eye. This instrument makes about 40,000 tiny vibrations per second and aspirates (sucks) the cataract material out of the eye like a small intraocular vacuum. This sophisticated technique has been associated with a high success rate for many cataract surgery patients. The major limitation of this procedure is the high cost of the equipment.

Prevention

If a dog is determined to have a hereditary cataract it should be removed from the breeding program.

COLLIE EYE ANOMALY

Collie eye anomaly (CEA) is the incomplete development of the eye. It is found in Rough and Smooth Collies, Border Collies, Shetland Sheepdogs, Boykin Spaniels, Chow Chows, German Shepherd Dogs and Australian Shepherds, and all coat colors are involved. Not all dogs are equally affected. There is a spectrum of malformations present at birth, ranging from inadequate development of the choroid (choroidal hypoplasia) to defects of the choroid, retina, or optic nerve, and complete retinal detachment. In collies, CEA is a simple recessive defect and therefore it is only seen when a defective gene is inherited from both parents.

Clinical Signs

Most collies (80-90%) with CEA do not demonstrate vision problems. Both eyes are affected but not necessarily to the same extent. Vision tends to be normal except when there is hemorrhage from the retina or detachment of the retina. Very large defects of the optic nerve (colomboma) can also cause vision abnormalities. These colombomas, sometimes referred to as scleral ectasia, may involve the area adjacent to the optic nerve, the areas entirely around the nerve, or around the optic nerve but with normal sclera between the nerve and the defect.

Diagnosis

Because the disorder is present in the newborn puppy, eyes can be checked as early as five to six weeks of age, although six to ten weeks of age is preferred. Unfortunately, carriers of the genetic defect cannot be determined by ophthalmic examination.

Diagnosis of the condition in merle-colored animals can be difficult and the examination should include the non-pigmented zone to the side of the optic disk. It should also be mentioned that some puppies have poorly formed choroid at an early age that later becomes pigmented, creating a more normal appearance.

Therapy

There is no treatment for this inherited condition. The only certain way to reduce or eliminate the problem is to avoid breeding affected animals.

GLAUCOMA

Glaucoma remains one of the leading causes of blindness in animals. The condition is caused by any underlying problem that increases the fluid pressure inside the eye. The increased pressure within the eye eventually destroys visual capability.

Obviously, too much fluid within the eye could result from either too much being produced or inadequate drainage of the fluid from the eye. At this time, it appears that most if not all cases are due to inadequate drainage. Increased production of intraocular fluid does not appear to be a problem. Therefore, glaucoma does not represent just one disorder but is the final result from any process that interrupts the delicate fluid balance within the eye.

Primary glaucoma is known to occur within certain purebred dog breeds and is thought to have an inherited basis. The types include open-angle glaucoma, as seen in Beagles and Norwegian Elkhounds, and narrow-angle glaucoma, as seen in American and English Cocker Spaniels. A third type of primary glaucoma results from abnormal development of the filtration angle (called goniodysgenesis). Goniodysgenesis occurs most commonly in the Basset Hound, American Cocker Spaniel, Samoyed and Chow Chow. Secondary glaucoma is the result of some other disease that interferes with the natural flow of fluid within the eye.

Clinical Signs

Early signs of glaucoma may be subtle. The conjunctival lining of the eyes may be reddened (red eye) or they may be weeping (epiphora) or sensitive to light (photophobia). Glaucoma should be considered in any dog with a red, painful eye. As pressure within the eye worsens, the pupil becomes fixed and dilated, the cornea becomes cloudy, and the eye may actually enlarge (buphthalmos) as it fills with fluid.

Diagnosis

The diagnosis of glaucoma requires careful inspection by a veterinarian and perhaps even a veterinary ophthalmologist, a specialist in problems of the eye.

Confirmation requires measuring the pressure within the eye with an instrument called a "tonometer." Often, an additional technique called gonioscopy is used to actually look at the place where fluid drains from the eye. This procedure is usually done by a specialist using a special dome-shaped contact lens, a goniolens.

incorporates the use of a surgical YAG laser was developed. Early clinical trials suggest that this method may provide excellent long-term control of glaucoma. There are many other surgical procedures currently available for the management of glaucoma.

If glaucoma is due to an underlying cause (secondary

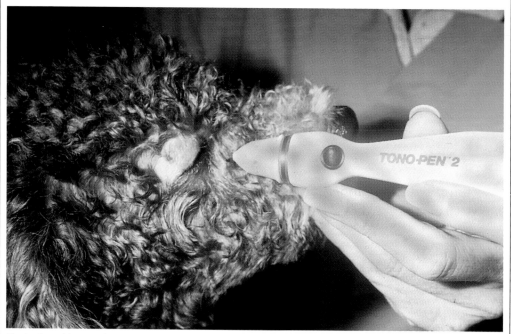

Evaluation of intraocular pressure with a Tonopen tonometer.

Therapy

The treatment of glaucoma aims at lowering the fluid pressures within the eye. There are several ways of doing this, some with medications and some with surgery. However, if sight has already been lost, it is unlikely to be restored with either process. That is why early, exact diagnosis is critical.

Recently a technique that

glaucoma), and that cause is removed, many times glaucoma can be "cured."

PROGRESSIVE RETINAL ATROPHY (PRA)

Progressive retinal atrophy (PRA) refers to several inherited disorders affecting the retina that result in blindness. PRA is thought to be inherited with each breed, demonstrating a specific age of

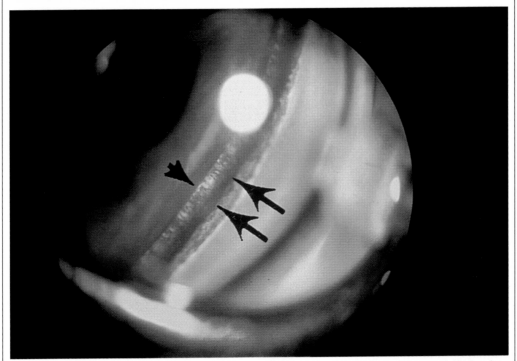

Above: Gonioscopic image of the eye. Courtesy of Dr. Dan Lavach, Eye Clinic for Animals, Garden Grove, California.

Below: A Yorkshire Terrier suspected of having PRA. The external appearance of the eyes is not diagnostic. Courtesy of Dr. Dan Lorimer, Michigan Veterinary Specialists, Southfield, Michigan.

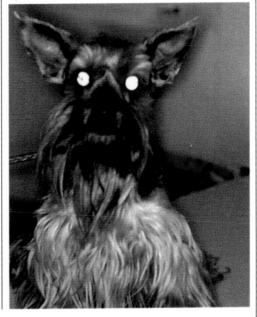

onset and pattern of inheritance. For example, a blind Collie with PRA bred to a blind Irish Setter with PRA will produce pups with eyesight but that are carriers for both forms of the disorder. The disease affects many breeds of dogs, each in a specific manner. Some breeds at increased risk include the Collie, Irish Setter, Cairn Terrier, Dachshund, Norwegian Elkhound, Samoyed, Cocker Spaniel, Miniature Poodle, Miniature Schnauzer, Akita, Standard Schnauzer, Golden Retriever, and Labrador Retriever.

All of the conditions described as progressive retinal atrophy have one thing in common. There is progressive atrophy or degeneration of the retinal tissue. Visual impairment occurs slowly but progressively. Therefore, animals often adapt to their reduced vision until it is compromised to near blindness. Because of this, owners may not notice any visual impairment until the condition has progressed significantly.

Progressive retinal atrophy encompasses both degenerative and dysplastic varieties. This distinction may seem confusing to owners, but it is important to remember that there are many distinctly different disorders that can result in PRA. Retinal dysplasia refers to malformation in the retinal tissue during fetal development. Breeds at risk for inherited retinal dysplasia include Bedlington Terriers, Sealyham Terriers, English Springer Spaniels, Gordon Setters, Samoyeds, Beagles, Collies, Cocker Spaniels, German Shepherd Dogs, Pembroke Welsh Corgis, Golden Retrievers, Samoyed, English Mastiffs, Rottweilers, Giant Schnauzers, and certain lines of Labrador Retrievers.

Retinal degeneration implies that the retina was normal at birth and later developed problems. Breeds at risk for inherited retinal degeneration include Miniature Poodles, English Cocker Spaniels, American Cocker Spaniels, and Labrador Retrievers. To complicate matters further, PRA may be subdivided further based on age of onset and pattern of progression.

Miniature Schnauzers have yet another form of PRA called photoreceptor dysplasia (PD). Affected dogs have defects in the differentiation of the rods and cones after birth. The result is that they have a rapid degeneration of the rods and cones but they maintain their vision longer than other breeds.

Clinical Signs

There are rarely any changes to the eyes that can be seen visually. That's what makes the condition so pernicious. In time, dogs will become blind and then the condition is obvious. In the early stages of PRA, night blindness occurs first. Affected dogs may have difficulty navigating themselves at night, or once the lights have been turned off. With progression, some pet owners may notice a characteristic shine from the eye, due to an increased reflectivity of the back of the eye.

Because dogs have many other well-developed senses, such as smell and hearing, their lack of sight is usually not immediately evident. The loss of vision is slow but progressive, and blindness eventually results.

Diagnosis

The diagnosis of PRA can be made in two ways: direct visualization of the retina, and electroretinography (ERG). An ophthalmoscope can be used to visualize the retinal tissue at the back of the eyes. The use of indirect ophthalmoscopy requires a great deal of training and expertise and is more commonly performed by ophthalmology specialists than general practitioners. When the ophthalmologist views the retina with this instrument, they can frequently see changes in the pattern of retinal blood vessels, the optic nerve, and the reflective tapetum that provides "eye shine." In some breeds, however, the early changes may not be clearly visible and the eyes may appear normal until the later stages of the disease. Cataracts may form as a consequence of progressive retinal atrophy in some dogs, especially late in the course of the disease. These cataracts may interfere with direct visualization of the retina and thereby confound an accurate diagnosis. Fortunately, there are other diagnostic options.

An additional highly sensitive test is electroretinography or ERG. This instrument measures electrical patterns in the retina the same way an ECG measures electrical activity of the heart. The procedure is painless, but usually available only from specialty centers. This instrument is sensitive enough to detect even the early onset of disease.

Therapy

Unfortunately there is no treatment available for progressive retinal atrophy. Since most dogs are presented very late in the course of the disease they are often blind at the time of diagnosis. Fortunately, PRA is not a painful condition and dogs do have other keen senses upon which they can depend. In time, they will acclimate to their living environment and can do quite well with the help of their owners. They can continue to go for walks, albeit always on a lead or halter. Indoors, they are usually fine, especially if owners are content not to constantly rearrange the furniture.

There has been much speculation about the role of nutrition in the management of PRA in dogs. Undoubtedly this is because research has determined that taurine retinopathy in cats, a related condition, can be successfully managed with the amino acid taurine. Other research in dogs has shown that vitamin E deficiency can result in conditions similar to PRA. At this time, however, no association has been made between any nutrient (or drug for that matter) and the successful resolution of PRA.

Prevention

Identification of affected breeding animals is essential to prevent spread of the condition within the breed. Dogs from breeds at increased risk should be examined annually by a veterinary ophthalmologist. Ideally pups should be screened at six to eight weeks of age, before being sold. Unfortunately, screening exams are not a sensitive method for early detection in many breeds. The mode of inheritance and extent of disease is different for most breeds. For example, Rough Collies usually develop rod-cone dysplasia (Type I) that starts at less than a year of age. The dogs are often night-blind by six weeks of age and functionally blind by six to eight months of age. The Miniature

Poodle develops a rod-cone degeneration that typically starts as night blindness at three to five years of age. In between, the Norwegian Elkhound may develop rod dysplasia and cone degeneration; night blindness is evident by six weeks of age while day vision is preserved until two to three years of age. Therefore, recommendations for ophthalmic evaluation differ for each breed because progressive retinal atrophy differs with each breed. Contact a breed club, veterinary ophthalmologist, or CERF for details on individual breeds.

ADDITIONAL READING

Bistner, SI: Recent developments in comparative ophthalmology. *Compendium for Continuing Education of the Practicing Veterinarian,* 1992; 14(10): 1304-1323.

Brooks, DE; Dziezyc, J: The canine glaucomas: Pathogenesis, diagnosis, and treatment. *Compendium for Continuing Education of the Practicing Veterinarian,* 1983; 5(4): 292-298.

Lorimer, D: Understanding Glaucoma. *Pet Focus,* 1989; 1(1): 24-26.

Dr. Paul Jackson using an indirect ophthalmoscope to view the retina.

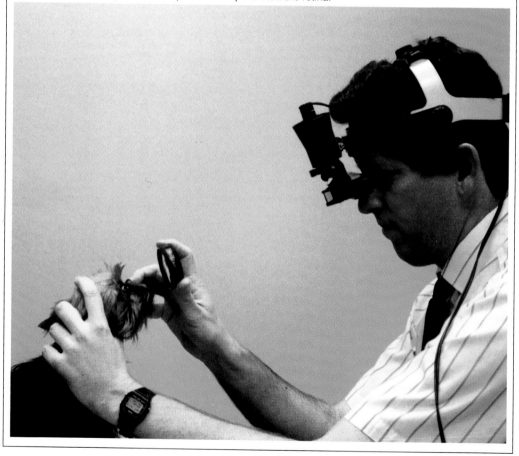

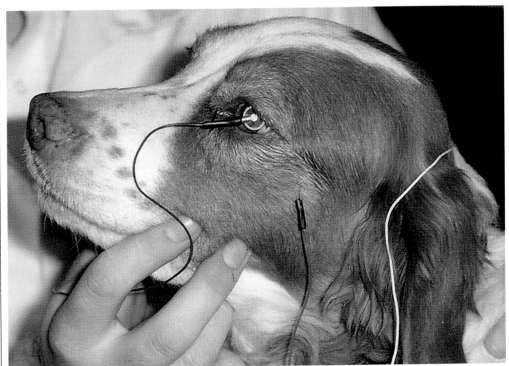

Electroretinographic (ERG) examination. Courtesy of Dr. Dan Lorimer, Michigan Veterinary Specialists, Southfield, Michigan.

Retina of an English Springer Spaniel with PRA.

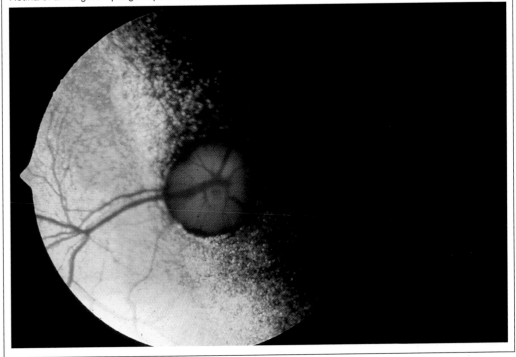

Lorimer, D: Progressive Retinal Atrophy. *Pet Focus,* 1990; 2(1): 4-6.

Lorimer, D: Cataracts. *Pet Focus,* 1990; 2(4): 55-57.

McWhirter, K: Keratoconjunctivitis sicca. *Pet Focus,* 1990; 2(2): 21-22.

Nasisse, MP: Canine ulcerative keratitis. *Compendium for Continuing Education of the Practicing Veterinarian,* 1985; 7(9): 686-701.

Peiffer, Jr., RL: Inherited ocular diseases of the dog and cat. *Compendium for Continuing Education of the Practicing Veterinarian,* 1982; 4(2): 152-165.

Rubin, LF: *Inherited eye diseases in purebred dogs.* The Williams & Wilkins Co, Baltimore, MD, 1989, 363pp.

Wilkie, DA: Management of Keratoconjunctivitis sicca in dogs. *Compendium for Continuing Education of the Practicing Veterinarian,* 1993; January: 58-63.

Disorders of the Heart and Respiratory System

The heart and lungs function so that oxygen can be inhaled, transferred through the lungs to the red blood cells, and distributed to all the tissues of the body. Without this action, we would quickly die.

The heart is an amazing organ, pumping every minute of every day for an entire lifetime. But what happens when the heart can no longer do its job? There are no other organs in the body that can do the job of the heart and so when it fails, life fails as well. It thus behooves us to learn as much as we can about this marvelous organ and the problems that may affect it.

THE MECHANICS OF HEART FUNCTION AND HEART FAILURE

The heart is a pump, and like any pump, it is prone to a number of plumbing problems. However, the heart is also the subject of much mystery and medical mysticism, and so heart disease often seems more confusing than it is. As if this isn't bad enough, the subject of cardiology has its own language that is foreign to the average person. If you truly have a desire to learn about heart disease, make an attempt to understand this language and its implications to treatment.

To understand the dynamics of this process, it is first important to understand some key terms used by cardiologists, namely cardiac output, heart rate, preload, afterload, and contractility. These terms may seem daunting, but they are basic to our understanding of how the heart can and cannot compensate for heart disease.

Cardiac output is a measure of the heart's ability to pump blood efficiently. Like any pump the heart can only pump faster or harder to move fluid throughout the network. The volume of blood moved also depends on how much blood was in the heart at the time of pumping, and any obstruction down the line that might increase the pressure in the system. Veterinarians estimate the cardiac output (CO) by multiplying the heart rate (beats per minute) by the ability of the ventricle to pump a volume of blood (stroke volume).

The heart rate refers to the number of times per minute that the heart beats. This can be measured by taking the pulse, or by listening with a stethoscope and counting. When the heart beats slower than normal, it is referred to as bradycardia. Tachycardia is the term used when the heart is beating faster than normal. Either can be evidence of heart disease. It should be evident that just because a heart is beating faster, does not mean it is pumping blood efficiently. The efficiency of

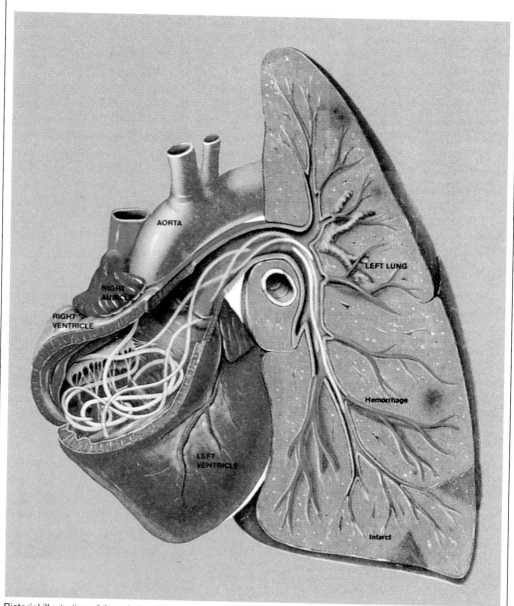

Pictorial illustration of the relationship of the heart and lungs. Notice the heartworms. Courtesy of Petcom, Inc.

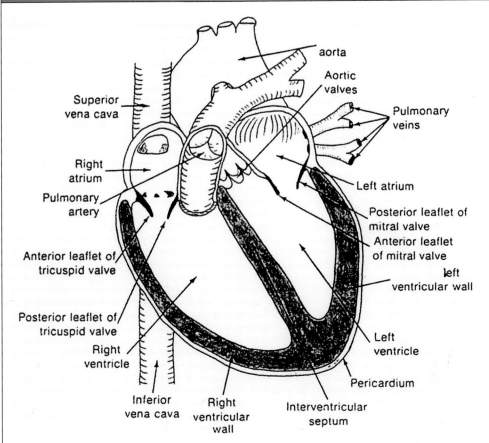

aorta

Aortic valves

Superior vena cava

Pulmonary veins

Right atrium

Left atrium

Pulmonary artery

Posterior leaflet of mitral valve

Anterior leaflet of mitral valve

Anterior leaflet of tricuspid valve

left ventricular wall

Posterior leaflet of tricuspid valve

Right ventricle

Left ventricle

Pericardium

Inferior vena cava

Right ventricular wall

Interventricular septum

Line drawing of the normal anatomy of the heart showing the different regions. Courtesy of Dr. Laura DeLellis, Michigan Veterinary Specialists, Southfield, Michigan.

pumping (stroke volume) is determined by the ability of the heart to fill completely and then empty the ventricles completely. Rapid fluttering of the heart muscle is not an effective way to pump blood. Imagine you are pumping up a bicycle tire with a hand pump. The most efficient way to inflate the tire is to fill the pump completely with air and then expel the air completely into the tire before repeating the motion. If you only pull the plunger part way out, it fills incompletely, and inflates incompletely. The same is true for the heart muscle.

The ability of the heart to fill completely with blood before pumping is known as preload. Imagine this as using pails of water to fill a swimming pool. The most efficient way to fill the pool is to carry pails completely filled with water, not partially filled. The same is true for the heart. If the heart pumps when the chambers (ventricles) are only half full, there is a lot of wasted effort. When blood completely fills the chambers of the heart, the walls of the heart are stretched, and this encourages a more forceful pumping action.

On the other side of the heart,

afterload measures the tension that develops in the wall of a contracting ventricle. This is affected primarily by the pressure within the ventricle and the chamber size. When diseases result in increased afterload, the muscular walls of the heart become thickened, in an attempt to compensate. This is referred to as myocardial hypertrophy. When the walls of the heart become overly thickened, it doesn't leave enough room for enough blood to fill the chamber.

Contractility is the function of the heart muscle to compress and forcefully eject blood from the heart chambers. Increasing the preload increases the force of contractility as the heart muscle stretches to fill completely with blood. Chronic overloading, however, taxes the heart muscle beyond its ability to compensate and, in the end, leads to a decrease in contractility.

ATTEMPTS TO COMPENSATE

The heart does what it can to treat its own ineffectiveness. It may seem that compensating for heart problems is a good thing but the benefits are only temporary. Eventually the compromises made cause even more problems. When there is a drop in cardiac output or blood pressure, the first compromise is made by the sympathetic nervous system. This causes the release of chemical stimulants (norepinephrine) for the heart and helps divert blood supplies away from peripheral tissues to those considered most

important. Unfortunately, the heart becomes more and more dependent on this artificial support, and progressively less receptive. Just like a drug addict, the heart needs more of these chemicals to get the same effect that it used to get from smaller doses. As the heart failure worsens, so do the side effects of this temporary form of compensation.

The next body system to try to help is the kidney. When heart disease causes a decrease in preload, the heart may not fill enough to contract effectively. When cardiac output drops, the kidney gets less blood flow. It responds by saving sodium and water and recycling them back into the blood stream. The kidney also releases an enzyme (renin) that acts on other proteins (angiotensin I & II) to help regulate sodium (salt) content. In a cascading effect, angiotensin II stimulates the secretion of a hormone (aldosterone) from the nearby adrenal gland. This hormone also encourages the kidney to save sodium. Keeping sodium in the bloodstream may temporarily fool the heart into thinking it's really filled with blood but the effect is short-lived. The high sodium (salt) content of the blood cannot provide oxygen to the tissues that need it. Also, the salt water dilutes the concentration of blood proteins whose job is to keep fluid within the blood vessels. As the blood becomes more dilute, the fluid portion seeps out of the blood vessels and into the tissues

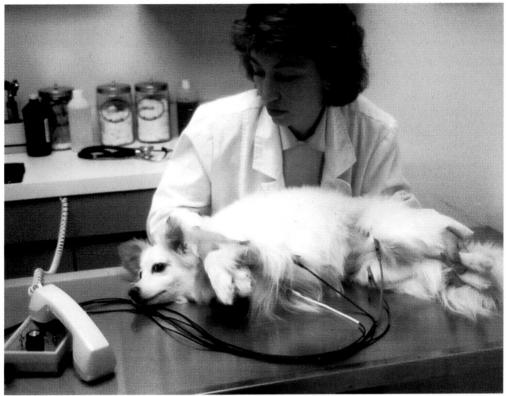

Electrocardiograms can also be transmitted to specialists via telephone lines. Courtesy of Cardiopet, Inc., Consultants and Educators in Cardiology, Internal Medicine and Radiology.

resulting in congestion, and swelling (edema). The damage becomes progressive because the body does not know enough to turn off this mechanism. As long as the kidney perceives a decrease in cardiac output, it continues to save sodium.

The final compromise made in cases of heart failure is by the heart itself. In response to chronic pressure or volume troubles, the heart increases the size of its muscular walls. This is referred to as cardiac hypertrophy. This handles the stress on the heart muscle initially but is detrimental in the long term. The increased thickness of the heart walls leads to decreased cardiac output. This becomes a critical factor in the progression of decompensated heart failure.

DIAGNOSTIC TESTING OF CARDIAC FUNCTION

Electrocardiography (ECG)

Each year there are hundreds of thousands of ECGs performed on dogs and cats. With ECGs, the electrical impulses can be traced throughout the conduction system of the heart. If problems exist within this conduction system, they become evident in the waves and intervals of the ECG. If there is an abnormal heart rhythm (arrhythmia), its location can often be determined quite accurately on an ECG. If necessary, electrocardiograms can be transmitted to cardiologists over telephone lines for interpretation (trans-telephonic electrocardiographic assessment); computerized electrocardiographic analysis is also available.

Echocardiography

Echocardiography, which uses sound waves, can provide much more information that can the electrical impulses of the electrocardiogram. A transducer is used to bounce sound waves off the interior of the heart and other structures so they can be translated (as echoes) by a computer. The computer maps the location of the echoes and displays them on a television screen. M-mode (motion) echocardiograms permit the cardiologist to make measurements of cardiac dimensions and a detailed analysis of complex motion patterns of valves and walls. A two-dimensional (2-D) ultrasound image (real-time ultrasound) provides moving, anatomically correct images of the heart. These appear like a motion picture on the television screen.

Doppler echocardiography is an even more precise diagnostic tool. The emitted ultrasound strikes red blood cells moving toward and away from the transducer. This provides valuable information about blood flow, including blood

With transtelephonic electrocardiography, an electrocardiogram can be received from patients located anywhere in the world. Courtesy of Cardiopet, Inc., Consultants and Educators in Cardiology, Internal Medicine and Radiology.

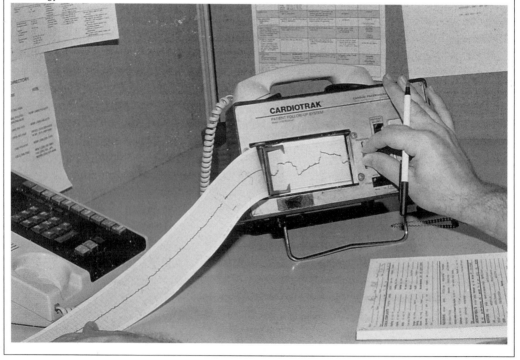

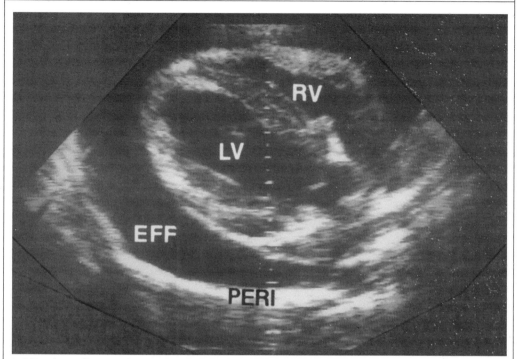

A 2-D echocardiogram of a dog with fluid within the pericardial sac (pericardial effusion = EFF, PERI = pericardium, LV—left ventricle, RV = Right ventricle). Courtesy of Dr. Laura DeLellis, Michigan Veterinary Specialists, Southfield, Michigan.

flow within the chambers of the heart. This simple, noninvasive technique can provide information that previously was only available by angiography, the technique whereby catheters were inserted into the heart and dye released to map the flow of blood. The technique allows for the diagnosis of narrowed or insufficient heart valves, the determination of pressure gradients across valves, measurement of cardiac output, and a very specific diagnosis of congenital heart defects.

CONGESTIVE HEART FAILURE

When the heart can't or doesn't pump the blood efficiently enough to meet the body's needs, the result is known as heart failure. If the heart can't do its job well enough, the body does try to accommodate. Thus, heart failure is the result of an inability to adequately compensate for decreased cardiac function. How long this takes to occur depends on the extent of heart damage and the body's ability to compensate.

It must be stressed that heart failure is not a diagnosis. It is the final common pathway for many different diseases that affect the heart and circulatory system.

Congestive heart failure is a term used to describe what happens when the heart is unable to effectively pump blood. Blood enters the right side of the heart through veins, and leaves the left side of the heart though arteries. In between, the blood is oxygenated in the lungs. If the left side of the heart is the cause of the problem, fluid tends to back up into the lungs. If the right side of the heart is the problem, fluid may collect in the liver and abdominal organs. It is this fluid load that is referred to as "congestive" in heart failure. However, in time, the distinction between right-side and left-side heart failure is lost; regardless of where the problem started, malfunction of one side eventually has a negative impact on the other.

Another way of describing heart diseases is in terms of compensated and decompensated heart failure. The body tries to compensate when the heart is not pumping effectively. If this effort is successful, heart function is maintained (for a time) even though there is still heart disease. The body can't fix the heart problem, but it tries to keep it working as best it can. Eventually, this noble effort is not enough and the body can no longer hide the fact that the heart is not doing its job. This is referred to as decompensated heart failure. This is important because during the compensated phase a dog can have heart problems that won't be evident to an owner. This is called congestive heart disease and leads to congestive heart failure. Some telltale signs can provide veterinarians with important clues if the animal is routinely examined.

Clinical Signs

Heart failure is usually slow and insidious. The body will try to compensate as best it can and as long as it can before there is clear evidence of trouble. One of the first signs noticed by owners is exercise intolerance. The dog seems fine when it's playing or sleeping around the house, but it tires quickly on walks or during play, or wants to go inside sooner than before. These animals are in compensated heart disease.

Other problems are attributed to the compensatory mechanism discussed above. When the kidney recycles sodium into the bloodstream, there is a tendency for fluid to seep out into the tissues. Early in the course of decompensation, there may be a moist cough after the dog lies down. This is because the fluid settled in the lungs. Dogs with right-side heart failure may have accumulation of fluid in the abdomen (ascites).

Owners are often surprised that devastating heart disease in dogs rarely causes a heart attack. They might attribute exercise intolerance to old age or arthritis and a moist cough to a viral infection. Most of the cardiac damage that occurs is only measurable by diagnostic tests.

Diagnosis

It is best to diagnose heart disease in its compensated stage before permanent damage is done to the heart muscle. Unfortunately, owners may not be aware of any problems at all at this stage since their pet shows little if any signs of impairment. Early diagnosis is usually made during routine veterinary examinations, where subtle abnormalities may be identified. For example, listening with a stethoscope (auscultation) may reveal an enlarged heart field, a rapid heart rate, and/or fluid sounds in the lungs. This should prompt the need for radiography (x-rays), electrocardiograms (ECG), and even ultrasound examinations of the heart (echocardiography).

Therapy

Heart failure cannot be cured but animals can be effectively managed with appropriate treatment. The first priority of therapy is to correct the side effects caused by the body's attempt to compensate. The first order of business is to counteract the good intentions of the kidneys. This is accomplished by using diuretics (water pills) such as furosemide

Chest radiograph from a dog with congestive heart failure. Courtesy of Dr. Kenneth Jeffery, Mesa Veterinary Hospital, Ltd., Mesa, Arizona.

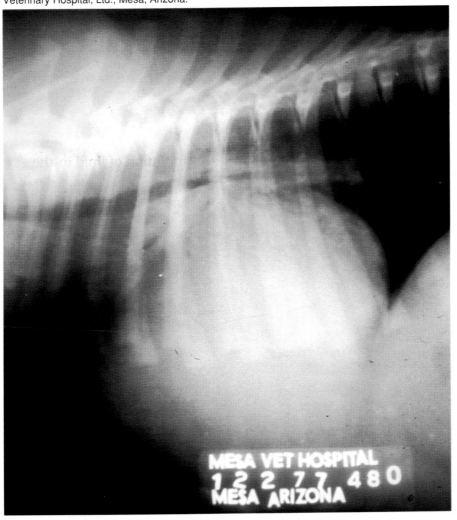

(Lasix) and salt-restricted diets to reduce the preload. Nitroglycerine can also be used to help remove fluids collecting in tissues but is rarely needed in veterinary medicine except to control acute pulmonary (lung) edema. These medications lessen the stress on the heart and the tendency of fluid to seep into the tissues that cause congestion. Drugs that cause blood vessels to dilate (venodilators) also help reduce preload and congestion. This is helpful but it still doesn't help the heart pump more efficiently. Also, since the blood volume is reduced, the ventricles of the heart also have less blood to pump.

To make the heart pump harder, drugs such as digitalis are sometimes used to increase the force of heart muscle contraction (positive inotropes). Positive inotropes increase the force of cardiac contraction and slow the heart rate. However, drugs like digitalis also have many side effects and so must be used carefully. Milrinone and amrinone are new positive inotropes being used experimentally in dogs.

Drugs that dilate small arteries (arteriolar vasodilators) reduce the afterload, which increases the stroke volume. This family of medications includes drugs such as hydralazine (Apresoline), calcium-channel blockers such as diltiazem and new drugs such as enalapril (Enacard™) and captopril (Capoten). These drugs were recommended to be used in patients in the late stages of heart failure, but many cardiologists are now using them earlier, when the heart muscle is healthier. The combined use of positive inotropes and arteriolar vasodilators has the greatest potential for increasing heart performance when heart muscle contractility is depressed and preload is high.

Another interesting therapy for dogs with heart failure is antibiotics. Some researchers suggest that heart failure worsens with infections such as pneumonia. Others contend that infection may pose a sort of stress on an already overworked heart. Because of this, antibiotics are often administered if infection is suspected, although they have no direct effect on the heart itself.

CONGENITAL HEART DISEASES

Cardiovascular abnormalities account for approximately 10% of all cases presented to most small animal hospitals. Most of these cases are acquired conditions that develop during a dog's lifetime. These are usually diagnosed at five to eight years of age or older. On the other hand, congenital disorders occur in newborn puppies, although they may not be diagnosed until much later. Many congenital defects are hereditary, meaning they are caused by a genetic defect that may be transmitted to the offspring.

In most cases of congenital cardiac abnormalities there is a single malformation, although multiple defects in the same puppy are not uncommon. The severity of

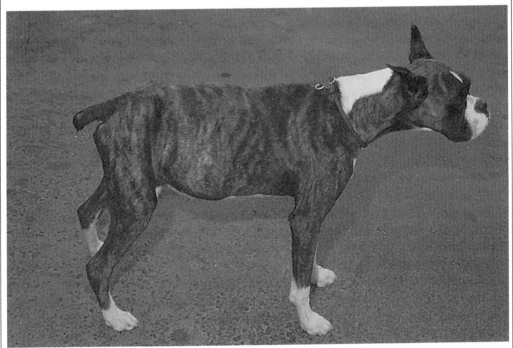

A nine-month-old-dog with fluid accumulating in the abdominal cavity (ascites). Courtesy of Dr. Kenneth Jeffery, Mesa Veterinary Hospital, Ltd., Mesa, Arizona.

the defects varies considerably amongst different patients and therefore the life expectancy or prognosis is also variable. Purebred puppies have a higher incidence of congenital heart defects than mixed-breed puppies, and certain cardiac anomalies occur more often in specific breeds or are more common in male or female puppies. Of the congenital defects, approximately 81% are one of the following: patent ductus arteriosus, pulmonic stenosis, aortic stenosis, vascular ring anomaly, and ventricular septal defects.

Congenital heart defects are prevalent problems in dogs. For this reason it is highly recommended each puppy be examined by a veterinarian at six to nine weeks of age. Although most puppies at that age do not show obvious signs of heart disease, if a defect is present a heart murmur can usually be heard. With better diagnostic methods now available by your veterinarian or at a referral center, the exact nature of a cardiac murmur in a puppy can now be determined. Early detection of these problems is important for the life and prognosis of the puppy as well as the overall effect on the breeding programs.

SPECIFIC DISORDERS

Patent ductus arteriosus (PDA) is the most common congenital defect seen in dogs. This is inherited as a polygenic threshold trait with a high degree of heritability in Poodles. This means that the trait is controlled by a number of

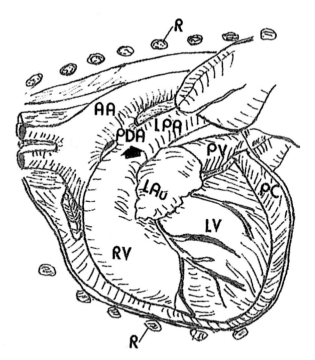

A schematic drawing showing a patent ductus arteriosus (PDA) between the pulmonary artery (PA) and aorta (AA). Left ventricle (LV), Right Ventricle (RV), Ribs (R), Pulmonary Vein (PV), Pericardial sac (PC), Left pulmonary artery (LPA), Left auricle (LAu). Drawing by Cathy Wilson.

different genes and has a threshold, since clinically there can only be a hole (patency) or no hole, no clinical intermediate. It frequently occurs in Pomeranians, Collies, Shetland Sheepdogs, Pembroke Welsh Corgis, Maltese and German Shepherds, but may be found in any breed. This defect occurs when the normal fetal communication between the nonfunctional lungs and the aorta (major blood vessel leaving the heart) fails to close after birth. This results in the shunting of blood into the pulmonary artery (major vessel to the lungs) and flooding the lungs. At the same time the rest of the body is getting an inadequate amount of circulation.

Pulmonic stenosis is the second most common congenital heart defect in dogs. This is a stricture or incomplete opening through the pulmonic valve within the heart. The valve is located between the right ventricle and the pulmonary artery, which delivers the blood from the heart to the lungs. This condition is seen most frequently in Beagles, Chihuahuas, English Bulldogs, Fox Terriers, Samoyeds, Schnauzers, and Cocker Spaniels. It can also be seen in most other breeds. Pulmonic stenosis in English Bulldogs has been found to be assiciated with, and probably caused by, a defect in the coronary artery.

The third most common

congenital heart defect in dogs is subaortic stenosis (SAS). This malformation is a narrowing or stricture just below the aortic valve. The stricture is usually an abnormal fibrous ring of tissue which results in a reduction of blood flow pumped from the heart. This causes an overworking of the left ventricle. This condition causes excessive workload of the cardiac muscle and thereby increases the oxygen needs of the heart itself. Congenital SAS is observed most often as a polygenic trait in larger breeds, including Newfoundlands, and is strongly suspected to be so in Boxers, German Shepherds, and Golden Retrievers. Other reported breeds include Pugs, English Setters, Boston Terriers, Fox Terriers, Schnauzers, and Basset Hounds.

Vascular ring anomalies are the fourth most common congenital cardiovascular abnormality. This is a group of defects that result from abnormal development and maturation of blood vessels in the fetus. This causes a physical external compression and stricture of the esophagus since in this condition, the abnormally directed vessels trap the esophagus between them. Vascular ring anomaly is found most often in Irish Setters and German Shepherds. A genetic cause is suspected, although the mode of inheritance is unclear.

Ventricular septal defect (VSD) is also a common cardiac abnormality in dogs. This is an abnormal opening or hole in the wall between the left and right ventricles or lower chambers of the heart. This creates a communication between the two ventricles. The exact cause or etiology of this defect is incompletely understood, but a genetic cause is suspected and has been demonstrated as a polygenic trait in Keeshonden. English Bulldogs also have an increased risk but the condition may occur in many other breeds.

Tetralogy of Fallot (TOF) is a four-part anatomical defect of the heart caused by the development of the great vessels of the heart to the right rather than the left side of the chest. The four components of this disorder are a ventricular septal defect, overriding of the right-left division of the heart by the aorta, pulmonic stenosis, and enlargement of the right side of the heart. This causes blood to be shunted from the right ventricle into the aorta, rather than from the left ventricle.

Clinical Signs

The diagnosis of a congenital heart disease may be made during a routine veterinary visit or only after an animal has begun to experience difficulties associated with the problem. The development of symptoms may be acute (developing within hours or days) or chronic (developing over a period of weeks or months). The length of time prior to development of signs and the age at which they occur is often an extremely important part of the patient's history and helps contribute to an accurate diagnosis.

The development of a cough is often the first indication of illness noted by the owner. It may be a mild cough at first and over a period of weeks or months progressively worsen. The cough is usually due to an accumulation of fluid within the lungs (pulmonary edema) or compression of the bronchi by an enlarged heart.

Other signs include shallow rapid respirations or difficulty in breathing. This may be more evident with exercise and affected animals may become prematurely fatigued. Some patients are uncomfortable and frequently shift body positions. An abnormal increase in heart rate (over 160 per minute) or a slow heart rate (below 60 per minute) may also indicate a cardiovascular abnormality.

Some patients will faint (called a syncopal episode), especially with exercise or excitement. This is due to a sudden decrease in oxygen supplied to the brain. The observation of a bluish discoloration (cyanosis) of the tongue or gums may also be seen, which suggests a possible cardiovascular problem.

In other patients, the only signs may be a loss of appetite or an increase in drinking and urinating. Some patients will show swelling or enlargement of the abdomen due to fluid accumulation internally, and/or occasional swelling (edema) in the limbs.

Most puppies with PDA show no clinical signs early in life but a heart murmur is detected upon examination during the first vaccination. Other puppies may develop acute heart failure and have difficulty in breathing, exercise intolerance, or develop a cough. The cardiac murmur detected is described as a machinery-type or continuous murmur which is characteristic for this particular cardiac defect.

Many dogs with pulmonic stenosis are asymptomatic but do have a cardiac murmur. As they get older or if the condition is severe, there may be evidence of exercise intolerance, fainting (syncope), coughing, or fluid accumulation within the body.

Most puppies with SAS do not develop signs of illness until approximately 6 to 18 months of age. Signs usually observed may include coughing, fainting, exercise intolerance, irregular heart rate, or lethargy. A pronounced cardiac murmur will be heard upon auscultation (examination with a stethoscope) by a veterinarian.

Pups with vascular ring anomaly are usually asymptomatic until weaning, after which time regurgitation or vomiting of solid food becomes apparent. Retarded growth of the animal and regurgitation of undigested food within minutes or hours of eating are typical clinical signs. Other clinical signs may include respiratory distress, wheezing, coughing, or bluish discoloration of the tongue or gums. In most cases of vascular ring anomaly, the diagnosis is made before the puppy reaches maturity.

Ventricular septal defect patients

have a pronounced heart murmur. Animals with a small uncomplicated opening may be asymptomatic. If the hole is large, clinical signs usually develop by one year of age and include a cough, exercise intolerance, and poor growth. Some patients show cyanosis (blue tinge to mucous membranes) and abnormal blood counts.

Tetralogy of Fallot is the most common cause of cyanotic heart disease in dogs. The mucous membranes of the gums and eyelids are often discolored with a blue tinge. This is because the shunting of blood from the right side of the heart to the left side of the heart does not allow the blood to become fully oxygenated. These animals are not usually very energetic and even mild exercise may worsen the condition.

Diagnosis

The diagnosis of PDA is normally made by the characteristic murmur, electrocardiogram (EKG) and chest radiographs (x-rays). There are specific criteria in the above tests which indicate the correct diagnosis for PDA.

An accurate diagnosis of pulmonic stenosis is made by the use of physical examination, radiographs, electrocardiogram, and either echocardiogram or cardiac catheterization. Quite often it is necessary to inject a medical dye solution during a catheterization of the heart to visualize the defect on a series of radiographs. This is known as an angiogram.

The diagnosis of congenital SAS is based upon physical examination (i.e., heart murmur), radiography, electrocardiography, and echocardiography. Cardiac catheterization with blood pressure measurements and angiography can also help determine the severity of the defect.

The diagnosis of vascular ring anomaly is made by radiographs of the thorax. Most often the pet is fed a mixture of a radiopaque dye (a dye that will show up on radiographs) with soft food and additional radiographs reveal an accurate diagnosis.

Diagnosis of ventricular septal defect is made by the detection of a heart murmur, electrocardiography, radiography and echocardiography. Cardiac catheterization with angiography is sometimes done to determine accurate pressure changes and ascertain the exact size of the opening.

Diagnosis of Tetralogy of Fallot can be accurately diagnosed with echocardiography or with cardiac catheterization and angiography.

Management

The treatment for PDA involves surgical correction. The surgery should be done as soon as possible, ideally before five months of age to minimize secondary damage to the heart and lungs. There is over a 90% success rate with the surgery and if completed early enough, the prognosis is excellent that the dog will be able to

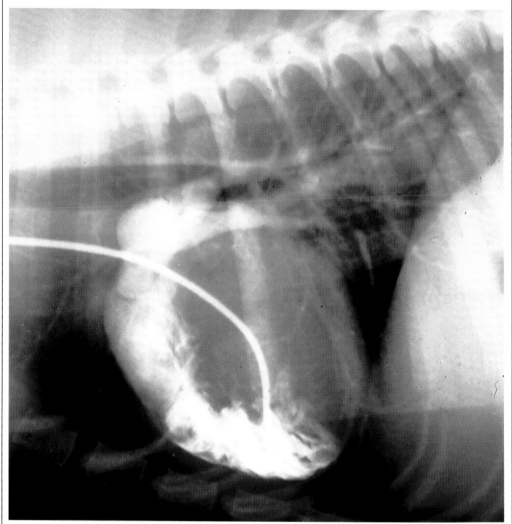

An angiogram revealing a pulmonic stenosis. Courtesy of Dr. Kenneth Jeffery, Mesa Veterinary Hospital, Ltd., Mesa, Arizona.

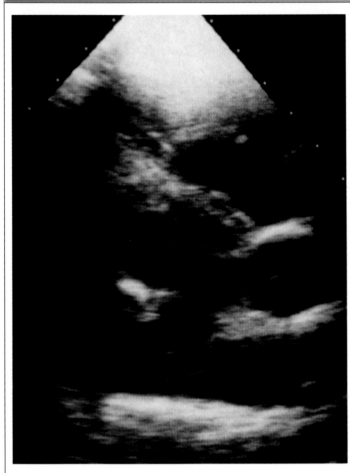

Two-dimensional echocardiogram revealing a subaortic stenosis caused by a fibrous ring just below the aortic valve. Courtesy of Dr. Kenneth Jeffery, Mesa Veterinary Hospital, Ltd., Mesa, Arizona.

live a normal life expectancy. If left uncorrected, the puppies usually do not live more than the first year or two. Medical management may be attempted for those pups that are poor anesthetic or surgical risks. Standard therapy should consist of diuretic administration (water pills), exercise restriction, and dietary sodium (salt) reduction. When heart failure occurs, drugs such as digoxin are used.

Treatment of SAS is difficult and often discouraging because many of these dogs either die suddenly or develop heart failure. Acute death, often without previous clinical signs, commonly occurs at one to three years of age. Certain medications, such as propranolol or nadolol, have been prescribed to reduce the oxygen demands by the heart muscle. The ultimate usefulness of such treatment is still unproven. Surgical correction of the problem is seldom attempted because a heart/lung bypass procedure is required. Recently the use of balloon valvuloplasty catheters has been suggested to relieve SAS and pulmonic stenosis, thus alleviating the need for the expensive and risky surgery. The results of this procedure are not as good in dogs as in humans so far. The reason is that many stenotic lesions in dogs have substantial obstruction below the level of the valve. They open with surgery but tend to re-obstruct within three months in most cases.

Treatment of the vascular ring anomaly is surgical correction of the abnormal vessel within the chest. The success of therapy is quite variable. Residual signs such as occasional regurgitation commonly occur postoperatively, due to the dilated condition of the esophagus.

The treatment for ventricular septal defect depends upon the clinical signs and size of the defect. Dogs with very small defects often remain normal and occasionally the defects close spontaneously. Definitive closure requires cardiopulmonary bypass surgery to close the defect. Alternative surgery includes restricting the overperfusion of blood into the lungs by suturing a band around the pulmonary artery, thereby better equalizing the pressures within the cardiac chambers. If the band is placed too tight, a right-to-left shunt or right heart failure might result. This can be corrected by loosening or removing the band. Many of these patients still develop congestive heart failure or cardiac rhythm disturbances and require additional medical therapy.

A radiograph showing an accumulation of food mixed with barium in front of the stricture in the esophagus caused by a vascular ring anomaly. Courtesy of Dr. Kenneth Jeffery, Mesa Veterinary Hospital, Ltd., Mesa, Arizona.

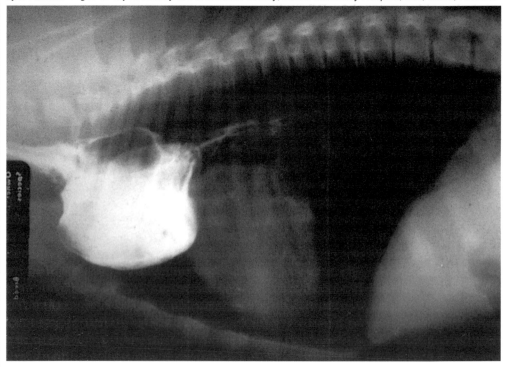

The treatment for Tetralogy of Fallot is heroic at best because of the number of defects involved. Medical therapy includes cage rest and periodic administration of oxygen. In an attempt to improve oxygenation, these dogs produce too many red blood cells (polycythemia). This is bad because it can result in "sludging" of the blood. Therefore, phlebotomy is used periodically when the red blood cell count gets too high. This removes blood and replaces it with intravenous fluids. Surgery is sometimes attempted, but the mortality rate is very high; only 25% of dogs survive the surgery.

CARDIOMYOPATHY

Cardiomyopathy is a descriptive term for a defect of the heart muscle. Two forms are recognized, dilated and hypertrophic. Dilated cardiomyopathy (DCM) is the form most commonly seen, especially in large breeds such as the Doberman Pinscher, Golden Retriever, German Shepherd Dog, Standard Poodle, and Great Dane. Smaller breeds, such as the American Cocker Spaniel and English Springer Spaniel, are also at risk.

In dilated cardiomyopathy, the heart muscle becomes thin and stretched, much like a balloon. In that condition, it is not a very effective pump and, eventually, affected dogs succumb to heart failure. Hypertrophic cardiomyopathy is rare in dogs and results when the heart muscle becomes too thick to allow efficient pumping.

The cause of dilated cardiomyopathy has been the subject of much debate because of its association with certain breeds. Although a genetic tendency is suspected, long-term studies are not yet available. In some breeds, especially the Doberman Pinscher and American Cocker Spaniel, a nutritional mechanism has been proposed. Some Boxers and Doberman Pinschers with dilated cardiomyopathy have a defect in L-carnitine (an amino acid) levels in the heart muscle. These dogs occasionally respond to carnitine supplementation. Although the underlying cause of dilated cardiomyopathy in these dogs remains unknown, an inherited defect resulting in carnitine deficiency of the heart muscle may be important, especially in Boxers. Whether or not this is true in other breeds has yet to be determined. Recent studies in the American Cocker Spaniel seem to suggest that taurine (another amino acid) may be implicated, as it is in the feline form of the disease. As if this isn't confusing enough, some researchers suspect that viruses might also be involved since there is some human research indicating that this might be the case in people.

Clinical Signs

Early in the course of dilated cardiomyopathy, affected animals seem normal. It is only when they show signs of heart failure that most owners seek veterinary attention. Early signs might

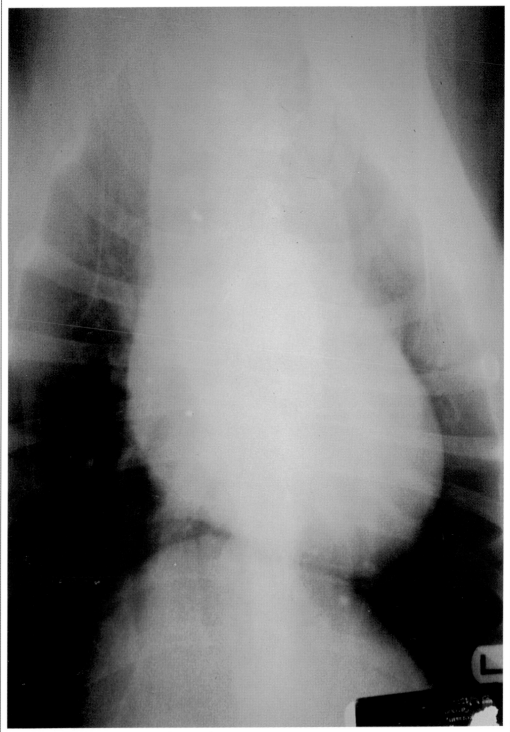

Chest radiograph of a dog with cardiomyopathy.

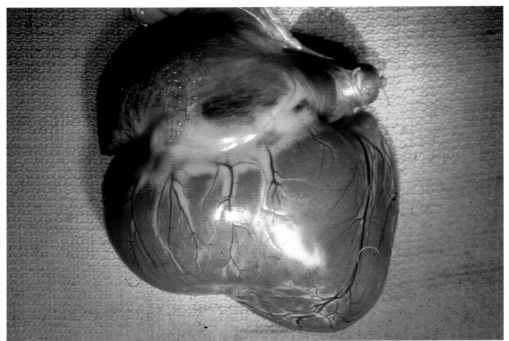

Swollen heart—cardiomyopathy. Courtesy of Dr. Kenneth Jeffery, Mesa Veterinary Hospital, Ltd., Mesa, Arizona.

An M-mode echocardiogram of a dog with cardiomyopathy. Courtesy of Dr. Kenneth Jeffery, Mesa Veterinary Hospital, Ltd., Mesa, Arizona.

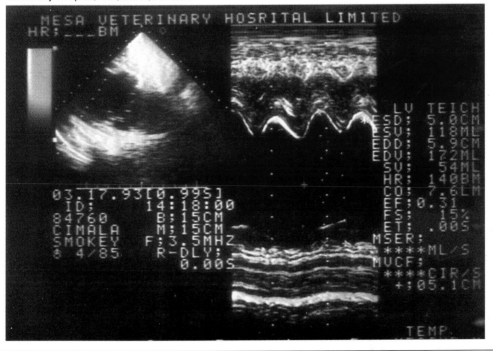

include depression, coughing, exercise intolerance, weakness, respiratory distress, decreased appetite, and even fainting.

Diagnosis

Dilated cardiomyopathy can usually be suspected on the basis of a thorough veterinary examination. By use of a stethoscope (auscultation), the heart rate is often increased. Atrial fibrillation may be suspected if the heart rate is rapid and irregular. However, this clinical diagnostic evaluation is not specific for DCM.

Taking radiographs (x-rays) and electrocardiograms (ECGs) help fill in the diagnostic gaps but the most specific test available is an ultrasound examination of the heart (echocardiography). This painless and precise method allows a definitive diagnosis because it allows the structure and function of the heart to be evaluated on a monitor, and analyzed by computer equipment.

For those dogs that responded to carnitine therapy, surgical biopsies were needed, not blood tests. It is important to note that the deficiency of L-carnitine was reported from biopsy of the muscular wall of the heart; blood levels were often normal. Diagnosis can thus only be made from facilities capable of performing this specialized procedure.

Management

Digoxin (a digitalis derivative) is often used to help the contractions of the heart muscle. Milrinone, an experimental drug, has been very effective in dogs with myocardial failure but is not yet available for dogs or people. Vasodilators such as captopril (Capoten), hydralzine (Apresoline), prazosin (Minipress), and enalapril (Enacard™) are also used to help reduce afterload and the stress on the heart muscle.

Animals with dilated cardiomyopathy are known to have reduced numbers of certain cardiac receptors (beta-1) and increased numbers of other receptors (beta-2). Therefore, certain drugs known as beta-1 blockers are important medicines that help strengthen the heart. The principal reason why these drugs work is complex but it is important that the dose be sufficient to "up-regulate" the beta-1 receptors but not high enough to block them.

In certain breeds, such as the Boxer, a nutritional supplement, L-carnitine, has been found to be very beneficial in affected animals. It is presumed that these dogs have a carnitine deficiency in their heart muscle which results in a defect in the contractions of those heart muscles. These dogs respond to L-carnitine (a non-prescription nutritional supplement) when appropriately dosed and administered three times daily. Similarly, affected dogs of some breeds, such as the American Cocker Spaniel, may have a heart muscle deficiency of taurine, similar to the situation in cats. These dogs might respond favorably to non-prescription taurine supplementation.

L-carnitine is a natural substance found in the heart and liver of normal animals and appears to be an important carrier of activated fatty acids. In the case studies reported, a family of Boxer dogs was found to be suffering from dilated cardiomyopathy and had low levels of L-carnitine in their heart muscles. This normally fatal condition was reversed with the oral administration of L-carnitine to these dogs. When the L-carnitine supplementation was stopped, the heart failure reappeared, and once again improved when the supplementation was reinstituted.

DISORDERS OF THE HEART VALVES

Valves separate the different chambers and outflow vessels of the heart and when they have problems, it is frequently referred to as valvular insufficiency. The most common valve to be affected with problems is the mitral valve, which separates the flow of blood between the left ventricle and the left atrium. Obviously, the purpose of the valves is to allow a watertight (blood-tight) seal so that the beating heart pumps blood in only one direction. With valvular insufficiency, there is a backwash of blood through the valve which results in less-than-efficient pumping action.

Chronic valve disease or endocardiosis is the most common form of heart disease in dogs and is associated with aging. There are many different causes for valvular insufficiency. In some small and medium-sized breeds of dogs, there is thought to be a genetic tendency to experience degeneration of the collagen in the heart valves. These same degenerative changes may be seen in other structures of the body, such as the ligaments. However, the most common causes of valvular disease are chronic wear and tear on the valves, heart diseases, bacterial infections, amyloidosis, and some cancers.

Clinical Signs

Mitral insufficiency is seen most commonly in small breeds such as Toy and Miniature Poodles, Chihuahuas, Yorkshire Terriers, Toy Fox Terriers, Cavalier King Charles Spaniels, Whippets, Miniature Pinschers, Maltese, Japanese Chins, and Cocker Spaniels. The insufficiency increases in frequency and severity with advancing age and it is estimated that chronic mitral valve insufficiency is present in over half of dogs nine years of age and older.

Mild forms of valvular insufficiency likely result in few if any clinical signs. Many older pets will have mild heart murmurs which develop as a consequence of aging. As the valvular incompetence increases, so does the murmur, and the result is various degrees of congestive heart failure.

Diagnosis

Early valvular insufficiency is usually a clinical diagnosis based on detecting a heart murmur. In the early stages, there are few if any changes to be noticed on radiographs (x-rays), electrocardiograms (ECG) or echocardiograms. As impairment increases, there will be gradual accumulation of fluid in the lungs or abdomen, which may be noted on radiographs (x-rays). In time there will also be enlargement of the heart itself. Echocardiography will eventually detect thickened heart valves and dilated heart chambers. Electrocardiography (ECG) does not usually detect problems until the condition is quite advanced since the electrical conduction pattern of the heart is not compromised until late in the course of the condition.

Therapy

Since valve replacement surgeries are not routinely performed in dogs, most treatment options involve a variety of different medications. In the very early stages, no treatment is often given, not even low-salt diets. Tranquilizers such as phenobarbital and diazepam (Valium) are sometimes given to highly stressed animals to help prevent further degeneration of the valves. Isosorbide dinitrate helps improve coronary circulation and is given in some cases.

As the condition progresses, it is managed more intensely. Diuretics (water pills) such as furosemide (Lasix) are given to help reduce fluid accumulation in tissues as heart failure advances. A low-salt diet is indicated at this time as well. Angiotensin-converting enzyme (ACE) inhibitors such as captopril (Capoten) may be needed

in animals not responding satisfactorily to isosorbide dinitrate, and other medications are also used as heart function deteriorates further (ultrasound).

ATRIAL FIBRILLATION

Atrial fibrillation is a common cause of abnormal heart rhythms (arrhythmias). It is very common in large breeds of dogs (e.g., Doberman Pinschers, Great Danes, and Irish Wolfhounds) but rare in small breeds and cats. Most dogs with atrial fibrillation have serious underlying heart disease and are in congestive heart failure.

With atrial fibrillation the atria (upper heart chambers) contract rapidly and not in a logical sequence. This, in turn, results in the ventricles beating too rapidly, which leads to ineffectual pumping of blood. Even though the heart is beating rapidly, it does not have enough time to fill completely with blood between beats, and therefore blood is inefficiently moved throughout the body.

Clinical Signs

Dogs with atrial fibrillation are usually not diagnosed until they have advanced heart disease and behavior that leads owners to seek veterinary advice. On the other hand, early atrial fibrillation may be detected by veterinarians on routine physical examinations and confirmed by diagnostic tests.

Diagnosis

A diagnosis of atrial fibrillation is suspected when a veterinarian listens to the chest with a stethoscope (auscultation). The condition results in a rapid, irregular heart rate.

The diagnosis can be confirmed by an electrocardiogram (ECG). There is an absence of p waves noted, which is very suggestive of this disorder. Abnormal or irregular intervals are also detected.

Management

There is no specific cure for atrial fibrillation. If there is no underlying disease, a cardiac defibrillator may convert atrial fibrillation to normal sinus rhythm. Most dogs with atrial fibrillation, however, have an underlying heart disease, such as cardiomyopathy, valvular disease, or a congenital heart defect. These dogs usually have very high heart rates, often exceeding 200 beats per minute.

Digoxin (a digitalis derivative), propranolol, and diltiazem can be used to lower the heart rate and improve the cardiac output, but they do not cure the condition. Verapamil, a human product, is generally considered too dangerous to use in dogs. Although it has been used successfully in dogs, it can result in severe lowering of blood pressure in patients with congestive heart failure.

Quinidine has been used to convert atrial fibrillation to normal sinus rhythm but it can result in an increased heart rate (ventricular tachycardia), which is an undesirable effect.

HEARTWORM DISEASE

Heartworm disease is caused by the worm *Dirofilaria immitis*, which is transmitted by mosquitoes and then resides within the lungs and great blood vessels of affected dogs. Although heartworm disease was

Electrocardiograph showing changes consistent with atrial fibrillation. Courtesy of Dr. Kenneth Jeffery, Mesa Veterinary Hospital, Ltd., Mesa, Arizona.

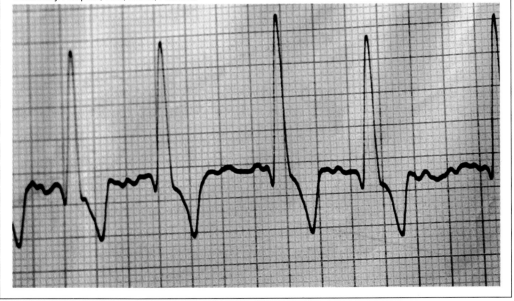

once thought to only affect dogs in the southeastern Atlantic and Gulf Coast states, it has now been reported in every state of the United States (including Alaska) and every province in Canada.

An infected dog has adult heartworms present within the heart and within the blood vessels leading from the heart to the lungs. The female heartworms produce baby worms, better known as microfilariae. The microfilariae are quite small, requiring magnification (100 times) with a microscope to be seen. These microfilariae float around in the bloodstream (where they can circulate for up to two years), while the adults stay put in the heart, the lungs, and the major blood vessels.

The adult heartworms occupy space in the heart and lungs and damage the blood-vessel lining and walls. The microfilariae pose a risk because if they are ingested when a mosquito bites the dog, that mosquito can then serve to transmit the infection to other unsuspecting dogs. The infection is only transmitted by mosquitoes, not by direct contact with infected dogs.

Mosquitoes play an important role in heartworm infection because the microfilariae change within the mosquito from harmless baby worms to infective larvae. When a mosquito bites a dog, the infective larvae migrate down the stinger and penetrate through the skin, introducing the parasite. The larvae remain under the skin for approximately two months. Then,

the larvae enter into the bloodstream and make their way to the heart. Once in the heart, the larvae will grow to be adults and will produce microfilariae to start the cycle all over again.

The complete process, from the time the larvae penetrate the skin until the microfilariae are produced by adults, takes approximately six months. Outdoor dogs in areas of heavy vegetation, which offers excellent mosquito cover, have the greatest risk of infection. The dusk to dawn hours, when mosquitoes are most numerous, are especially dangerous.

Clinical Signs

Signs of heartworm disease can include a chronic cough, loss of appetite, weight loss, and fatigue. These signs, however, generally do not appear until the disease is well advanced, by which time severe damage may have occurred.

During the early stages of infection, most dogs appear normal. Clinical signs develop slowly and may not be evident for up to three years after exposure. Thus, not all dogs affected with heartworm are clinically ill. Some dogs may have heartworms for months or possibly years, and the owners may not be aware of it. Eventually, in most cases, signs will start to become evident. Most of the clinical signs are a result of increased work for the heart (cardiac workload) associated with increased pressure (hypertension) in the arteries supplying blood to the lungs (pulmonary arteries).

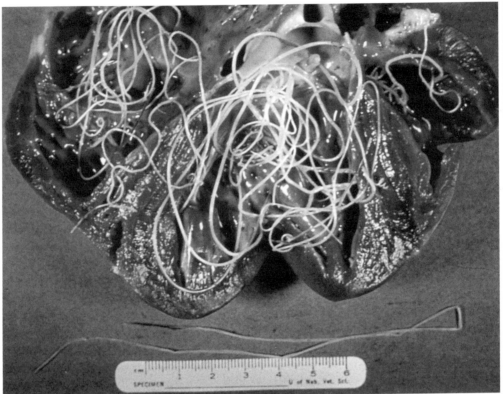

A canine heart infected with heartworms. The actual length of an adult heartworm is evident at the bottom of the picture. Courtesy of MSD/Agvet.

Some of the first clinical signs are lack of energy and/or exercise intolerance. Other signs include coughing, poor appetite, abdominal distension (pot-bellied appearance) and weight loss. More severe signs include heavy breathing, falling over, and coughing up blood.

Diagnosis

Heartworm disease usually cannot be diagnosed in entirety with only one laboratory test. Different tests measure different aspects of infection. For example, microfilarial tests measure the presence of larval (immature) forms in the blood, but not adults. Antigen tests measure the presence of adult forms, but not circulating larvae.

One of the simplest and best initial screening tests available is to check blood for microfilariae. The two best ways of doing this are the Knott's (concentration) test and the filter test. Filter tests have become popular because they can be performed quickly, with an answer often available even before the pet leaves the clinic. Most microfilarial tests involve taking a blood sample from your dog, processing the sample with filters and dyes, then looking for the microfilariae with a microscope. If microfilariae are present, there will be an extremely high chance that adult heartworms are present. But, that still doesn't

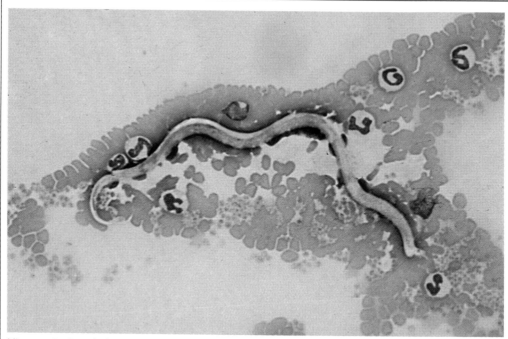

Microscopic view of microfilariae detected by a rapid in-house diagnostic test.

Life cycle of heartworm. A mosquito, having bitten an infected dog, is capable of transmitting the infection to a susceptible dog within about two weeks. Courtesy of MSD/Agvet.

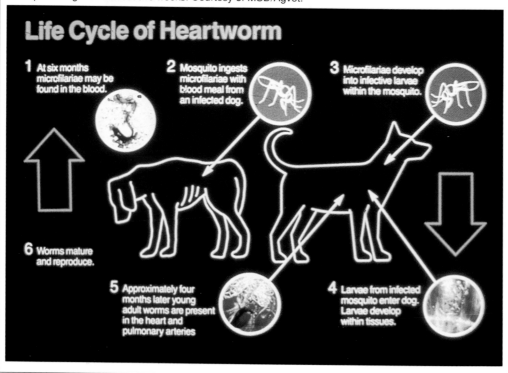

Life Cycle of Heartworm

1 At six months microfilariae may be found in the blood.

2 Mosquito ingests microfilariae with blood meal from an infected dog.

3 Microfilariae develop into infective larvae within the mosquito.

6 Worms mature and reproduce.

5 Approximately four months later young adult worms are present in the heart and pulmonary arteries

4 Larvae from infected mosquito enter dog. Larvae develop within tissues.

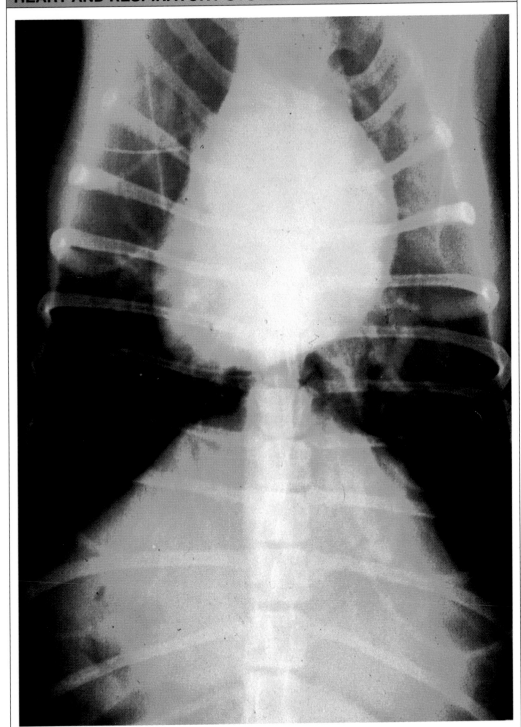

Chest radiograph from a dog with heartworm infection.

mean that there is 100% certainty that adult heartworms are present. Other problems with this test include the fact that not all heartworm-positive animals have circulating microfilariae and that other worms (e.g., *Dipetalonema reconditum*) have subtle differences on microscopic evaluation, and must be considered.

In the early 1980s, antibody blood tests were developed but were associated with many problems, including giving positive results in dogs that didn't have heartworm. These tests have now been abandoned in favor of antigen tests.

Antigen blood tests use more sophisticated means to detect bits and pieces (antigens) of the actual adult heartworms. Actually, these tests measure circulating uterine antigens discharged by female heartworms. Usually, at least five or six female heartworms must be present to give a positive result. Any dog older than six months of age should be checked by both microfilarial concentration and antigen tests before any preventive program is begun. After that, blood tests are recommended on a yearly basis. It must be emphasized that a large number of heartworm-positive dogs may not have detectable microfilariae in their blood (occult infection) and therefore a negative test does not definitively prove the dog does not have heartworm. A new antigen test, the VetRed test, is a rapid in-clinic test of whole blood. It is quite specific, but positives should still be confirmed by other antigen tests before treatment is commenced. Additional tests, such as taking radiographs of the chest and running immunologic tests for heartworm antigen, are important in patient assessment.

Once animals are on regular heartworm preventive therapy, they should be monitored yearly. For dogs on monthly therapy (e.g., Interceptor, Heartgard), the preferred annual screening test is the antigen blood test. For those on daily preventive therapy, the microfilarial (e.g., filter, Knott's) tests are recommended.

Treatment

Although there are treatments for heartworm disease, clearly prevention is the preferred alternative. Not only can heartworm disease be fatal but the treatments used can also be dangerous. Since heartworm disease is so easy to prevent, it is a pity that some pets remain unprotected and may contract this terrible disease.

There are many ways of treating heartworm disease. Most treatments consist of killing the adult heartworms first and therefore we often use the term "adulticide" therapy. This is most often done by injecting thiacetarsamide (Caparsolate: Sanofi, an arsenic compound) intravenously for several treatment periods. This portion of the treatment is best accomplished by hospitalizing the patient since the arsenic compound is not only toxic to the heartworms but to the dog itself. A new medication, melarsomine dihydrochloride (RM340: Rhone Merieux), is currently being evaluated. It appears to be an effective and potentially practical treatment for dogs with severe pulmonary artery disease and a large number of heartworms.

The most common and serious complication of adulticide therapy is blood clots in the lungs (pulmonary thromboembolism) caused from circulating dead worms. Another major complication is that the adulticide treatment is toxic and can cause damage to the liver and kidneys. Signs we see from this are lethargy, depression, hard and rapid breathing, severe coughing and possibly death. It is important that the dog remains quiet and its activity level is kept to a minimum throughout the heartworm treatment and for three to four weeks afterward. If we can do that, then we are less likely to encounter the severe complications of heartworm treatment.

The second phase of the treatment consists of killing the microfilariae. Remember, the first phase of the treatment only killed the adult worms living in the heart; now it is necessary to kill the young forms, the microfilariae. To accomplish this, the patient is reevaluated between the third and fourth week following the initial treatment. This "microfilaricide" treatment is a one-time treatment and usually requires no overnight hospitalization for the patient. The patient then returns two weeks later for a blood test to make sure there are no more microfilariae present in the bloodstream.

The third phase of therapy is directed at preventing reinfection. This treatment is an at-home treatment the owner can give orally to help prevent the dog from ever acquiring heartworm disease again.

For those dogs that cannot tolerate arsenical therapy, there are other options. Although not approved for this use, ivermectin or milbemycin is sometimes given to heartworm-positive dogs. Although these drugs will not kill adult heartworms at preventive doses, they do decrease the number of microfilariae and the damage they might cause. Dogs should be hospitalized and closely monitored on the day the preventive is given. This might be an alternative if regular treatment is not a viable option. However, whenever possible, a cure should be pursued with adulticidal therapy.

Prevention

The three most popular heartworm preventatives on the market today are Heartgard (Merck), Interceptor (Ciba-Geigy), and Filarabits (Norden-SmithKline Beecham). All of these medications are given orally.

Filarabits has diethylcarbamazine (DEC) as the active ingredient. They must be given every day to enhance effective heartworm prevention. Filarabits are flavored chewable tablets that most dogs will like and take quite freely.

Heartgard's active ingredient is

ivermectin. This is a tablet that only has to be given once a month, which is one of the reasons for its popularity with owners. Ivermectin should be cautiously used in the Collie, although it appears that the extremely low dose used in Heartgard is unlikely to cause toxicity.

The newest heartworm preventative on the market today is called Interceptor. The active ingredient is milbemycin oxime and this product also only needs to be administered (orally) once a month. It has the added benefit of being effective at controlling hookworms, roundworms, and whipworms as well as heartworm. Research conducted by the company suggests that at even 15-20 times the normal dose, no toxicities were seen in dogs, including Collies.

All of these products are very effective, and, if used properly, will prevent heartworm disease. They are not treatments. It is very important to have dogs tested for heartworm disease before using these preventatives as they have the potential to make a dog very sick if administered to a heartworm-positive dog. Interceptor is particularly effective and can kill the microfilariae, making it more difficult to detect active infection while on this preparation. Ideally a heartworm test should be done two to four weeks after commencing treatment with this preventative.

Prior to giving any preventative medication for heartworm, an antigen test should be performed with negative results. If owners are using diethylcarbamazine citrate (DEC) and it has not been given faithfully every day, a microfilarial test should be performed before

The SNAP heartworm antigen test kit. Courtesy of IDEXX Laboratories, Inc., Westbrook, Maine.

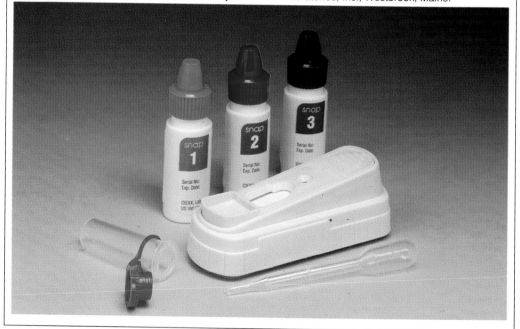

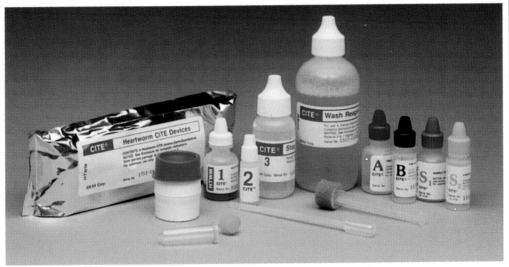

The CITE® Heartworm antigen test kit. Courtesy of IDEXX Laboratories, Inc., Westbrook, Maine.

DEC therapy is started again. A microfilarial examination should also be used before animals are placed on milbemycin oxime because the preventative dose kills microfilariae. Antigen tests are preferred on all cases because there is evidence that ivermectin and milbemycin oxime administration reduces the concentration of microfilariae in the blood enough to make microfilarial concentration tests inaccurate. They appear to make female heartworms sterile so the microfilariae are harder to find even if there are still adult heartworms present.

The length of time the heartworm preventatives must be given depends on the length of the mosquito season. Dogs should probably be started on preventatives when about eight weeks old, even though adult heartworms are not found in dogs less than six months of age. After that, it is generally held that animals should be on preventatives from one to two months prior to mosquito season until one full month past the end of mosquito season. Since mosquitoes will emerge when temperatures climb to 40°F or above, predicting the mosquito season can be difficult. In many cases, year-round preventative treatment is recommended. Once again, it is critical that all dogs be heartworm tested with negative results before commencing any preventative.

Heartworm vaccines may soon be on the horizon. This was once believed near-impossible because dogs do not appear to become naturally immune to heartworm infection. Therefore, it was suspected that it might not be possible to induce immunity through vaccination. Another concern was that the parasite may be too large to be killed by antibodies. Most research today is focusing on specific antigens (small parts of the heartworm larvae) as the targets for vaccine- induced parasite control. The biggest hurdle that vaccines will have is that they will need to be more effective than the once-a-month preventatives to be acceptable to most owners. This is a big task, because the preventatives are highly effective, very safe, and reasonably priced. Vaccines aren't ready yet, but it just may be a matter of time before they are.

CARDIOPULMONARY RESUSCITATION

Cardiopulmonary arrest is an emergency situation in which breathing stops and malignant dysrhythmias (e.g., ventricular fibrillation, heart stoppage) occur. It can result from many different causes, including traumatic accidents (e.g., hit by car), pneumonia, drug reactions, heartworm disease, drowning, electrocution or other underlying diseases.

Clinical Signs

Medically, cardiopulmonary arrest is when an animal is not breathing and no pulse or heartbeat can be detected. Respiratory arrest occurs when the animal is not breathing but there is still a pulse. Both are emergency situations that will result in death if action is not taken promptly.

Diagnosis

The distinction between cardiopulmonary arrest and respiratory arrest is easy when a stethoscope is used to listen to chest sounds. More specific diagnostic tests (e.g., blood pressure) are useful but may not be performed immediately because of the emergency nature of the condition. Where available, blood gases (oxygen and carbon dioxide) can provide an important measure of the level of oxygen deprivation experienced.

Management

Cardiopulmonary arrest is managed by prompt basic and advanced life support. Basic life support consists of establishing an open airway for breathing together with cardiopulmonary resuscitation (CPR) to provide circulatory support. This is an emergency procedure that should only be performed by experienced individuals. Pet CPR courses are available to those owners that are interested.

The ABC's of CPR are reiterated to remind rescuers the order in which they should be performing their duties. The A stands for Assess and Airway; it is imperative that the animal have a method by which it can receive oxygen. The B stands for Breathe, which means that oxygen must be provided to that animal. Finally, C stands for Circulation, the movement of oxygen-rich blood throughout the body. This is achieved by compressions of the chest wall.

The best way to establish an airway is with an endotracheal tube, but this is only available in veterinary hospitals. These tubes can be inserted directly into the trachea and, if available, connected to mechanical breathing machines (respirators), including anesthetic devices which have oxygen tanks.

Breathing can be instituted with the oxygen from tanks on an anesthetic machine or mouth-to-tube resuscitation. Two initial breaths of 1–1.5 seconds' duration are recommended. Then small dogs should be ventilated at 12–24 breaths per minute and large dogs should receive 20–25 breaths per minute.

Chest compressions are applied according to body weight; small dogs (15 kg) receive 120 compressions per minute compared to 100 compressions per minute for larger dogs. Most researchers recommend that the dog be laying on its side and that the compressions be directed over the heart between the fourth and fifth rib space. Some researchers recommend that CPR is more effective in large dogs if they are laying on their back. This maximizes the pressure exerted when compressions are performed on the breastbone (sternum). How much pressure should be applied? This is impossible to describe in practical terms, but enough pressure is needed to compress the thorax (chest) by 25-33% of its diameter. This technique is best practiced on resuscitative models. Simultaneous compressions and ventilation (SCV) are more effective if two experienced rescuers are involved.

The use of various drug treatments at the same time as CPR may be beneficial in some cases but is not without controversy. Fluid therapy appears to increase total blood flow (which is good) but decrease blood flow to the brain and heart (which is bad). Epinephrine (adrenaline) is often given to humans and dogs during CPR and this stimulates the heart. High-dose administration may be more successful than the conservative dosing once recommended. However, cardiac arrhythmias and aberrations of blood glucose and potassium levels could be complicating factors. A new medication, methoxamine, has recently been recommended for use during CPR in dogs which increases the diastolic pressure in the aorta. Further study is needed before it can be routinely recommended.

Despite all the positive press about CPR, it must be remembered that it is a last-ditch heroic procedure and many dogs will not survive, even with expert attention. Recent studies have suggested a survival rate of approximately 10%, for dogs that arrest while already in a veterinary hospital. Delays in performing CPR, which is common following an accident, would likely have even lower success rates.

PACEMAKER IMPLANTATION

No discussion of cardiology would be complete without mention of cardiac pacemaker implantation. The cardiac pacemaker is a device that induces the heart muscle to contract by stimulating it with an electrical impulse. Today cardiac pacemaker implantation is commonly used in human medicine and is no longer a rare occurrence in veterinary medicine.

Indications

Pacemakers will not correct congestive heart failure, cardiomyopathy, or most other cardiac ills. The main indication for using them is "heart block," a collection of disorders in which the normal electrical conduction system of the heart has become dysfunctional. The conditions most amenable to successful management are: complete atrioventricular block; second-degree atrioventricular block; and sick sinus syndrome. Candidates for implantation should have low cardiac output that has not responded adequately to conventional medical therapy.

Technique

There are now several different techniques whereby permanent placement of a pacemaker can be performed. All require general anesthesia. The electrical lead is inserted through a vein or through an incision made between the ribs until it is implanted in the heart. Once the lead is in a satisfactory position it is tested, and the correct stimulation threshold determined to ensure that the electrical current provided is only that necessary to do the job. It is then connected to a pulse generator which is usually placed in the abdominal wall.

Monitoring

There is no point performing a pacemaker implantation if regular

Pacemaker implantation surgery. Courtesy of Dr. Kenneth Jeffery, Mesa Veterinary Hospital, Ltd., Mesa, Arizona.

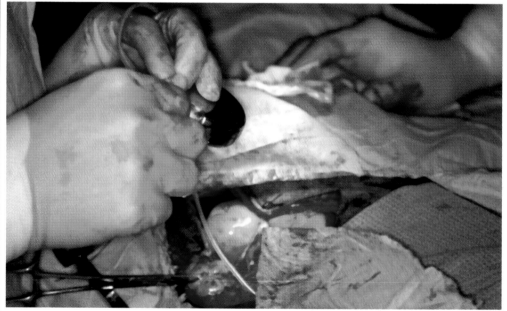

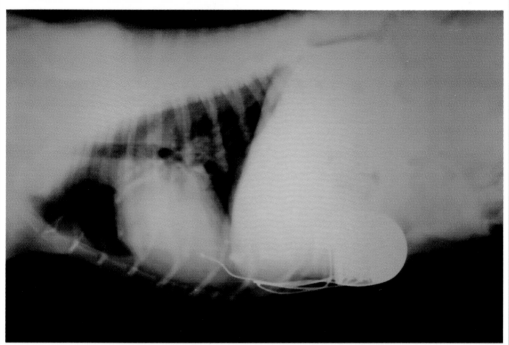

Radiograph showing pacemaker implantation in a dog. Note the lead running from the pacer in the abdomen to the heart. Courtesy of Dr. Kenneth Jeffery, Mesa Veterinary Hospital, Ltd., Mesa, Arizona.

follow-up examinations are not feasible. Evaluations are often necessary every week for the first month or so, and then every three to six months. More careful monitoring may be necessary as the battery powering the pacemaker reaches the end of its anticipated lifespan. Evaluations are needed to fine tune the settings on the pacemaker, including the threshold output, sensitivity, rate and mode. It is also important to make sure that the pacemaker is doing what it's supposed to—make the animal symptomatically better. Also, from time to time, the pacemaker may need adjustments.

BLEEDING DISORDERS

Bleeding disorders in dogs can be either inherited or acquired. The inherited conditions result from inbreeding and line breeding; they are common in breeds in which particular affected animals are popular show winners and are sought after for breeding purposes. The acquired conditions are actually more common but are usually given less attention because they are not passed on to successive generations.

The body has developed a complex mechanism involved in proper blood clotting. Most blood vessels develop leaks from time to time and the body patches them quickly and efficiently. This conserves the blood supply (hemostasis) so that hemorrhages do not occur routinely. The body accomplishes this in several different ways. When blood vessels are damaged, the vessels themselves constrict, platelets are summoned to plug the leak, and "clotting factors" are produced to finish the job.

Most inherited bleeding disorders result from defective platelet function, or deficiencies of a variety of "factors" from either of two different but interrelated clotting systems (the intrinsic and extrinsic clotting systems). The most common inherited bleeding diseases are von Willebrand's disease and two forms of hemophilia. The most common acquired bleeding defects are low numbers of platelets (thrombocytopenia), vitamin K deficiency, and disseminated intravascular coagulopathy (DIC).

Von Willebrand's disease (vWD) is the most common, mild inherited bleeding disorder of dogs. It is an autosomal (non-sex-linked) trait with two forms of clinical and genetic expression. In the most common form (type I vWD), the gene can be inherited from either or both parents. Not all pups will be equally affected; it is highly variable. This form of the disease has been reported in over 50 breeds of dogs. If a defective gene is inherited from both parents, the condition is usually lethal. Type II vWD is quite rare but is inherited in German Shorthaired Pointers. The parents are clinically normal but if they are both carriers, the pups will be affected. Type III vWD is recessive and has been recognized in Scottish Terriers and Chesapeake Bay Retrievers. A similar variant has

been seen in Shetland Sheepdogs. In addition to the inherited form of vWD, this disorder can also be acquired in association with familial hypothyroidism. There appears to be some significant differences between breeds with respect to age and concentration of von Willebrand's factor in the blood. Most Doberman Pinschers are older (about five years of age) when affected, compared to Scottish Terriers and Shetland Sheepdogs (about two years of age). Affected Dobermans also have more residual von Willebrand's factor in their blood (15%), compared to Shetland Sheepdogs (8%) and Scottish Terriers (0%).

The following dog breeds exhibit a high incidence of von Willebrand's disease:

Basset Hound
Corgi (Pembroke Welsh)
Dachshund (Standard and Miniature)
Doberman Pinscher
German Shepherd Dog
Golden Retriever
Keeshond
Manchester Terrier (Standard and Toy)
Poodle (Standard and Miniature)
Rottweiler
Schnauzer (Miniature)
Scottish Terrier
Shetland Sheepdog.

Hemophilia A is a sex-linked recessive disease carried by the female and manifested in the male. Females are only affected if a hemophiliac male is mated to a carrier or hemophiliac female. Male hemophiliacs can be produced by two normal carrier parents. Hemophilia A is the most commonly reported, severe inherited coagulation defect of animals and has been recognized in many breeds of dogs, as well as mongrels.

Hemophilia B is less common than hemophilia A but has been reported in several different breeds of dog. It involves a different clotting factor defect than hemophilia A.

Inherited disorders of platelet function such as thrombasthenia (weak platelets) and thrombopathia (diseased platelets) are rare in dogs, and it's a good thing. Thrombasthenia has only been recognized in Otterhounds but similar conditions have been seen in other hound breeds. Animals with thrombopathias have defective platelet function but normal platelet numbers. These have been recognized in Basset Hounds and American Foxhounds. Thrombopathia can also be an acquired condition, especially in dogs that have been receiving drug therapy such as aspirin, estrogens, or sulfonamides. It can even occur in animals with internal diseases (e.g., liver disease, kidney disease) and occasionally as an adverse reaction to vaccination with modified live-virus products.

Another common platelet disorder which is important but not inherited is thrombocytopenia. In this condition, there just aren't enough platelets present to form a sufficient clot. The most common cause of this condition is an aberration of the immune system, in which the body targets the platelets and sets out to destroy them. Most commonly the condition is a reaction to a variety of other entities such as autoimmune diseases, drugs, toxic agents, chemicals, live-virus vaccines and even incompatible blood transfusions. Often the circulating platelets get caught up as innocent bystanders in battles conducted by the immune system against a variety of real or imagined opponents. In a small number of cases, thrombocytopenia can occur in conjunction with internal diseases or problems in the bone marrow.

Vitamin K is needed for the liver to manufacture clotting factors. It is highly unlikely that dogs would ever develop vitamin K deficiency through poor diet. However, vitamin K is inhibited by many rodent poisons that are made with warfarin (coumarin). Therefore, vitamin K deficiency is often associated with rodenticide poisoning. Also, any disease that affects the liver will affect the levels of vitamin K in the body.

Disseminated intravascular coagulopathy (DIC) is the final common result when the clotting system has run amok. It is confusing to many people because it does not result from a lack of clotting elements exactly. The blood clots too quickly, and then bleeding results because all the needed clotting factors are "used up" and not available for further clotting.

Common causes include whelping problems (obstetrical complications), cancers, and severe infections. There is always an underlying cause when animals develop this life-threatening condition.

Clinical Signs

Clinically, bleeding disorders are quite variable in their presentation. Pinpoint hemorrhages in the mouth or skin may be noted. Bleeding episodes from the nose, mouth or rectum may be apparent. These animals are more prone to bruising and they may have swollen joints, caused by the accumulation of blood in the joint space. Blood may also be found in the stool or urine. The presentation is highly variable because animals may have different degrees of clotting abnormalities. For example, a dog with a clotting factor defect of 45% of normal will fare better than a dog with a clotting factor level only 10% of normal. Therefore, some animals will appear entirely normal until they undergo routine surgery, such as neutering or spaying, in which they have a tendency to bleed more than usual.

The majority of dogs with vWD (von Willebrand's disease) have a relatively mild form of the disease. They may experience bleeding problems that tend to be worsened by stress and other diseases. They may have some blood loss into the bowels or urine or have a tendency to develop nosebleeds. More severely affected dogs may have pronounced bleeding, especially following surgery, even minor procedures. Dogs with 30% or less of the normal level of von Willebrand factor are at risk of hemorrhage.

Hemophilia A (factor VIII: C deficiency) can also vary greatly in clinical presentation. Since it is sex-linked, most affected animals are male. Mild cases are frequently undetected until the animal reaches young adulthood, unless it is a dog breed whereby tail docking and dewclaw removal are routine procedures. In other cases, the defect is discovered following elective surgeries such as castration.

Basically the clinical signs of platelet function disorders are similar to those of vWD because patients have a tendency to bleed. The disease in Basset Hounds is quite widespread among North American breeding stock and is unique. Most of the bleeding is limited to the mucosal surfaces, such as the gums, prepuce, and nose.

Diagnosis

A bleeding disorder is usually not suspected until there is a crisis. A safe, elective surgical procedure results in pronounced bleeding that is difficult to stop. There is blood found in the stool or the urine, for no apparent reason. Pups are stillborn or fail to thrive after birth (fading puppy syndrome).

A thorough physical examination is needed to determine the location and severity of the bleeding and to identify any underlying disease that may be present. The next task at hand is to perform blood tests (coagulation profiles) to help identify the source of the problem (e.g., platelets, clotting factors). Routine screening blood tests of clotting activity, such as the activated partial thromboplastin time (APTT), prothrombin time (PT), and thrombin clotting time (TCT), are basic screening tests used to test the overall effectiveness of the clotting mechanism. It is important to realize that they will not uncover the majority of inherited bleeding disorders. These first tests are used to determine the extent of the bleeding tendency, not necessarily to identify the exact cause. Specific tests are usually run later, unless there is a breed tendency to suggest the most likely diagnosis. For example, a Doberman Pinscher with a bleeding problem might be screened initially for von Willebrand's disease because the condition is so prevalent in this breed.

When a pet is identified with a specific inherited bleeding disorder, the job is not yet done. Diagnostic blood testing of relatives to uncover carriers is important since the responsible position is to limit the spread of the disorder in related animals. In general, these tests must be performed by specialty veterinary laboratories knowledgeable and experienced in providing coagulation tests for animals. The blood samples require special handling procedures, special blood tubes, and very exacting testing procedures to be valid.

The most common inherited bleeding disorder, von Willebrand's disease, is detected by measuring levels of von Willebrand's factor (vWF) in the blood. In the most common form (vWD I), levels are usually 1-60% of normal. Animals with the recessive type III disease have zero levels of vWF, whereas their carrier parents have reduced levels of this protein (15-60% of normal). Unfortunately, the incidence of von Willebrand's disease is increasing, especially in certain breeds, such as the Doberman Pinscher.

Results of diagnostic screening tests for hemophilia A and hemophilia B are similar and an exact diagnosis requires measurements of factor VIII:C (hemophilia A) and factor IX (hemophilia B). Affected animals have low levels of those specific factors; carriers often have reduced but adequate levels for their own health concerns.

Diagnosis of platelet function defects is very difficult because the samples cannot be shipped to diagnostic laboratories for processing. These specialized tests need to be performed immediately on blood samples. This requires that the dogs actually go to the testing facilities to have the samples drawn and processed.

Management

There are no cures for any of the inherited bleeding disorders but some animals may lead relatively normal lives if they are only mildly or moderately affected. Of the acquired bleeding disorders, vitamin K deficiency can usually be successfully managed if treatment is begun in time. Disseminated intravascular coagulopathy (DIC) is a life-threatening disorder that requires emergency intervention.

The treatment of inherited bleeding disorders needs to be individualized for each case. Severe bleeding requires transfusions with plasma or whole blood. Dogs with von Willebrand's disease usually also benefit from supplementation with thyroid hormone (thyroxine). Another drug, deamino 8-D-arginine vasopressin, has been used experimentally in dogs but is less useful in canines than it is in people. Hemophiliac dogs often require frequent (twice daily) transfusions during bleeding episodes because the factors are so short-lived within the body. These have to be given from cross-matched and type-compatible blood donors. Treatment and management considerations for pets with hemophilia (both A and B) require special consideration. The larger the dog, the potentially more serious the condition. In some cases it is almost impossible to maintain these animals in a near-normal condition, making them unsuitable as housepets.

Treatment of dogs with platelet function disorders requires transfusion with whole blood or platelet-rich plasma. There may also be some benefit to supplementing these animals with therapeutic doses of thyroid hormones.

Treatment for vitamin K deficiency or liver disease requires supplementation with vitamin K. This therapy must be used cautiously and only as necessary because levels higher than recommended can produce secondary side effects of their own. If the animal has liver disease, the underlying cause of the liver disease needs to be treated.

Many severe cases of DIC are fatal, despite the best efforts to treat them. Because these conditions result in overactive clotting, treatment is often instituted with aspirin or other products designed to thin the blood by inhibiting the clotting process. Obviously this type of therapy would be disastrous in other cases of clotting disorders and therefore correct diagnosis is critical.

Prevention

The best way to prevent the inherited bleeding disorders is to purchase puppies that have been screened for prospective diseases that are most common in the breed. This is particularly important for von Willebrand's disease, which can be easily diagnosed with screening tests. Carriers of these diseases should not be used for breeding, even if they appear clinically normal. Since hypothyroidism can be linked with von Willebrand's disease, thyroid profiles can also be a useful part of the screening procedure.

For the acquired bleeding

disorders, prevention involves good routine veterinary medical care. Internal disorders such as liver disease, kidney disease, cardiopulmonary disease, and cancers need never result in bleeding tendencies if addressed early. The likelihood of vitamin K deficiency can be greatly reduced if dogs are kept away from rat poisons which contain anti-coagulants.

ANEMIA

Anemia occurs when there are not enough red blood cells or hemoglobin to carry oxygen to the tissues of the body. It is a description, not a diagnosis, and can be the final common result of many different disease processes. Anything that hampers the manufacture of hemoglobin, causes loss of blood, or results in red-blood-cell destruction can cause anemia.

Iron deficiency anemia results from chronic blood loss. Rarely is it caused by an actual nutritional deficiency of iron. Animals with intestinal parasites (especially hookworm) or those with chronic bleeding diseases are most likely to suffer from iron deficiency. Although nutritional deficiencies (e.g., vitamin B_{12}, copper) can result in anemia, these are rare in dogs.

The most common cause of anemia in dogs not associated with internal or external bleeding is hemolytic anemia. This form of anemia results when red blood cells are destroyed. This destruction may occur in the bloodstream or in other areas, such as the liver, spleen, or bone marrow. The most common cause of hemolytic anemia is the destruction of red blood cells by the animal's own immune system. This is referred to as immune-mediated hemolytic anemia. Hemolytic anemia can also result from eating onions, exposure to excessive amounts of zinc, infections (e.g., babesiosis, ehrlichiosis), inherited disorders (e.g., pyruvate kinase deficiency), and from other diseases (e.g., heartworm).

Hereditary red-blood-cells disorders have been documented in a number of dog breeds. Phosphofructokinase deficiency has been reported in English Springer Spaniels. Pyruvate kinase deficiency has been observed in Basenjis, Beagles, and West Highland White Terriers. The second disorder mentioned is more severe and often results in death of affected animals by four years of age. The effects of phosphofructokinase deficiency are relatively mild but may be potentiated by exercise.

Clinical Signs

The cardinal signs of anemia include weakness, a bounding pulse, pale gums, and increased heart rate. However, in the early stages of anemia, animals will appear outwardly normal. In fact, no problems may be noticed at all until about one-third of the blood volume has been lost.

Dogs with hemolytic disease may appear jaundiced (icteric) and have

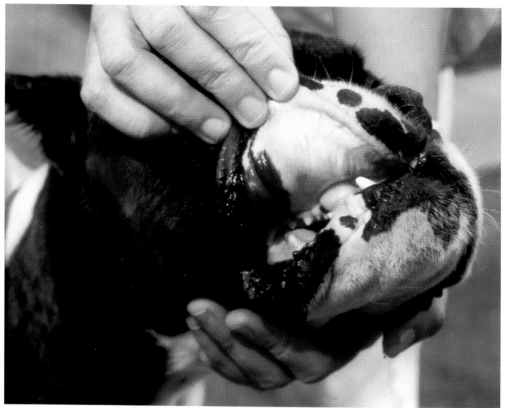

Anemia, as evidenced by pale gums. Courtesy of Dr. Kenneth Jeffery, Mesa Veterinary Hospital, Ltd., Mesa, Arizona.

an enlarged spleen and/or liver. Other causes of anemia may be associated with their own particular clinical signs. When severe anemia is present, shock and death result.

Diagnosis

The diagnosis of anemia can be confirmed by measuring red-blood-cell and hemoglobin levels but finding the underlying cause can involve many different tests. Fecal examinations are warranted to look for internal parasites.

The basic workup for anemia used by most veterinarians includes blood-cell counts, analysis of urine (urinalysis), and function tests for different internal organs. Tests for blood-cell parasites *Babesia* and *Ehrlichia* are performed in geographic regions where they are prevalent. Radiographs (x-rays) should be taken if an enlarged liver or spleen is palpated (felt) by the veterinarian during the clinical examination. Tests for inherited disorders can be done at specialized facilities.

The blood cell counts usually provide the most important clues to diagnosis. Small red blood cells may be associated with iron deficiency. Spherical red blood cells may suggest an immune-mediated disease. Large blue-staining red blood cells indicate increased production to compensate for blood-cell loss. Peculiar figures such as Heinz bodies may suggest onion toxicity.

HYPERTENSION (HIGH BLOOD PRESSURE)

We are all familiar with high blood pressure (hypertension) and its risks in people, but did you know that pets can be affected with high blood pressure as well? In pets, high blood pressure has been associated with kidney disease, heart disease, hormonal disorders (including Cushing's disease, diabetes mellitus, and thyroid disorders), obesity, and other conditions.

Hypertension is defined as a sustained elevation in either systolic or diastolic blood pressure. It is classified as essential hypertension if no underlying cause can be found. Although essential hypertension accounts for 90% of cases in people, this is not true in the canine. In dogs, the vast majority of cases are secondary to a variety of other diseases.

Clinical Signs

As in humans, many cases of hypertension cause no noticeable abnormalities of their own. The diagnosis may be made by routine screening tests or when other problems are detected. For example, some hypertensive dogs may show signs of eye, heart, or nervous-system abnormalities. Some signs might include acute blindness, nosebleeds, heart failure, kidney disease, head tilt, and even seizures.

Diagnosis

The biggest problem facing veterinarians is finding a convenient method of measuring blood pressure in animals, because currently the technology is quite sophisticated and expensive. The most accurate method requires placement of a measuring device directly into a peripheral artery; this may be suitable for measuring blood pressure in animals already affected but is not convenient for routine use.

The traditional indirect measures of blood pressure as used in human medicine were not initially suitable for dogs. Some of these problems have been circumvented by using an ultrasonic Doppler; this appears to satisfactorily measure systolic pressure but is unsatisfactory for the routine diagnosis or monitoring of patients with diastolic hypertension. With the Doppler device, ultrasound waves are directed at the artery of a leg and are reflected back to a receiver. An inflatable cuff is placed above the transducer and inflated; as the cuff is slowly deflated, the systolic and diastolic pressures are measured.

Newer oscillometric techniques which use an inflatable cuff can provide rapid, convenient measurements in medium and large breeds of dogs, but are slightly less reliable when used in small dogs and cats.

If hypertension is diagnosed, a veterinarian will likely need to search for potential underlying causes before starting treatment.

Since hypertension can be worsened by a high-salt diet, restricting the level of sodium in the diet, as is done in people, would be significantly helpful.

Therapy

Since essential (primary) hypertension is rare in dogs, treatment is always more effectively directed at the underlying cause. However, steps should also be taken to directly lower blood pressure. This can conservatively be achieved by weight reduction, and restricting salt and processed sugars in the diet. Diuretics (water pills) may be necessary if diet changes alone are not sufficient.

A second phase of blood-pressure control might involve heart drugs classified as beta-blockers (e.g., prazosin) and calcium channel antagonists (e.g., diltiazem). However, life-threatening consequences of hypertension are much less common in dogs than in people.

RESPIRATORY SYSTEM DISORDERS

Primary Ciliary Dyskinesia

Primary ciliary dyskinesia, also known as immotile cilia syndrome and Kartagener's syndrome, refers to a condition in which the hair-like cilia in the respiratory passages cannot perform their needed defense mechanisms. The result is chronic respiratory infections.

Primary ciliary dyskinesia is believed to be inherited in people as an autosomal recessive trait, and the condition has been reported in the English Springer Spaniel, Chinese Shar-Pei, Doberman Pinscher, English Setter, Golden Retriever, Border Collie, and Old English Sheepdog.

Clinical Signs

The most common clinical manifestation of ciliary dyskinesia is recurring chronic respiratory infection. Therefore, affected dogs often cough, and may develop a runny nose, poor exercise tolerance, and sometimes fever. The result is often bronchitis and pneumonia.

The tails (flagellae) of sperm are modified cilia, so it is not surprising that many dogs with primary ciliary dyskinesia are infertile. Many other defects have also be seen in association with this condition. Hydrocephalus is seen in some dogs with this condition, presumably because modified cilia are involved with the circulation of cerebrospinal fluid (CSF). A bizarre condition, situs inversus, has also been seen in association with ciliary dyskinesia. Approximately half of affected dogs have internal organs that are transposed to the wrong side of the body. Some affected individuals also have hearing loss, middle-ear infections, and dysfunction of some of their white blood cells (neutrophils) to fight off infection.

Diagnosis

The best way to confirm a diagnosis of primary ciliary dyskinesia is to submit biopsies from the nasal cavities or trachea (windpipe) to a pathologist to be evaluated with an electron microscope. This is definitive because the defective cilia can be visualized and counted. This is a specialized diagnostic procedure and not available from every laboratory. Similarly, mucociliary clearance can be evaluated using the radionuclide 99 technetium macroaggregated albumin technique. However, this procedure involves radiation so the animal needs to be isolated for one to two days, and often anesthetized during the procedure.

Because the above diagnostic procedures listed above are so specialized, most animals don't get definitive diagnoses. In most cases, the diagnosis is suspected when a young animal gets recurrent respiratory infections that respond to antibiotics, but recur soon after the drug is discontinued. With mature intact males, sperm can be evaluated for defective sperm motility. This is not an absolute test, because some dogs may have apparently normal sperm yet still have the condition. In about 50% of cases, chest radiographs will reveal the heart on the right (instead of the left) side of the chest.

Therapy

There is no cure for primary ciliary dyskinesia. Symptomatic therapy includes periodic antibiotics based on culture results. Cough suppressants should not be used since they further impede normal defense mechanisms. If the infections can be maintained under reasonable control, affected dogs stand a chance of living a relatively normal existence.

CANINE COUGH (TRACHEOBRONCHITIS)

Canine infectious tracheobronchitis is called by many names, including canine cough and kennel cough. The term kennel cough is falling into disfavor, because kennel operators are not the cause of the problem. The disorder is the result of infectious agents in an environment where dogs are kept in close quarters. Therefore, canine cough is a problem wherever dogs congregate, including kennels, pet stores, grooming parlors, training classes, and even veterinary clinics.

There are many different viruses and bacteria that have been implicated in canine cough, but the condition appears to be more complicated than just a simple infection. Dogs often need to be stressed before they are susceptible and, of course, this is not unusual in situations where many dogs are maintained. They then seem to contract one of a variety of respiratory viral infections (e.g., parainfluenza) that then sets the stage for an imposing bacterial infection. The bacterium that is responsible for the clinical signs seen is called *Bordetella bronchiseptica.*

Clinical Signs

It's not usually difficult to spot a dog with canine cough. Of course, the classic feature is a cough, but they may also have discharges from the eyes and nose. The infection usually takes five to ten days to take hold, so may not be evident immediately. More severely affected dogs can develop bronchitis and pneumonia, but this is uncommon. Some affected dogs, especially puppies, may run a fever and lose their appetite.

Most affected dogs have a dry, hacking, nagging cough that persists for several weeks and then slowly clears. Dogs that are repeatedly boarded at the same kennel are usually not as susceptible, since they develop a degree of resistance to the infection.

Diagnosis

It is always important to distinguish a cough associated with a respiratory infection from more serious underlying problems, such as heart disease or respiratory fungal diseases. However, this is usually not difficult if dogs have the classic history of exposure to other dogs, a five-to-ten-day incubation period, and the dry, hacking cough so common to this condition.

Routine laboratory tests such as blood counts are usually normal since most affected dogs are not systemically "sick." Swabs and bronchial washings can be used to isolate viruses or bacteria but these are rarely indicated in routine cases. However, a chest radiograph is helpful if there is risk that the infection is moving deeper into the respiratory tract.

Treatment

There are no specific treatments for canine cough. In most cases, the condition will improve on its own, over the course of several weeks. Antibiotics are frequently prescribed for this condition but there is little evidence that they are helpful, unless a deeper bronchitis or pneumonia develops. Most oral antibiotics do not reach high concentrations in the bronchial tree or the trachea (windpipe), which is where the infection is located in most cases. On the other hand, antibiotics administered by nebulizer (vaporizer) or by direct injection into the trachea can be very helpful but need to be administered daily for several days.

Cough medications are indicated if the coughing is painful, since they allow the respiratory tract to rest and have a chance to heal. However, a dry, nonproductive cough can be suppressed with regular cough medicines if recommended by a veterinarian. Good nursing care is the best medicine.

When many dogs in a facility are affected, it may be advisable to close areas for one to two weeks and disinfect them with appropriate chemicals, such as diluted chlorine bleach, chlorhexidine, or benzalkonium chloride. Then, only dogs that have been properly vaccinated and are in good health should be allowed into the facility. Kennel personnel should be aware that they can transmit infectious organisms to susceptible dogs via hands and clothing.

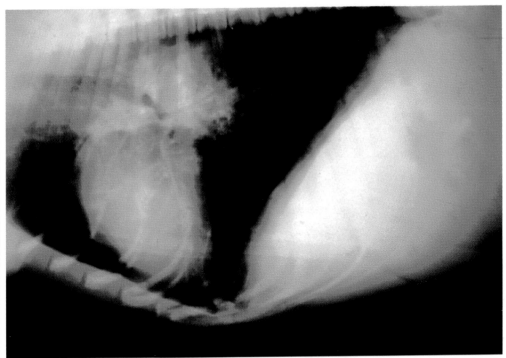

Localized pneumonia in a dog with a systemic fungal infection known as coccidioidomycosis (valley fever). Courtesy of Dr. Kenneth Jeffery, Mesa Veterinary Hospital, Ltd., Mesa, Arizona.

Prevention

There is no foolproof way to prevent canine cough. Most annual vaccines contain parainfluenza and adenovirus, which are the most common instigators of infection, but there are countless other respiratory viruses that could be involved. It is impossible to protect against all of them.

Recently, a *Bordetella bronchiseptica* bacterin has become available, which is administered as a spray into the nose. It has been known for many years that injections of this bacteria failed to stimulate protective antibodies in the blood. However, when the bacterin is squirted into the nose, a "local immunity" is created which is quite effective.

Dogs that are to be boarded, groomed, sent to shows or any other activity that exposes them to other dogs might benefit from this intranasal vaccination. However, to be most effective, it should be administered one to two weeks before anticipated exposure, although protection starts within the first 24 hours. In addition, brachycephalic (squat-faced) and toy breeds should be vaccinated because they are more prone to chronic bronchial disease and chronic obstructive pulmonary disease. The intranasal vaccine is also safe for puppies as young as two weeks of age. Vaccination with this agent should be repeated every six months to be effective.

PNEUMONIA

Pneumonia refers to an infection in the lungs, but it is not specific for just one malady. There are many different causes for pneumonia in dogs.

Most cases of pneumonia are caused by respiratory infections that manage to penetrate deeper than the bronchioles and respiratory passages. Although bacteria are frequently implicated, there are other situations that can result in pneumonia as well.

Clinical Signs

Most dogs with pneumonia are noticeably sick. They may have fever, lack of energy, and lack of appetite. In many cases, there is a history of an upper-respiratory infection that did not get better. Once the pneumonia has taken hold, dogs often have a productive cough, in addition to their other complaints.

Diagnosis

It is often difficult to confirm a diagnosis of pneumonia with a clinical examination alone. The telltale signs that may be ascertained with a stethoscope include abnormal lung sounds, such as crackles and rales.

Chest radiographs are necessary to confirm the diagnosis and the extent of lung involvement. This usually allows the diagnosis to be further refined as bronchopneumonia, lobar pneumonia or interstitial pneumonia based on the areas of the lungs involved.

Many other tests are usually performed, including blood-cell counts and the analysis of respiratory secretions. Cultures may also be performed to determine the types of microbes involved and the treatments most likely to be successful.

Therapy

For most cases of pneumonia, antibiotics are prescribed to treat infection. These are usually continued for a minimum of two weeks, but at least until the problem has been resolved based on clinical examination and repeat radiographs.

Other treatments are introduced, depending on the extent of the problem. It is important that dogs maintain their hydration; this will be provided by intravenous or subcutaneous fluid replacement if necessary. Nebulizers can be effectively used to loosen respiratory secretions and make them easier to cough up. However, cough suppressants are usually counterproductive and not recommended in most cases.

It is critical that dogs with pneumonia be closely monitored to make sure they are recovering completely. If they are not, more diagnostic tests should be utilized and more aggressive therapy may be needed.

ADDITIONAL READING

DeLellis, L: Echocardiography. *Pet Focus,* 1990; 2(1): 11-14.

Beardow, AW; Buchanan, JW: Chronic mitral valve disease in Cavalier King Charles Spaniels: 95 cases (1987-1991). *Journal of the American Veterinary Medical Association,* 1993; 203(7): 1023-1029.

Brooks, M; Dodds, WJ; Raymond, SL: Epidemiologic features of von Willebrand's disease in Doberman Pinschers, Scottish Terriers, and Shetland Sheepdogs: 260 cases (1984-1988). *Journal of the American Veterinary Medical Association,* 1992; 200(8): 1123-1127.

Buchanan, JW: Changing breed predispositions in canine heart disease. *Canine Practice,* 1993; 18(6): 12-14.

Crager, CS: Canine primary ciliary dyskinesia. *Compendium,* 1992; 14(11): 1440-1444.

Dodds, WJ: Bleeding disorders of dogs and cats: Part I. *Pet Focus,* 1991; 3(2): 12-15.

Dodds, WJ: Bleeding disorders of dogs and cats: Part II. *Pet Focus,* 1991; 3(3): 5-7.

Goodwin, J-K; Cooper, Jr., RC: Understanding the pathophysiology of congenital heart defects. *Veterinary Medicine,* 1992; July: 650-668.

Goodwin, JK; Cooper, Jr., RC; Weber, WJ: The medical management of pets with congenital heart defects. *Veterinary Medicine,* 1992; July.

Grieve, RB: Progress toward a vaccine to prevent canine heartworm infection. *Compendium for Continuing Education of the Practicing Veterinarian,* 1992; 14(5): 613-617.

Henik, RA; Basic life support and external cardiac compression in dogs and cats. *Journal of the American Veterinary Medical Association,* 1992; 200(12): 1925-1931.

Jeffery, K: Congenital cardiovascular diseases. *Pet Focus,* 1990; 2(2): 15-17.

Kass, PH; Haskins, SC: Survival following cardiopulmonary resuscitation in dogs and cats. *Veterinary Emergency and Critical Care,* 1992; 2(2): 57-65.

Keene, et al: Myocardial L-carnitine deficiency in a family of dogs with dilated cardiomyopathy. *Journal of the American Veterinary Medical Association,* 1991; 198(4): 647-650.

Kirberger, RM: Doppler echocardiography: Facts and physics for practitioners. *Compendium for Continuing Education of the Practicing Veterinarian,* 1991; 13(11): 1679-1686.

Klag, AR: Hemolytic anemia in dogs. *Compendium for Continuing Education of the Practicing Veterinarian*, 1992; 14(8): 1090-1098.

Klement, P; Del-Nido, PJ; Wilson, GJ: The use of cardiac pacemakers in veterinary practice. *Compendium for Continuing Education of the Practicing Veterinarian*, 1984; 6(10): 893-902.

Manohar, M; Smetzer, DL: Atrial fibrillation. *Compendium for Continuing Education of the Practicing Veterinarian*, 1992; 14(10): 1327-1333.

Meyers, KM; Wardrop, KJ; Meinkoth, J: Canine von Willebrand's disease: Pathobiology, diagnosis, and short-term treatment. *Compendium for Continuing Education of the Practicing Veterinarian*, 1992; 14(1): 13-22.

Newland, T: Heartworm disease update. *Pet Focus*, 1991; 3(2): 8-11.

Rawlings, CA; Calvert, C; Hribernik, T; Dillon, R: Answers to typical questions on heartworm problems. *Compendium for Continuing Education of the Practicing Veterinarian*, 1993; 15(5): 711-724.

Snyder, PS: Canine hypertensive disease. *Compendium for Continuing Education of the Practicing Veterinarian*, 1991; 13(12): 1785-1792.

Van Pelt, DR; Wingfield, WE: Controversial issues in drug treatment during cardiopulmonary resuscitation. *Journal of the American Veterinary Medical Association*, 1992; 200(12): 1938-1944.

Wingfield, WE; Van Pelt, DR: Respiratory and cardiopulmonary arrest in dogs and cats: 265 cases (1986-1991). *Journal of the American Veterinary Medical Association*, 1992; 200(12): 1993-1996.

Disorders of the Digestive System

The digestive system is an amazing complex of tubes and organs that allows us to ingest foods, digest them, absorb them, and use the nutrients to fulfill bodily needs.

When food is first ingested, it is mixed with compounds in the saliva that start the digestive process. In the stomach, acids are produced that break down the foods into smaller units that can be absorbed. Most of this absorption takes place in the small intestines, with the help of secretions from the pancreas and liver. The final absorption of water and nutrients takes place in the large intestines and the remainder is excreted as waste.

ORAL PAPILLOMATOSIS

Oral papillomatosis is a viral disease of young dogs caused by a contagious papovavirus (wart virus). It is characterized by multiple growths in the mouth but is not a cancer. It is not related to skin papillomas and does not spread to the skin or genital areas. Dogs pick up the infection from other infected dogs and it takes about a month to become clinically evident. Although it has been reported where the oral warts have transformed into malignant cancers (squamous-cell carcinoma), this should be considered a very rare event.

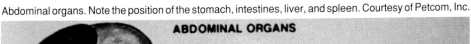

Abdominal organs. Note the position of the stomach, intestines, liver, and spleen. Courtesy of Petcom, Inc.

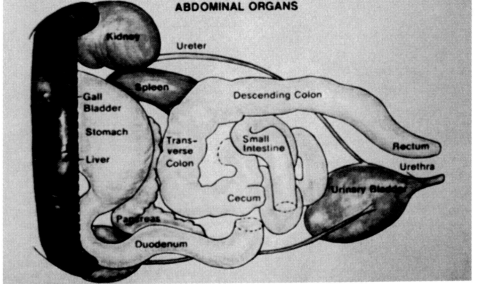

Clinical Signs

The diagnosis is not easy to miss because affected dogs have nodules and cauliflower-like growths in their mouth and throat (pharynx). As the growths start to regress, they appear small and dark.

Diagnosis

The diagnosis of oral papillomatosis is confirmed by removing a nodule surgically and submitting it in formalin to a pathologist for evaluation.

Therapy

Oral papillomatosis resolves on its own, without any treatment, in two to three months. Removing one or two growths (e.g., for pathological evaluation) usually hastens the process. Additional surgery is only indicated if the growths interfere with breathing or swallowing. Once recovered, affected dogs are considered immune for the rest of their lives.

GASTRIC ULCERATION

Gastric (stomach) ulcers are small defects in the wall of the stomach that occur from several underlying causes. Anything that causes inflammatory reactions in the stomach (gastritis) can result in ulcers. The true underlying cause is often difficult to determine because so many different conditions need to be considered. Not all causes need to be associated with increased production of stomach acids. Many result from conditions that compromise the integrity of the stomach lining. Gastric ulcers can be associated with liver disease, kidney disease, hypoadrenocortism (Addison's disease), and many other metabolic illnesses. Also, many different drugs, including aspirin, naproxen, phenylbutazone, corticosteroids, and flunixin meglumine can cause gastric ulcers.

Clinical Signs

The most common manifestation of gastric ulceration is vomiting, usually most profound at the time of eating. With chronic vomiting, dehydration and electrolyte imbalances occur and this can result in shock. Affected animals may spit up blood, but more often the blood passes through the intestines, is digested, and appears as black, tarry stools (melena). There may be appetite and weight loss, but this is very variable. If the ulcer perforates the wall of the stomach, animals can bleed into the abdominal cavity. This can lead to collapse and even death.

Diagnosis

Gastric ulceration may be suspected if routine blood counts and biochemical profiles reveal anemia and protein loss. These tests might also detect abnormalities associated with an underlying disease process, such as conditions affecting the liver or kidneys.

Regular radiographs are not usually helpful at pinpointing a gastric ulcer but contrast studies and endoscopic examinations can

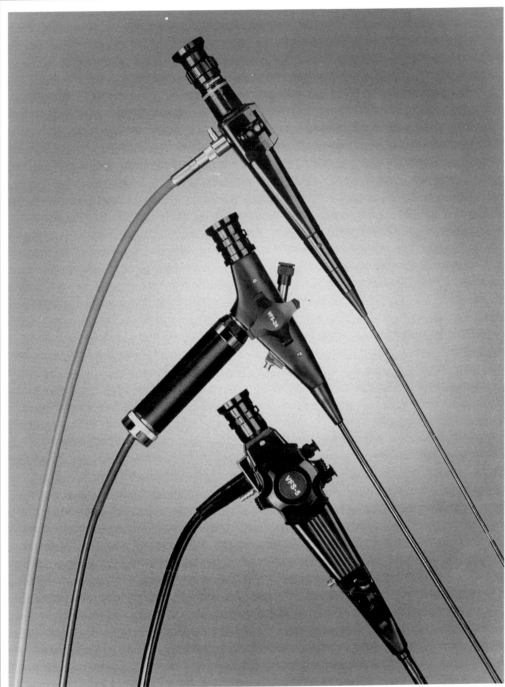

Examples of flexible fiberoptic endoscopes with many diagnostic uses in veterinary medicine. Courtesy of Schott Fiber Optics, Southbridge, Massachusetts.

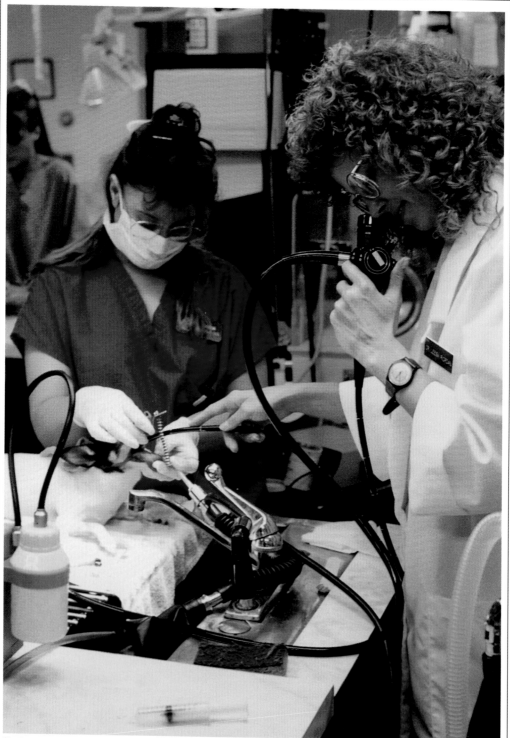

Dr. Leesa Riordan of Northern Animal Hospital, Phoenix, Arizona, performs an endoscopic examination.

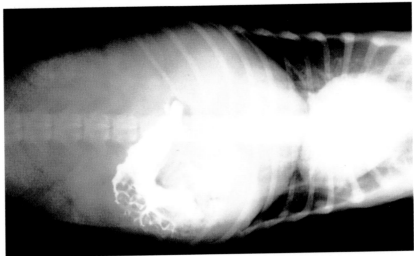

Contrast radiographs using barium to outline the contours of the stomach.

Endoscopic view of a gastric ulcer (double arrows). Single arrow marks the pylorus, the part of the stomach that connects with the duodenum of the small intestine. Courtesy of Dr. M.D. Willard, Texas A&M University, College Station, Texas.

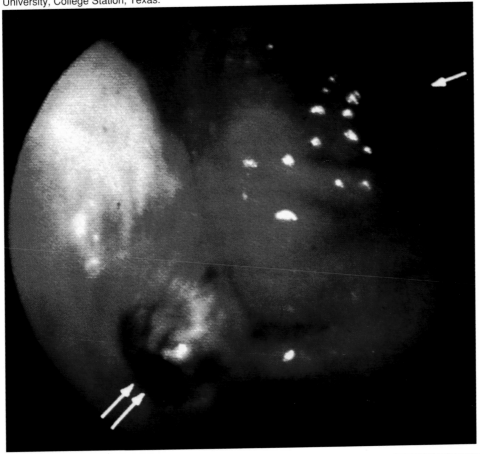

be very beneficial. Barium is often used for contrast studies unless it is suspected that the ulcer may have perforated through the wall of the stomach. In these cases, organic iodine compounds are usually used instead. Endoscopic examination often permits visualization of the defect, and biopsies can be taken if warranted.

Therapy

As in human medicine, the most successful way to manage gastric ulcers is to identify and correct the underlying cause. Otherwise, symptomatic therapy or surgery are the only other options.

Initial treatment is often commenced with antacids but they need to be given frequently or they result in an increased secretion of stomach acid. All have some potential side effects with continuous use.

Specific antihistamines are as commonly used in dogs as they are in people. The most common are famotidine (Pepcid), ranitidine (Zantac), and cimetidine (Tagamet). Sucralfate (Carafate) is a sugar derivative that helps form a protective barrier on the stomach lining against the effects of acid. Because of its effects on digestion and absorption, other drugs should not be given at the same time as sucralfate. Even the antihistamines listed above should be given 30-60 minutes later.

Supportive care is important for the ulcer patient. It is critical to stop any drugs that may be promoting ulcers, especially corticosteroids and the nonsteroidal anti-inflammatory agents. Intravenous therapy may be needed to correct dehydration and electrolyte imbalances. Blood transfusions may even be needed if there has been significant blood loss. During initial treatment, food and liquids are withheld until bleeding and vomiting have been effectively controlled.

In severe cases, surgery may be used to remove the part of the stomach where the ulcers are. If the ulcers have perforated the wall of the stomach, exploratory surgery may be needed to correct the situation. Antibiotic therapy is indicated when perforation has occurred since the damage done could result in peritonitis and shock.

GASTRIC DILATATION-VOLVULUS SYNDROME (GDV)

The gastric dilatation-volvulus syndrome (GDV) is a life-threatening condition characterized by marked distension of the stomach with gas (bloat) and varying degrees of twisting of the stomach around its long axis. GDV can lead to shock, infection, clotting abnormalities and heart problems. If not treated rationally and vigorously, GDV will ultimately lead to the death of the patient.

Gastric dilatation (bloat) results from the stomach being distended by swallowed air (aerophagia), not gas produced by the stomach. Air may be swallowed as a consequence of stress, exercise, or gulping of food or water. This is often referred to as "bloat" because the stomach can enlarge like a balloon. If the stomach cannot empty its contents into the small intestine, the result can be disastrous. Gastric volvulus implies complete obstruction of the flow of stomach fluid, gases and food as a result of the twisting of the stomach on its long axis. This twisting kinks the digestive tract where the stomach narrows to the small intestines as well as twisting the blood vessels that supply the area and the spleen which is attached to the stomach by a ligament. In fact, the process puts a strangle hold on the stomach, intestines, spleen and their blood supplies, which will cause death if not corrected quickly.

GDV is primarily a condition of large to giant deep-chested canine breeds, including the Great Dane, German Shepherd, Irish Setter, Irish Wolfhound, Borzoi, and St. Bernard. The exact etiology (cause) of GDV is unknown but likely many factors are important. Possible incriminating factors include: delayed emptying of the stomach, laxity of the supporting ligaments of the stomach, diet, and abnormal smooth muscle motility.

At one time or another various theories have been proposed but none have been completely satisfactory. However, recently it has been shown that aerophagia (swallowing of air) plays the primary role in the production of gas in GDV. This means that any factor inducing dogs to swallow air, such as eating food rapidly, may increase the risk of bloat. Dogs fed one huge meal per day (and allowed to drink large quantities of water with their meal) experience marked gastric distension, which may result in a lack of tone of the smooth muscle of the stomach (gastric atony) and a looseness or laxity of the supporting ligaments of the stomach, duodenum and liver. One might then conclude that the weakening of the stomach's smooth muscular activity results in delayed emptying, and combined with stretched supporting ligaments, may predispose to a twisting of the stomach.

Clinical Signs

With severe GDV, torsion (twisting) of the splenic attachments and blood vessels is common and the compromise of the blood supply is deadly. The tissues of the stomach and spleen become starved for oxygen and the tissues begin to die and release toxins. Rotation of the stomach also obstructs blood flow in the vein that delivers nutrients from the small intestine to the liver (the portal vein), which produces congestion of the blood vessels, lack of oxygen supply to the tissues, and eventual death of these and other abdominal organs (liver, pancreas, small intestines and spleen).

The dramatic effects of gastric dilatation and volvulus result in shock, diminished cardiac output and an accumulation of acid in the bloodstream (acidosis). These events, if allowed to progress, will usually result in death to the patient within four to six hours.

The earliest clinical signs exhibited by dogs with GDV include

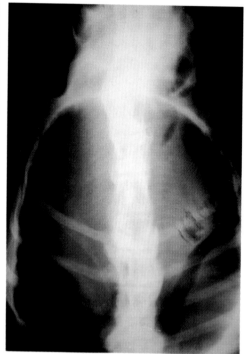

Greatly enlarged gas-filled stomach evident on radiographs of a German Shepherd Dog with gastric dilatation/volvulus. Courtesy of Dr. Frederick H.I Drazner, Animal Specialty Services of Cook County, Des Plaines, Illinois.

restlessness, drooling, rapid shallow breathing, depression, weakness and, of course, marked abdominal distension. The femoral pulse (femoral artery located on the inner surface of the thigh) may be weak, rapid and irregular. The gums may be pale (shock due to low blood volume), very red (due to shock from bacterial toxins) or blue (due to lack of oxygen perfusing the tissues).

Diagnosis

The diagnosis of GDV is usually not difficult and is usually suspected based upon the breed of dog, history given by the pet owner and careful inspection and examination of the patient. Radiographs help confirm the diagnosis.

Since GDV can adversely affect so many body systems, routine evaluations are wise. Blood may be collected for blood tests (e.g., blood counts, organ function, electrolytes, acid/base balance). Heart function can be assessed by electrocardiography (ECG).

Rarely, some patients will have only occasional bloating and may actually have a mild chronic gastric torsion. In these patients an upper GI series (using barium sulfate for contrast) will aid in distinguishing uncomplicated bloating from torsion.

Therapy

When dogs are diagnosed with uncomplicated gastric dilatation, a stomach tube is usually passed so that their stomach can be pumped out. Of course, this is only a temporary measure and the problem will quickly recur if the underlying problem is not addressed. If necessary, radiographs can be taken to differentiate uncomplicated "bloating" from torsion.

When it is known that the problem is GDV, the stomach is decompressed with a stomach tube or a large needle is inserted through the skin and into the stomach to release trapped gas and fluid. A catheter is used to introduce fluid therapy to help correct fluid, electrolyte, and pH imbalances and to aid in preventing or managing shock.

Antibiotics are frequently administered to prevent absorption of bacteria from the damaged gastrointestinal tract. Even with quick and comprehensive treatment, about 40% of dogs with GDV do not survive.

The best chance for long-term control of GDV is surgical intervention. This can be done in one-step or two-step procedures, depending on the skill of the surgeon and the ability of the animal to tolerate anesthetic risks. The two-step approach is used when animals are presented in an emergency situation and need to be stabilized first, before the corrective surgery can be performed.

Surgical techniques to prevent recurrence of GDV are numerous and success varies with the individual surgeon. At present suturing the stomach wall to a flap of peritoneum (lining of the abdominal cavity) and inner abdominal muscular wall (gastropexy) is preferred, thus permanently securing the stomach to the inner abdominal surface. This procedure is effective in preventing future torsion and volvulus of the stomach. The chances of recurrence after this surgery is less than 20 percent. Following surgery, it is important to follow the veterinarian's advice regarding feeding until the surgical area has healed.

Abnormal heart rhythms (dysrythmias) are relatively common during and after surgery, especially if the patient's blood potassium levels drop below normal (hypokalemia). The use of the electrocardiogram will identify accompanying dysrythmias. Correction of hypokalemia and

Distended stomach obvious in the surgical site. Courtesy of Dr. Gary Moody, Moody Mobile Surgical Services, Mesa, Arizona.

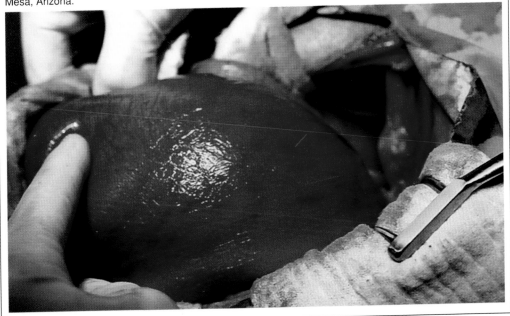

acidosis is essential if such dysrhythmias are to be controlled. Therapy for cardiac irregularities is usually continued for seven to 14 days following the surgery.

Prevention

It is important to feed large breed dogs three small meals daily instead of one large meal to prevent stretching of gastric smooth muscle and gastric ligamentous attachments. Likewise, drinking large volumes of water should be discouraged, as should vigorous exercise.

PERITONITIS

The peritoneum is the thin lining layer of the abdominal cavity. There is a small amount of fluid in the peritoneal cavity that acts as a lubricant so the internal organs can slide past each other. Most diseases of the peritoneum result from accumulation of fluid in the perito-neal cavity. Fluid can seep into this cavity as a result of liver disease, protein-losing conditions, and severe malnutrition. Fluid can also accumulate in the abdomen as a result of heart disease, abdominal cancers, and blood loss into the region.

Peritonitis refers to inflammatory diseases of the peritoneum, and the most common causes are microbial infections that somehow get inoculated into this area. This can result when there is penetration of an abdominal organ so the contents are released into the abdomen and from contamination of other conditions affecting the peritoneum.

Clinical Signs

Peritoneal disease usually results from some other problem (e.g., gastric ulceration) so the clinical picture often reflects the underlying cause. There is often abdominal enlargement as fluid accumulates in the peritoneal cavity.

Peritonitis, the inflammatory reaction in the peritoneal cavity, is often painful and is one of the causes of acute abdomen syndrome, an emergency situation. If the peritonitis results from an organ rupture, shock, collapse and even death might come quickly.

Diagnosis

Since diseases of the peritoneum are likely secondary to some underlying disease process, it is important to perform routine cell counts, biochemistry profiles, and urinalysis.

Peritonitis is an emergency situation and diagnostic efforts must be aggressively pursued. Peritoneal fluid is collected with a needle and syringe and is quickly evaluated for cell content, microbes, and protein.

Samples are prepared for microbial culture, but treatment can not be suspended for the 24-48 hours it would take for identification of the organism. Ultrasonography (ultrasound evaluation) and radiography are used to try to pinpoint the site of the problem.

Therapy

Since peritoneal disease is usually a feature of some other

problem, the underlying disease must be identified and corrected. Symptomatic therapy consists of fluid therapy to correct dehydration and electrolyte imbalances; blood transfusions are sometimes necessary depending on the condition. It is also sometimes necessary to flush the abdominal cavity (peritoneal lavage) to remove microbes, toxins, and foreign material, depending on the underlying cause of the problem.

PANCREATITIS

Acute pancreatitis is an inflammatory disorder of the exocrine pancreas. The distinction is made here between the exocrine pancreas that produces digestive enzymes and the endocrine pancreas that produces insulin and glucagon.

The exocrine pancreas produces several digestive enzymes that break down foods in the intestines so that they can be properly digested. Unfortunately, in some circumstances, those enzymes can also digest pancreatic tissue, creating an inflammatory reaction.

The pancreas protects itself from the digestive enzymes by maintaining them in an inactive state, and they get converted to their active forms when they reach the intestines. Blood plasma also contains several "inhibitors" that can deactivate small amounts of these enzymes if they should escape from the pancreas.

Dietary factors are the major cause of acute pancreatitis in dogs. The feeding of high-fat diets for extended periods is probably the most common cause. Dogs with pancreatitis also tend to be obese. Other potential causes of pancreatitis include viral and parasitic infections, obstruction of the pancreatic ducts, trauma, drug administration and metabolic disorders. The metabolic disorders that are most often implicated are hyperlipidemia (increased blood fats) and hypercalcemia (increased blood calcium).

Acute pancreatitis develops when the enzymes become activated within the pancreas itself and begin to digest the tissue. These enzymes then wreak havoc in the body by a number of mechanisms. Some of the enzymes cause vascular (blood vessel) injury and can lower blood pressure (hypotension). Marked hypotension is probably the main factor that contributes to death in some of these animals.

Clinical Signs

Most occurrences of acute pancreatitis involve middle-aged, obese female dogs, but any dog can be affected. There is usually a sudden onset of vomiting, anorexia, and depression. Diarrhea is only occasionally noted.

There is much variability in clinical presentation. Mildly affected dogs may have only mild depression and some abdominal tenderness. Severely affected dogs may have fever, depression, painful abdomen, an irregular pulse, low blood pressure, and considerable dehydration.

Diagnosis

The diagnostic approach to acute pancreatitis usually involves radiographs, ultrasonography (ultrasound examination), and biochemical profiles. The blood tests usually considered specific for pancreatitis are serum amylase and lipase, two pancreatic enzymes. Both of these tests are valuable in the diagnostic process, but neither are specific for pancreatitis. Conditions such as kidney disease, liver disease, and some cancers can also cause elevations of these enzymes.

Radiographs of the abdomen will not detect pancreatic inflammation, but are useful because it may show evidence that the inflammatory reaction has spread to the inner body lining (peritonitis). Ultrasound evaluation of the pancreas is also helpful.

Therapy

The most important aspect of medically managing dogs with pancreatitis is to restrict oral intake of food while providing fluids intravenously. In some severe cases, oral intake of food needs to be restricted for as long as two weeks. Fluid therapy is critical because it helps correct the low blood pressure (hypotension) that can be associated with pancreatitis as well as providing needed nutrition. In most cases, oral fluids, then bland foods, can be re-introduced within five to seven days. If animals need to be fasted longer than this, parenteral nutrition should be considered.

This provides all the needed nutrients (vitamins, minerals, amino acids, fats) in intravenous forms.

Many medications have been recommended for pancreatitis over the years but now it is understood that the fewer drugs given, the better. Drugs such as cimetidine (Tagamet) are sometimes still given, but antibiotics are usually reserved for moderately or severely ill patients. These animals are prone to systemic infections (septicemia), urinary tract infections, pneumonia, and pancreatic abscesses. Insulin treatments are necessary if blood glucose levels skyrocket, which they sometimes do as a result of pancreatic dysfunction. Long-term management involves feeding a low-fat diet, divided into two or three feedings per day, and managing diabetes mellitus, should it be a consequence of the pancreatic disorder.

Surgery is rarely needed for management of acute pancreatitis. It is used in moderately to severely ill animals to help remove some of the enzymes and toxins in the body cavity, or to manage a pancreatic abscess. In general this is only used when patients fail to respond to medical treatment after the first five to seven days of therapy. The body cavity is "washed" (peritoneal lavage) and internal organs are inspected for the possibility of bile-duct obstruction or tissue death in the intestines (bowel ischemia).

EXOCRINE PANCREATIC INSUFFICIENCY (EPI)

The exocrine pancreas produces several needed digestive enzymes. In some circumstances, dogs do not make enough enzymes for their digestive needs. This is what is referred to as exocrine pancreatic insufficiency.

The principal cause of exocrine pancreatic insufficiency is known as idiopathic pancreatic acinar atrophy. This implies that the exocrine pancreatic tissue atrophies or "wears out" for some unknown reason. A genetic predisposition is recognized in the German Shepherd Dog, but several other breeds are also affected.

It is also possible that processes that damage the pancreas, such as pancreatitis, could eventually result in pancreatic insufficiency, but this would be expected to be more common in older animals. The genetic form of the disorder is seen in younger dogs, usually less than two years of age.

Clinical signs

Animals with exocrine pancreatic insufficiency are usually recognized because they tend to eat a lot yet lose weight. They don't produce enough of the digestive enzymes to break down the nutrients in their diet to forms they can use. Also, most affected dogs have loose stools, if not actual diarrhea. The stools are semi-formed and some imaginative individuals have described them as "castle-building" stools. Because the fats in the diet don't get properly digested, the stools often smell much worse than usual. It is important to realize that early cases have relatively mild signs, which gradually worsen as long as the disease remains undiagnosed and untreated.

Diagnosis

Most of the routine laboratory tests performed for other internal diseases are not helpful in the patients with exocrine pancreatic insufficiency. It might seem reasonable that the pancreatic enzymes in the blood, namely amylase and lipase, should be reduced, but this is not the case.

The diagnostic test of choice for exocrine pancreatic insufficiency is the serum trypsin-like immunoreactivity (TLI) test. The serum TLI concentrations are dramatically reduced in affected dogs. Older tests, such as x-ray plate gelatin digestion, starch tolerance, and plasma turbidity, are all inferior to the TLI test. Fecal proteolytic (protein-digesting) activity using azocasein is more reliable than these older tests, but at least three fecal specimens should be tested because normal dogs also occasionally pass feces with low protease (protein-digesting enzyme) activity.

Therapy

Most dogs with exocrine pancreatic insufficiency can be managed successfully by simply supplementing each meal with pancreatic enzyme extracts. The powdered extracts are mixed with the dog food immediately prior to feeding. If animals do not show a good response to this regimen, raising the amount given is not likely to help.

Chopped healthy ox or pig pancreas (three to four ounces per meal) is sometimes an economical alternative to feeding the relatively expensive dried extracts. Pancreas can be stored frozen at -20°C for at least three months, while still maintaining its enzyme potency. Another alternative is to use a plant-based enzyme supplement (e.g., Prozyme™) that provides digestive enzymes derived from plants.

Other treatments sometimes needed include antibiotics, highly digestible low-fiber diets, and vitamin supplementation. The antibiotics are needed if the condition results in bacterial overgrowth in the intestines. The low-fiber diet is recommended because it is easily digested and requires less enzymes to reduce it to a form that can be absorbed by the intestines. Vitamin supplementation with vitamin B_{12} (cobalamin) and the fat-soluble vitamins (especially vitamins A and E) is useful because these vitamins may not be adequately absorbed from the diet. Beta carotene can be substituted for vitamin A, which can cause toxicities if it is oversupplemented.

LIVER AND GALLBLADDER DISEASES

The liver performs critical functions in the dog. The production of bile and bile salts is only one of its many important functions. The cells of the liver are active in the manufacture, storage, and metabolic conversion of many compounds. Most of the blood that perfuses the liver arrives through the portal vein that drains the stomach, spleen, pancreas, and intestines. It is then filtered through the canal-like sinusoids, where it is detoxified and modified before entering the general blood supply.

The liver is the sole site of albumin manufacture, an important protein in the blood. The liver also manufactures most of the globulins, other than the ones that become antibodies. The reserve capacity of the liver for proteins is large, and therefore liver disease must be severe before protein deficiency results.

The liver is also responsible for the manufacture of many of the factors responsible for blood clotting, including factors I, II, V, VII, IX, X, and vitamin K. Therefore, clotting abnormalities may be seen as a consequence of severe liver disease.

Hepatic (liver) disease may be due to processes centered in the liver or it may be secondary to other problems in other organs that can damage the liver. Therefore, the liver is susceptible to infiltrative, infectious, metabolic, toxic, or congestive disorders. For diagnostic purposes, it is often helpful to distinguish actual liver damage (hepatocellular degeneration) from bile-duct problems (hepatobiliary disorders) and blood-supply bypass of the liver (portosystemic shunting).

Damage to liver cells can happen in many ways, especially by toxins, viral infections, and inflammatory processes. It can also result from heart diseases (including heartworm disease) in which fluids "back up" into the liver and deprive the liver tissue of needed oxygen. Bacteria and fungi also affect the liver, and immune-mediated and cancerous processes can also be involved. Toxins are a major cause of liver dysfunction and include heavy metals, many drugs, anesthetic agents and even nutrients. Some breeds of dog (e.g., Bedlington Terrier, West Highland White Terrier, Doberman Pinscher, Cocker Spaniel, Labrador Retriever, German Shepherd Dog, Miniature Schnauzer, Pekingese, English Bulldog, and Skye Terrier) are prone to accumulating copper in their liver because of an inherited metabolic defect.

When the bile ducts become obstructed (cholestasis), bile can not flow from the liver to the gall bladder. This can be due to some local disorder that blocks the ducts or a diffuse problem in the liver that causes swelling and blockage. Eventually, bilirubin present in the bile backs up into the liver and bloodstream, and the result is known as jaundice or icterus.

Congenital problems are also possible. In fetal animals, the liver is bypassed by the blood supply from the mother. In some cases, these "shunts" (better known as portosystemic shunts) persist and therefore the portal blood from the abdominal organs does not get filtered by the sinusoids of the liver before entering the general circulation. This bypass of the liver is analogous to liver failure, because the liver is not performing its needed detoxifying role.

Chronic hepatitis (chronic inflammatory liver disease) is a confusing array of disorders that affect the liver. This is not the same as infectious canine hepatitis, which is caused by a specific virus. Potential causes of chronic hepatitis include infectious agents, drugs, toxins, metabolic disorders, and immune-mediated disorders. The cause of these disorders is largely unknown. The exception to this rule is copper-related hepatitis, which has been reported in several breeds of dogs. These animals accumulate dietary copper in their livers rather than excreting it into the bile. This is similar to Wilson's disease in people. Eventually, liver function becomes compromised.

Cholelithiasis (gall stones) are uncommon in dogs and most dogs that do develop them have few clinical problems. Clinical signs tend only to develop when the gall bladder becomes inflamed (cholecystitis), the bile ducts become obstructed (cholestasis), or there is rupture of the gall bladder and/or ducts.

Clinical Signs

Because the liver performs so many different functions, the clinical signs can differ significantly between patients, depending on the root of the problem. Patients with slowly progressive liver disease may not show clinical signs until late in the course of the disease because the liver has so many compensating mechanisms.

Often, the most common signs of liver disease are nonspecific and can be confused with many other ailments. There may be anorexia, weight loss and vomiting; many animals will also have increased thirst and urination.

Jaundice or icterus is a yellow discoloration of the blood serum and staining of soft tissue such as mucous membranes and skin. It results when the bilirubin content of the blood becomes significantly elevated. This happens when more bilirubin gets produced than gets excreted through the bile ducts. Jaundice is most commonly associated with bile-duct obstruction (cholestasis), liver-cell damage (hepatocellular degeneration) or disruption of red blood cells (hemolysis).

When dogs have little functional liver reserve, their ability to detoxify is severely compromised. For these dogs, even protein can become toxic, since it is broken down to ammonia once digested. Normally the liver processes the ammonia from the portal circulation so that it causes no problems. If liver function is severely compromised, the ammonia and other toxins accumulate in the bloodstream and can affect the brain. This is known as hepatic encephalopathy. These dogs may have abnormal behaviors, such as pressing their head against a wall, or even seizures.

Diagnosis

The diagnostic approach to liver disorders involves determining first that a liver problem exists, and then further defining the nature of the problem. The usual first approach is to perform blood cell counts and biochemical profiles. The biochemical tests that are of most significance are alanine aminotransferase (ALT, formerly SGPT), serum alkaline phosphatase (SAP), gamma-glutamyltransferase (GGT), and bile acids.

Increased ALT means that the liver-cell membranes have been damaged by some process. This enzyme is readily released by liver cells and elevations of even twice normal does not mean the liver is diseased. ALT levels that are four times normal are a good indication that liver disease is present. Increased SAP typically results when there is bile duct obstruction but various drugs and hormones, especially corticosteroids, can significantly increase levels in the blood. GGT is similar to SAP but may be more specific for the liver. In fact, ALT, SAP, GGT and bilirubin levels are commonly included in most biochemical profiles.

The clinical usefulness of measuring serum bile acid concentrations as a diagnostic test for liver disease has become more routine over the last few years. Blood samples are collected for bile acid determination after fasting; significantly elevated levels are highly suggestive of liver dysfunction. Other tests that can be done include bromsulphalein (BSP) dye retention and blood ammonia levels, but these add little to the picture provided by the basic biochemical profile and bile acids.

Radiography is used to determine the size and shape of the liver. This helps determine which processes may be involved. This can also be performed with ultrasound examinations. Biopsy sampling of the liver can provide very specific information of what's going on but is not without risk. Since the liver is responsible for making many clotting factors, clotting tests should be performed before any surgical biopsy techniques are utilized. Biopsies are needed for the diagnosis of chronic hepatitis and copper-related hepatitis.

Therapy

Most cases of liver disease never need treatment because they go unrecognized. The liver has a fantastic ability to regenerate itself and it has been estimated that a liver that is 80% compromised could regenerate itself within three weeks if the disease process had been arrested. Therefore, whenever possible, treatment should be specific for the exact cause of the problem.

The objectives of therapy are to eliminate the underlying causes of liver disease and to provide general supportive care, thus allowing time for the liver to heal itself and to prevent or manage the complications of liver failure. Thus, antibiotics are used to manage bacterial and fungal liver disease, a low-copper diet and chelation therapy (e.g., zinc acetate) are used for dogs with copper-associated liver disorders, and immune-suppressing drugs are needed for chronic active hepatitis. Surgery is used to correct portosystemic shunts found in young dogs.

General supportive care and management of complications are the only treatment available for many liver disorders. All drugs should be cautiously administered since the liver is responsible for detoxifying most drugs in the body. If the liver isn't working, the drugs may cause more problems than they treat. These dogs should be given rest and confinement to allow the liver time to regenerate and to spare the nutritional demands of other tissues. Fluid therapy is often indicated to correct dehydration and electrolyte imbalances. Once fluid, electrolyte, and acid-base balance has been corrected, liver management depends largely on nutritional support.

Nutritional support is critical because it is required for liver regeneration, and because it decreases the workload of the liver while supplying needed nutrients to other body tissues. Most of the calories in the diet need to be provided by carbohydrates, such as boiled white rice. Too much protein will cause ammonia accumulation in the blood and brain, and too much fat will contain short-chain fatty acids, which can also be toxic to the brain. Small amounts of high-quality proteins, such as eggs,

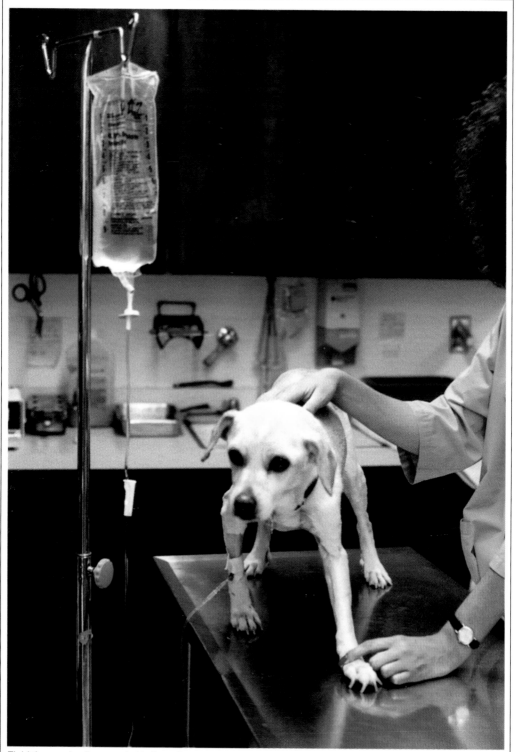

Fluid therapy is often needed in liver diseases, to correct dehydration and electrolyte imbalances.

lean meats, poultry, and cottage cheese, fulfill the amino acid requirements of dogs. Essential fatty acids and fat-soluble vitamins are also useful supplements.

Lactulose, a form of sugar that traps ammonia in the intestines, is often given to dogs with high blood ammonia levels and hepatic encephalopathy. Antibiotics may also be given to reduce the numbers of bacteria in the digestive tract that convert urea to ammonia. Also, animals with liver disease are more susceptible to infections.

SMALL-BOWEL DISEASES

The small bowel, or small intestine, provides a large surface area for absorbing nutrients from the diet. Just as the pancreas produces enzymes to digest foods, the small intestine is responsible for absorbing those nutrients that have been digested.

Motility of the small intestine consists of mixing and propulsive movements that provide for optimal contact of food items with digestive secretions and excretions, and to the absorptive surface area. When this system fails to work properly, the result is often diarrhea.

There are a great many disorders that can result in small-bowel diarrhea and only a few can be explored here. Although some are congenital, the vast number of conditions are acquired. Giant Schnauzers have a genetic predisposition toward malabsorption of cobalamin (vitamin B_{12}) while Irish Setters have a documented hereditary defect associated with a wheat-sensitive enteropathy.

Viral infections are common causes of small-intestinal disease (enteropathy) and the more common ones include parvovirus and coronavirus. Bacterial infections of the small intestines are also common (enteritis) and can result from microbes that either invade the intestine, or produce toxins. Some of the more common bacteria causing infections are *Salmonella* and *Escherichia coli* (*E. coli*). Parasites are also common invaders of the small intestine. Fungal infections of the intestines, such as pythiosis and histoplasmosis, are common in some geographic areas but otherwise are rare causes of intestinal infections.

Malabsorption describes the condition in which the intestines fail to absorb the needed nutrients from the diet. Any of the above-mentioned conditions can result in malabsorption. There are also a variety of poorly understood immune-mediated diseases that can result in malabsorption. These are described as lymphocytic-plasmacytic enteritis, eosinophilic enteritis, neutrophilic enteritis, and granulomatous enteritis based on the types of cells invading the intestines. Some cancers can also involve the intestines and result in malabsorption.

Clinical Signs

Despite the fact that so many different disease processes can affect the intestines, the result is usually the same—diarrhea. There are usually some features of diarrhea that help distinguish between diseases of the small intestines from those of the large intestines.

Diarrhea associated with small intestinal disease is usually more profuse and watery. Mucus is less likely to be a common finding. Blood in the stools can be seen with either small- or large-bowel diarrhea. The most common causes for bloody diarrhea in small-intestinal disease are parvovirus infection and a poorly understood condition known as canine hemorrhagic gastroenteritis. Vomiting, weight loss, and bad breath (halitosis) are more likely with diarrhea of small-bowel origin than large-bowel origin. Dehydration is much more profound when the small intestine has been compromised.

In some cases, the small intestinal disorder can profoundly affect protein absorption. The result is known as protein-losing enteropathy. The most common causes are inflammatory bowel diseases, fungal infections such as histoplasmosis, gastrointestinal ulcerations, some cancers, and lymphangiectasia. Lymphangiectasia is a condition in which the lymph vessels in the intestines dilate, and it can be congenital or acquired. This is the most common cause of protein-losing enteropathy in the dog. The result is chronic intermittent or persistent small-bowel diarrhea, weight loss, enlarged liver or spleen, and sometimes fluid loss into the chest or abdominal cavities. Breeds reported to be at risk for the development of lymphangiectasia are the Soft Coated Wheaten Terrier, Lundehund, and Basenji.

Diagnosis

For all cases of small-bowel diarrhea, it is critical to determine if dietary, viral, bacterial, fungal, or parasitic causes could be involved. This is important because these conditions can usually be quickly and effectively managed. Basic blood profiles, such as blood counts and serum biochemistries are warranted in all cases although only rarely do they provide critical information (e.g., protein-losing enteropathy). In addition, dogs with lymphangiectasia will also have low lymphocyte counts.

Samples of stool should be evaluated for internal parasites on several different occasions. Concentration techniques are often more useful than the flotation techniques, which are the most commonly used in practice. Bacteria and fungi can be recovered from the stool with special culturing techniques, and some blood tests are also available to diagnose specific infections.

Malabsorption can be diagnosed by determining the presence of nutrients in the stool that failed to get absorbed. Unfortunately, these diagnostic tests are usually not helpful until there is profound small-intestinal disease. Some of the more commonly used tests are d-xylose absorption and fecal evaluation for fat.

Sometimes, blood tests for nutrients are helpful at pinpointing the site of the trouble. Folic acid (folate) is normally absorbed in the upper small intestine and vitamin B_{12} (cobalamin) is normally absorbed in the lower small intestine. If blood has been collected after the animal has fasted for 12 hours, the nutrient levels can offer diagnostic information. Low serum folate concentrations indicate disease of the upper small intestine, while low serum cobalamin concentrations indicates disease of the lower small intestine. Tests for pancreatic function (TLI) should be performed at the same time.

Protein-losing enteropathy is usually characterized by low blood levels of protein (albumin and globulins) as well as cholesterol and lymphocytes. The fecal concentration of the plasma protein alpha-1-protease inhibitor is generally increased in dogs with PLE, but this test is not commercially available and the human test kits do not provide reliable information for the dog. The diagnosis is confirmed by biopsy findings.

Radiographs of the abdomen are sometimes helpful in small-intestinal disease. The radiographs may show subtle changes, such as thickened loops of bowel. Contrast agents such as barium can be administered and then a radiographic series taken. This might outline defects in the bowel such as ulcers, masses, or infiltrative diseases.

The use of fiberoptic endoscopes has greatly improved the diagnostic capabilities of veterinarians when it comes to intestinal diseases. The endoscope allows the bowel to be visualized and also permits biopsies to be taken. Since many conditions may appear nonspecific visually through the endoscope, the biopsies are often more important. These tissue samples can be entrusted to a competent pathologist who can then provide a wealth of information about the findings.

Therapy

To be effective, treatment should be directed towards the underlying cause. Therefore, parasites should be treated with specific anti-parasitic therapies; bacteria such as *Salmonella* should be treated with antibiotics; and fungal infections such as histoplasmosis should be treated with specific anti-fungal therapies such as ketoconazole (Nizoral).

All dogs with small-intestinal disease benefit from being fed a low-fat, low-fiber, highly digestible, and preferably hypoallergenic diet. This minimizes the demands on the intestine for nutrient absorption. Nutritional supplementation with cobalamin, folic acid, vitamin E, thiamine, and vitamin K may be indicated but oversupplementation is to be discouraged.

Medium chain triglyceride (MCT) oil is sometimes recommended for dogs with malabsorption because it can be absorbed intact without

weeks of age. Bitches should be treated at the same time as the pups since they are most often the source of the pups' infection. All bitches should be presumed to be carriers of roundworms even though they have had negative fecals prior to whelping, since the worms often persist in her system in a resting stage.

It is hoped that at some point in the future a vaccine will become available for roundworm control since current control measures seem to be only marginally effective. For the present, however, routine treatment of pups and bitch as well as environmental control are necessary and essential.

Hookworms

Hookworms are important because they not only are capable of causing disease in dogs and cats but are potential causes of infection in people as well. *Ancylostoma caninum* is the most common hookworm parasite of dogs throughout the United States and most of the world. The larvae of this worm can cause cutaneous larva migrans in humans.

Ancylostoma caninum have teeth and latch onto the intestines of dogs. Hookworm eggs are passed in the feces and develop into infective larvae in areas that are shady and sandy. The length of time involved in developing into infective larvae varies from three to 22 days. The optimum temperature for development is between 25°C and 30°C (77–86°F).

Dogs become infected by ingesting the infective larvae or when the larvae penetrate the skin. If the larvae are swallowed, they molt in the intestines. If they penetrate through the skin, they have to follow a circuitous route to get to the intestines. They first travel to the lungs, then to the trachea (windpipe) and enter the gastrointestinal tract via the esophagus. The larvae complete their development to adults in the intestines. Between two and four weeks later, eggs begin to appear in the stool. Adults tend to live for about six months in the intestines but can survive indefinitely as arrested larvae in the walls of the intestines.

Hookworms suck blood and can cause anemia, specifically iron-deficiency anemia. In their feeding habits, they change sites approximately six times each day; large amounts of blood are also lost from the attachment sites.

There are many safe and effective compounds that can be used to treat infected dogs. Also, for dogs on heartworm-preventative medication, the active agents used are highly effective against adult hookworms in the intestines.

Whipworms

Surveys consistently identify whipworms (*Trichuris vulpis*) as one of the most common parasitic worms of dogs in North America, while only infrequently being reported in cats or humans. They live in the lower aspects of the intestines (the cecum and colon) where they latch on to feed.

Sometimes they cause no problems at all but they may cause abdominal upset (colic) or diarrhea, often tainted by blood and mucus.

When eggs are laid in the intestines, they pass into the feces and become infective within nine to ten days. When consumed by dogs, the infective eggs hatch in the intestines and the larvae parasitize the intestines and mature further. Many people do not realize that dogs do not begin to shed whipworm eggs in their stool until about three months after being infected. At that time each female whipworm may pass from 1000 to 4000 eggs per day into the stool. Complicating matters further, female whipworms are long-lived, surviving for months or years in the intestines. The life cycle therefore includes a larval stage in the small intestine, an adult stage in the large intestine, and infective eggs that pass into the feces.

Diagnosis is not always easy since it depends on finding whipworm eggs in the feces. Remember that animals are infected for three months before they begin to shed eggs and you can appreciate the problem. Once females begin shedding eggs, they are usually recoverable by direct smears and centrifugal flotation. They are not as easily found with standard fecal evaluations. In some instances, the adult worms are actually seen attached to the lower bowel during endoscopic procedures.

Treatment is also not straightforward because of the peculiar life cycle of this parasite. Although many medicines are effective in removing adult worms, the larvae are less reliably cleared. Therefore treatment must often be repeated in three weeks and often, in three months as well, when the larvae have evolved into egg-producing adults. The biggest hindrance to effective treatment is that animals are often re-exposed to environments in which whipworm eggs are plentiful, and are thereby reinfected.

It can be difficult to control exposure to whipworm eggs on lawns or soil but concrete can be effectively disinfected. Proper disposal of egg-containing dog feces is critical.

Tapeworms

The main tapeworm affecting dogs is called *Dipylidium caninum* and is carried by the flea. Humans can get tapeworms, the same way dogs do, by ingesting fleas. Although this common tapeworm does not cause many health problems in people, infection should be discouraged by keeping pets flea-free.

One form of tapeworm infection, caused by *Echinococcus multilocularis*, is raising increasing concern. This tapeworm with its strange-sounding name is found throughout much of the northcentral United States and southcentral Canada. Studies indicate that the parasite is spreading southward and eastward in the United States.

Adult tapeworms of this species

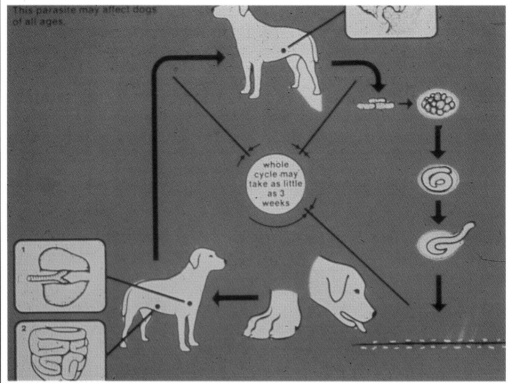

Hookworm cycle. Courtesy of Rogar/STB.

Hookworm in the pregnant bitch. Courtesy of Rogar/STB.

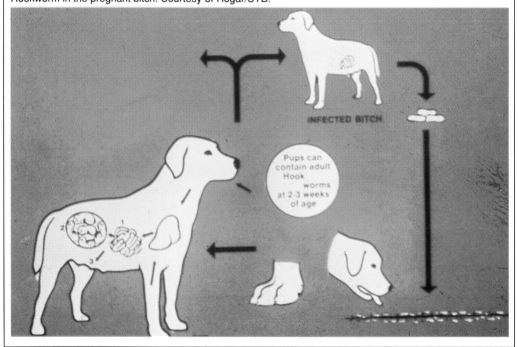

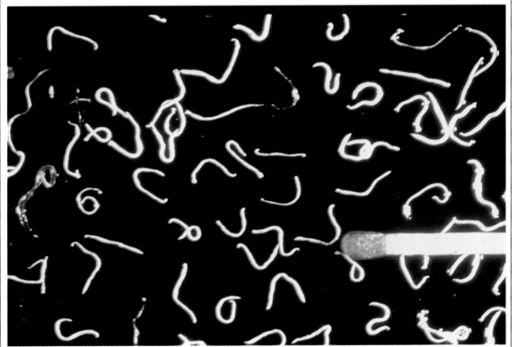

Hookworms. Courtesy of Rogar/STB.

Hookworms, close-up showing teeth. Courtesy of Rogar/STB.

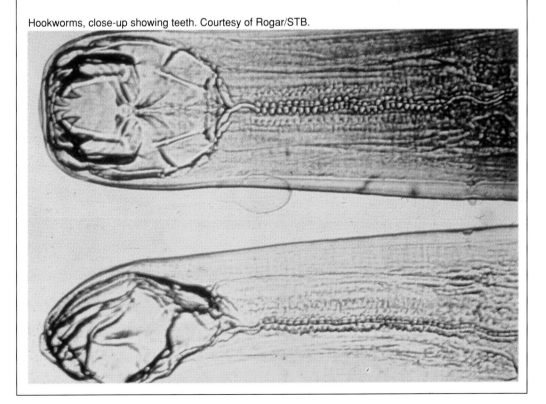

are found in wild foxes, coyotes, and wolves, where they live in the small intestine and produce eggs that are shed in the feces and subsequently contaminate the local environment. Rodents then become infected by ingesting these eggs, which then form hundreds or even thousands of hydatid cysts in the tissues. When dogs or their wild cousins eat these rodents, they can be infected with hundreds to thousands of adults. These adults latch onto the wall of the intestines and after about a month, start shedding eggs. These eggs are then immediately infective to other animals, including people. To complicate matters further, these tapeworm eggs can remain infective in the environment for several months.

Adult tapeworms of *Echinococcus multilocularis* appear to cause very few clinical problems in dogs. Infected dogs and cats therefore may seem clinically normal while shedding large numbers of infective eggs. This is the real point of concern because infected people are not as lucky. Alveolar hydatid disease in humans, caused by *Echinococcus multilocularis*, is a very serious infection that usually involves the liver. Early in the course of the infection, patients may be misdiagnosed with other liver ailments. Involvement of other tissues, including the lungs and brain, can also occur. Since over 50% of people with alveolar hydatid disease die, this is considered the most lethal worm infection that people get.

It is therefore important that all dogs and cats in high-risk areas be screened for tapeworm infection. This is more difficult than it sounds since infection with *Echinococcus* eggs can not be readily differentiated from the more common tapeworms which do not affect people. Veterinarians finding tapeworm eggs on fecal exams usually closely examine pets for the rice-like grains known as proglottids, which are found with common tapeworms but not the lethal variety. Occasionally more dramatic methods are necessary to try to recover worms from suspect pets. A more convenient blood test is available to diagnose infection in people and hopefully similar tests will soon become suitable for pets.

The best defense is increased public awareness of this condition. Personal protection and hygiene are important, especially to those individuals that may contact feces from potentially infected pets. Children are particularly at risk. Mulch that contains feces from dogs, cats, wolves or foxes should not be used on gardens. Pets should be discouraged from hunting and consuming wild rodents.

Fortunately for pets, there are medicines that are safe and very effective for treatment. People are not as lucky and surgery still remains the preferred treatment. In conclusion, *Echinococcus multilocularis* may cause a mild problem in pets but if people get infected, the results can be fatal. In order to minimize the risk of human infection, the public must increase its awareness of the potential complications that are associated with these parasites.

Wormers

Roundworms, hookworms, whipworms, and tapeworms are common parasites in pets. Roundworms and hookworms are potentially contagious to people and therefore they constitute a public health hazard. It is recommended that pets be dewormed according to the information provided above. Prophylactic deworming programs should be initiated two to three weeks after pups are whelped, and these programs should include the nursing bitch. Treatment should be repeated every two to three weeks until three months of age. Care should also be taken to reduce environmental contamination with eggs of roundworms and hookworms.

For animals that are on regular heartworm prevention, there is an added bonus in that most products also have effects against certain worms. For example, the once-a-month preparations work against adult roundworms, hookworms and whipworms. The daily preparations work against adult roundworms and hookworms but also significantly suppress egg shedding on a daily basis. The monthly treatments remove adult worms, suppress egg shedding by roundworms, and temporarily suppress egg shedding by hookworms.

It is natural that some pet owners should want to treat their pets for these pests, and sometimes products are purchased over-the-counter for this purpose. Although it is safe to buy many medicines from retail outlets, you should always check with a veterinarian first before they are administered to pets.

There are several veterinary products used in the treatment of internal parasites in dogs and cats. The mixture of febantel and praziquantel was first sold in the United States in 1985. It is effective against tapeworms, roundworms, hookworms, and whipworms but should not be given to pregnant bitches. Nitroscanate is available in several countries and has a similar spectrum of activity, as does mixtures of febantel, praziquantel, and pyrantel embonate. And, of course, individual medications can be selected when only one form of parasite is recovered. None of these medications is available for over-the-counter (OTC) use.

The combination of toluene and dichlorophen is available from retail outlets under a variety of names and is effective in the treatment of roundworms and hookworms and some tapeworms, although it is not considered the safest product available. Dichlorophen was shown in 1946 to be effective against some tapeworms, while toluene was found, a year later, to be effective against roundworms and hookworms, but not whipworms. Clearly much better products have

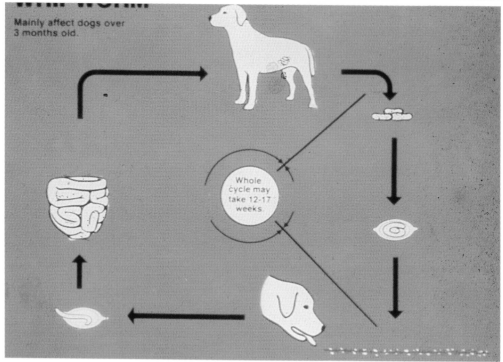

Mainly affect dogs over 3 months old.

Whole cycle may take 12-17 weeks

Whipworm cycle.

been developed over the last half century but are not available without a prescription.

What are the problems associated with buying a wormer in a supermarket or pet-supply store? It must be remembered that wormers are potentially dangerous chemicals and their indiscriminate use is to be discouraged. From 1973 to 1984 the FDA received adverse drug reaction reports involving 141 dogs and cats following administration of this combination (toluene/ dichlorophen). The Illinois Animal Poison Information Center (IAPIC) received over 100 calls from 1984 through 1987 relating to adverse reactions in dogs and cats to this combination product.

Side effects reported include awkwardness, altered behavior, vomiting, depression, increased salivation, dilated pupils, and muscle tremors. Most symptoms occur within six hours of administration.

Most animals can recover if given adequate supportive care. This may involve correcting any fluid or electrolyte imbalances, keeping the animal in quiet surroundings, and administering activated charcoal to decrease further absorption of the chemicals. Liver and kidney functions should be monitored in severely affected patients.

Coccidia

Coccidial parasites are commonly found in dogs and cats but only infrequently cause clinical disease. These microscopic

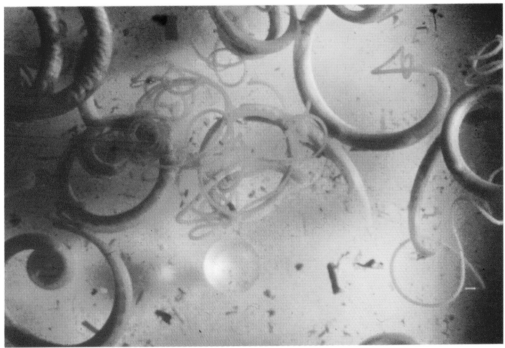

Adult whipworms. Courtesy of Rogar/STB.

Whipworm eggs, as seen on a fecal evaluation. The eggs will not hatch on the ground and the thick shell makes it the most resistant egg of all the dog parasites. The infective stage is reached when a dog swallows the eggs and they hatch in the small intestine. Courtesy of Rogar/STB.

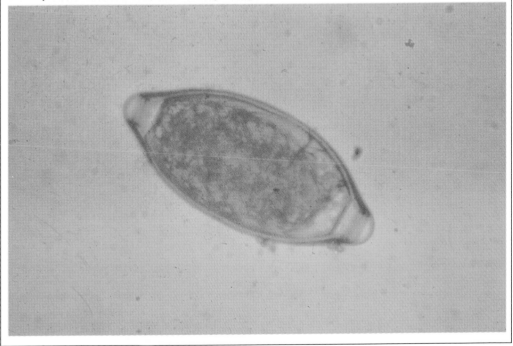

parasites may cause mucus-laden diarrhea, but in many cases, the pups show no outward signs of problems. Death may result in extreme cases. Pups that are nursing, recently weaned, or have a poorly functioning immune system are the ones most likely to have problems. Because they frequently only get problems when they are moved to a new location (such as to a new home), clinical coccidiosis is often considered to be stress-related.

The term "coccidia" is used loosely to include a number of organisms such as *Isospora, Eimeria, Toxoplasma, Besnoitia, Hammondia, Sarcocystis, Neospora,* and *Cryptosporidium. Isospora* species are the coccidia that are most often associated with diarrhea in dogs. This species can be identi-fied by microscopically examining oocysts (eggs) present in feces.

Coccidia can be effectively treated with a variety of medicines, especially sulfa drugs. Treatment of infected bitches soon after whelping may be beneficial in preventing the spread of infection to the young. Proper sanitation is helpful in preventing the spread of infection in kennels and catteries. Oocysts (eggs) in the feces are infectious and tend to be resistant to most disinfectants. Ammonia compounds tend to be effective when used on hard surfaces, and steam-cleaning removes most infectious oocysts from fabrics and carpets. The mature oocysts can survive for months or years in the environment.

Giardia

Giardia are protozoan parasites that can affect people as well as dogs. Whether or not *Giardia* is contagious from dogs to humans has always been a matter of some controversy. Many human infections of *Giardia* are acquired by drinking unfiltered municipal drinking water originating from *Giardia*-contaminated streams, rivers, or lakes. Children in day-care facilities also have a high risk of infection.

There are two different forms of *Giardia*, a motile form and a cyst form. The motile form is known as a trophozoite and it attaches to the wall of the intestines without actually penetrating the cells. The trophozoite reproduces itself and is eventually transformed into the cyst form which passes into the feces. When the cysts are consumed by a susceptible animal, the cysts open in the small intestine, and trophozoites become established once again. Dogs infected by a canine source of *Giardia* cysts show an average period of eight days between infection and cyst excretion.

Most infections with *Giardia* don't cause clinical problems. *Giardia* infects an estimated 10% of well-cared-for house dogs, up to 50% of pups, and up to 100% of kennel dogs. In dogs that develop clinical problems with infection, the most common sign is diarrhea. The stool may be soft, pale, and foul smelling, and the diarrhea may be acute and self-curing, or chronic. Some animals may experience weight loss and poor condition.

Giardiasis is diagnosed by finding characteristic organisms in the stool. However, these cysts are not often detected by routine fecal examinations. The preferred method for detecting *Giardia* organisms is the zinc sulfate fecal concentration technique. Because *Giardia* is known to produce cysts only intermittently, it is usually recommended that at least three samples be examined over a period of about one week before excluding the possibility of *Giardia* infection. If an animal is being examined with an endoscope, a duodenal aspirate can be collected and evaluated for the parasite. Recently, immunological test kits have become available in human medicine for the diagnosis of giardiasis and have also been used in dogs. The tests were developed for detection of *Giardia* infections in humans but also can detect similar infections in several animal species, including dogs. This ELISA (enzyme-linked immunosorbent assay) test relies on detection of antigens released from *Giardia* organisms during active infection. There is little benefit to selecting these tests over the standard fecal evaluation using zinc sulfate.

The drug most commonly used in North America to treat *Giardia* is metronidazole (Flagyl). Metronidazole is estimated to be effective in about two-thirds of treated cases. Albendazole, a drug used to treat giardiasis in people, appears to be highly effective in eliminating *Giardia* in dogs but four consecutive doses are required, and the drug is not licensed for this use. It is typically administered for five days and, although considered quite safe, may cause side effects in some animals. Common disinfectants (e.g., chlorine bleach, quaternary ammonium compounds) can also be used to kill cysts in the environment.

ADDITIONAL READING

Anderson, JG; Washabau, RJ: Icterus. *Compendium for Continuing Education of the Practicing Veterinarian*, 1992; 14(8): 1045-1059.

Barriga, OO: Rational control of canine toxocariasis by the veterinary practitioner. *Journal of the American Veterinary Medical Association*, 1991; 198(2): 216-221.

Bowman, DD: Hookworm parasites of dogs and cats. *Compendium for Continuing Education of the Practicing Veterinarian*, 1992; 14(5): 585-593.

Campbell, BG: Trichuris and other trichinelloid nematodes of dogs and cats in the United States. *Compendium for Continuing Education of the Practicing Veterinarian*, 1991; 13(5): 769-778.

Drazner, F: Gastric dilatation/volvulus syndrome. *Pet Focus*, 1990; 2(4): 63-66.

Gulbas, NK: Canine parvovirus infection. *Pet Focus*, 1989; 1(1): 15-17.

Harvey, JB; Roberts, JM; Schantz, PM: Survey of veterinarians' recommendations for treatment and control of intestinal parasites in dogs: Public health implications. *Journal of the American Veterinary Medical Association*, 1991; 199(6): 702-707.

Hubbard, B: Flatulence and Coprophagia. *Veterinary Focus*, 1989; 1(2): 51-53.

Jordan, HE; Mullins, ST; Stebins, ME: Endoparasitism in dogs: 221,583 cases (1981-1990). *Journal of the American Veterinary Medical Association*, 1993; 203(4): 547-549.

Kirpensteijn, J; Fingland, RB; Ulrich, T; *et al*: Cholelithiasis in dogs: 29 cases (1980-1990). *Journal of the American Veterinary Medical Association*, 1993; 202(7): 1137-1142.

Lieb, MS, Blass, CE.: Gastric dilatation volvulus in dogs: an update. *Compendium for Continuing Education of the Practicing Veterinarian*, 1984; 11:961.

Lindsay, DS; Blagburn, BL: Coccidial parasites of cats and dogs. *Compendium for Continuing Education of the Practicing Veterinarian*, 1991; 13(5): 759- 765.

Lovell, RA; *et al*: A Review of 83 reports of suspected toluene/dichlorophen toxicoses in cats and dogs. *Journal of the American Animal Hospital Association*, 1990; 26: 652-658.

Meyer-Lindenberg, A; Harder, A; Fehr, M; et al: Treatment of gastric dilation-volvulus and rapid method for prevention of relapse in dogs: 134 cases (1988-1991). *Journal of the American Veterinary Medical Association*, 1993; 203(9): 1303-1307.

Papageorges, M, *et al.* Gastric drainage procedures: effects in normal dogs—Clinical observation and gastric emptying. *Veterinary Surgery*, 1987; 16:5: 332-340.

Schaer, M: Acute pancreatitis in dogs. *Compendium for Continuing Education of the Practicing Veterinarian*, 1991; 13(12): 1769-1780.

Schulman, AJ, Lippincott, CL, et al. Muscular flap gastropexy: A new surgical technique to prevent recurrences of gastric dilatation volvulus syndrome. *Journal of the American Animal Hospital Association*, 1986; 22:339.

Simpson, KW: Current concepts of the pathogenesis and pathophysiology of acute pancreatitis in the dog and cat. *Compendium for Continuing Education of the Practicing Veterinarian*, 1993; 15(2): 247-253.

Zajac, AM: Giardiasis. *Compendium for Continuing Education of the Practicing Veterinarian,*, 1992; 14(5): 604-611.

Disorders of the Reproductive and Urinary Systems

ANATOMY AND PHYSIOLOGY OF THE MALE REPRODUCTIVE SYSTEM

The anatomy of the male reproductive system is similar in dogs and humans. There is a prostate gland located at the base of the bladder and this is also the area where the ductus deferens enter the urethra. These ducts serve as conduits or tubes for products produced in the testicles. The epididymis is a long tube that forms a cap on the testicles and stores spermatazoa before ejaculation. It is the tail end of the epididymis that leaves the testicle and becomes known as the ductus deferens. The canine penis has a bone, called the os penis, in its length, which is not found in humans.

Within the testicles are found seminiferous tubules that comprise 80-90% of the testis. Within these tubules are found germ cells that go on to produce sperm and Sertoli cells which surround and nurture the sperm. Interstitial cells

Schematic diagram of the male urinary and reproductive tracts. Courtesy of Petcom, Inc.

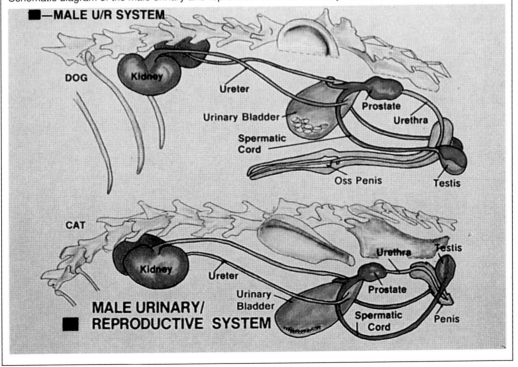

■—MALE U/R SYSTEM

DOG
Kidney
Ureter
Urinary Bladder
Prostate
Urethra
Spermatic Cord
Oss Penis
Testis

CAT
Kidney
Ureter
Urinary Bladder
Urethra
Testis
Prostate
Spermatic Cord
Penis

■ MALE URINARY/ REPRODUCTIVE SYSTEM

within the testes secrete testosterone and small amounts of other hormones. These cells typically comprise 5-10% of the normal testis.

Normal dogs typically produce between 400 million and 1.5 billion sperm in their ejaculate, depending on their size and health status.

ANATOMY AND PHYSIOLOGY OF THE FEMALE REPRODUCTIVE SYSTEM

The canine ovaries are located just behind the kidneys. The left ovary lies between the abdominal wall and the left colon, and the right ovary is above the descending colon. They are held in place by suspensory ligaments. Within the ovaries are a variety of important but complicated structures.

The primary "follicles" are actually specialized cells (granulosa cells) that surround an egg (oocyte). By 15 days of age, it is estimated that the ovaries in a bitch contain 700,000 follicles, but only about 250,000 remain by the time she actually reaches puberty. Only about 500 follicles remain by ten years of age.

Stimulating hormones (gonadotropins) induce the growth and maturation of follicles. Follicle stimulating hormone (FSH) induces the specialized granulosa cells to produce estrogens and to form receptors for luteinizing hormone (LH). The secretion of FSH increases slowly, beginning about five weeks before ovulation in the bitch. The luteinizing hormone (LH) stimulates the production of other hormones, including male sex

hormones (androgens). The secretion of LH increases approximately two weeks before ovulation of the growing ovarian follicles. Although all follicles are exposed to FSH and LH, less than 1% reach full development and ovulation. The hormones typically encourage four to six follicles to reach the point of ovulation.

After ovulation, the granulosa cell layer forms into the corpus luteum (plural is corpora lutea) which produces the female sex hormone progesterone. The cells then lose their ability to produce estrogens and male sex hormones (androgens). Ovulation occurs and corpora lutea form about 24-72 hours after the LH reaches peak blood levels.

THE ESTROUS ("HEAT") CYCLE

The estrous cycle in the bitch is significantly different than the hormonal cycles of women, although the same hormones are involved. Bitches are typically six to 12 months of age when they reach puberty and first start to cycle. Only one or two estrous cycles occur per year. With each new estrous cycle, there is the development of follicles on the ovaries that secrete estrogen. This is referred to as proestrus, and the result is swelling of the vulva, thickening of the vagina, and a clear to slightly bloody discharge.

During actual estrus ("heat"), the estrogen level actually starts to drop and the bitch is ready to receive the male for breeding. Before she ovulates, the follicles on the ovaries start to "luteinize" and her progesterone levels start to increase.

Luteinizing hormone (LH), which causes the follicles to luteinize and produce progesterone, is produced by the pituitary gland at the base of the brain. The eggs (oocytes) are ovulated within 48 hours of this LH peak. Two days later the eggs start to divide and form mature eggs capable of being fertilized. If, however, they are not fertilized in the next two to three days, the eggs begin to degrade. Thus, the bitch is capable of conceiving four to six days after the LH peak, and this is the best time for breeding or insemination with chilled or frozen semen.

WHEN TO BREED

In our high-tech world of dog breeding, it is often necessary to predict the best chances for conception. This can be done by carefully observing the bitch and her relationship to the stud or by performing a variety of tests. Canines have evolved so that they know the best times to breed. When a bitch is in estrus ("heat") she becomes receptive to the male. In general, ovulation occurs 12-24 hours after the onset of true estrus. This time can be determined if, during proestrus, a male is allowed to spend five minutes or so with the bitch. The bitch should wear some form of chastity belt if the dog used for testing is not the anticipated stud. When she's in heat the dog will attempt to mount and she will allow it. Even castrated males may attempt to mount a bitch in heat. For two days or so before estrus, the bitch may growl and snarl at the stud dog's attempts to mount.

The best ways of determining when to breed is to measure blood levels of luteinizing hormone (LH). Unfortunately, human test kits cannot be used and canine test kits are not widely available. Therefore, other tests are usually used to estimate the time of ovulation.

Vaginal cytology is the most common test used by veterinarians to estimate the stage of estrus and when ovulation is most likely to occur. Cell samples are taken from the vagina and examined microscopically. The presence or absence of red blood cells, white blood cells, superficial cells, parabasal cells, and intermediate cells is used in the estimation. Superficial cells are more prevalent when bitches are in estrus. When the sample is maximally cornified (more than 95% superficial cells), breeding is most likely to result in conception. However, it must be noted that the presence of superficial cells does not relate directly with luteinizing hormone (LH) levels. Maximal cornification can occur from eight days before until three days after the LH peak.

Progesterone levels can be used alone or with vaginal cytology to predict ovulation. The first rise in progesterone is closely related with the LH peak, but later increases cannot reliably be used to predict ovulation. Therefore, it is best to perform vaginal cytology until about 60% of the cells are

■—FEMALE U/R SYSTEM

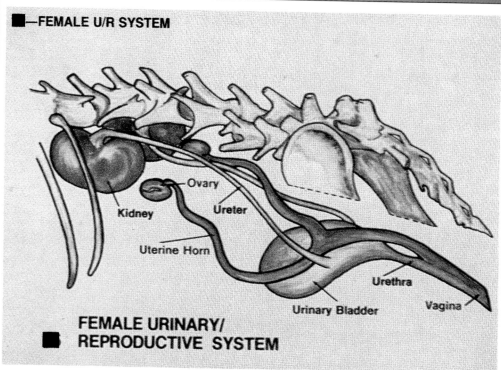

FEMALE URINARY/
REPRODUCTIVE SYSTEM

Schematic diagram of the female urinary and reproductive tracts. Courtesy of Petcom, Inc.

Bitch stands during estrus, allowing stud dog to sniff. Courtesy of International Canine Genetics, Inc, Malvern, Pennsylvania.

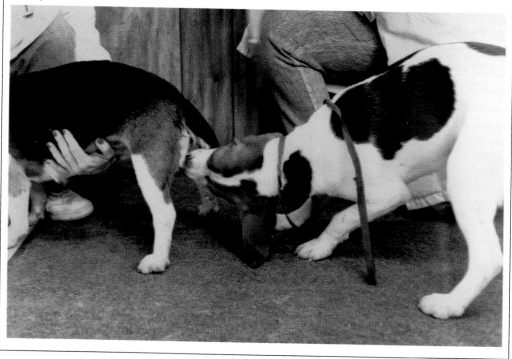

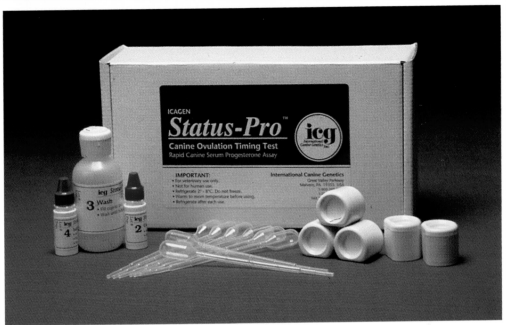

The Status-Pro™ canine progesterone test kit. Courtesy of International Canine Genetics, Inc, Malvern, Pennsylvania.

Stud dog mounts bitch. Assistant prepares to collect semen. Courtesy of International Canine Genetics, Inc, Malvern, Pennsylvania.

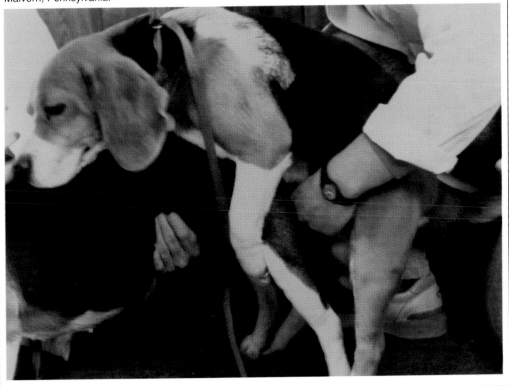

superficial (60% cornified) and then perform progesterone levels every one to two days until the "first rise" is noted.

Test kits were available to measure luteinizing hormone (LH) present in the urine but, unfortunately, they were taken off the market recently. The presence of LH in the urine corresponds to the first rise in progesterone levels. Therefore, urine LH is measured throughout proestrus until it becomes positive. On the day the test first becomes positive, a progesterone-level test can be performed. If the progesterone level is in the right range, it helps confirm a LH peak. Ovulation will then occur two days later and the eggs will be mature by two days after that.

Breedings are conducted during those days most likely to result in conception. To do this effectively, it is important to identify the time of the LH peak. This can be estimated by vaginal cytology, progesterone levels, or urine LH tests. The best times for the bitch to conceive are two to six days after the LH peak. Therefore, for most natural matings or artificial inseminations with fresh semen, breeding should begin two to three days after the LH peak and continue every two to three days until the end of the fertile period. When using chilled or frozen semen, or a stud dog with compromised semen quality, breedings should occur on the most fertile days (days four to six) after the LH peak.

ARTIFICIAL INSEMINATION

Canine semen is collected with appropriate equipment that is sterilized and lubricated. Some novice studs need a bitch in heat nearby to perform, but experienced dogs will perform without the benefit of such a stimulus. The ejaculate is collected and the quality of the semen is evaluated microscopically before insemination. The semen evaluation is most important when the male is suspected of being infertile. About 200 million sperm are necessary for a single insemination dose.

The semen is evaluated for the presence of abnormally shaped sperm as well as their motility. There are many different abnormal sperm shapes, but as long as 80% are normal they should be satisfactory for insemination. Healthy sperm move forward vigorously while those that swim slowly or in circles are considered abnormal. A sample of the semen can even be used to evaluate for communicable diseases such as brucellosis.

Collected semen can be used for immediate insemination or chilled or frozen for later use. For immediate insemination, the semen should be used within 20-30 minutes. For later use, the semen is mixed with a liquid extender and slowly cooled to about 4°C. This makes it viable for one to two days, in which time it can be sent across the country for insemination in a bitch thousands of miles away. For long-term storage, semen is placed

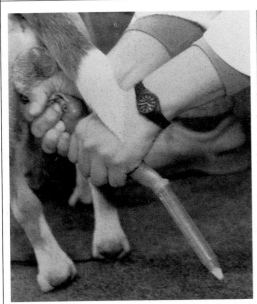

Collecting semen for use in artificial insemination. Courtesy of International Canine Genetics, Inc, Malvern, Pennsylvania.

in sterile straws and kept in a tank with temperatures below -70°C. At these temperatures, the semen can be maintained for years, and thawed and used as needed.

The best chances for conception are when collected semen is used within 30 minutes of collection. Conception rates in these cases are not appreciably different than those from natural breedings. Fresh-chilled semen used within 48 hours contributes to a conception rate of about 75-80% while frozen semen gives a conception rate of about 70%.

The use of fresh-chilled semen for insemination has been greatly simplified by the production of kits for this purpose (e.g., Fresh Express™ by International Canine Genetics, Inc.). After breeding arrangements are made, supplies are ordered and communications are made between collecting and inseminating veterinarians. On the basis of tests, the inseminating veterinarian determines when the semen is needed. The collecting veterinarian then collects semen from the stud dog, usually two collections on separate days, and the semen is evaluated, extended, packaged and shipped. The inseminating veterinarian then receives the semen within two days and performs the insemination procedure.

PREGNANCY

Pregnancy lasts from 58-69 days, with an average of 63 days. The length of the gestation (pregnancy) period varies with the criteria for a starting date. Diestrus is that period of sexual inactivity associated with increased progesterone levels. If onset of diestrus is used as a starting point, 85% of bitches will deliver 56–58 days later. If a single breeding is used as a starting point, most bitches will deliver about 63 days later. Since sperm are able to survive for six days in the female's reproductive tract and the exact day of ovulation is unknown in most cases, the length of gestation (pregnancy) is difficult to calculate exactly.

Among the current methods available to diagnose pregnancy, diagnostic ultrasound is one of the most valuable and accurate techniques. With this technique, the earliest that diagnosis of pregnancy is possible is 18 days after ovulation. The fetal heart is usually

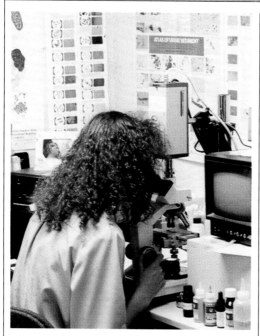

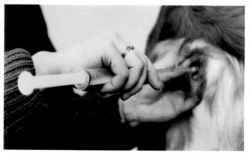

Above: Using collected semen for insemination. Courtesy of International Canine Genetics, Inc, Malvern, Pennsylvania.
Below: The Fresh Express™ used for collecting and shipping fresh chilled semen. Courtesy of International Canine Genetics, Inc, Malvern, Pennsylvania.

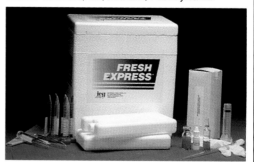

Above: After collection, a sample of the semen is evaluated for sperm quality.
Below: Dr. Paul Tackett of Mesa Veterinary Hospital, Mesa, Arizona performs an ultrasound examination on a bitch to see if she is pregnant.

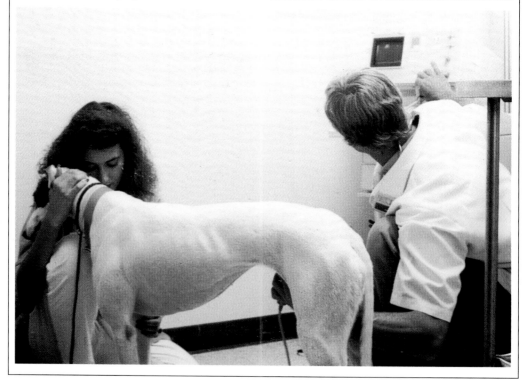

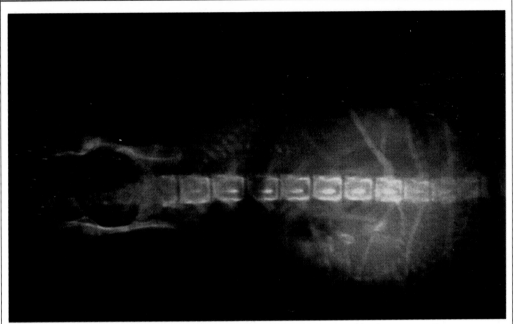

Radiograph of a pregnant bitch showing the presence of pups (skeletons evident).

Gloved hand inserted in the vagina to palpate the birth canal and stimulate contractions. Amniotic sac is present in the doctor's hand. Courtesy of Dr. Samuel L. Beckman, Tennessee Valley Veterinary Surgical Referral Center, Nashville, Tennessee.

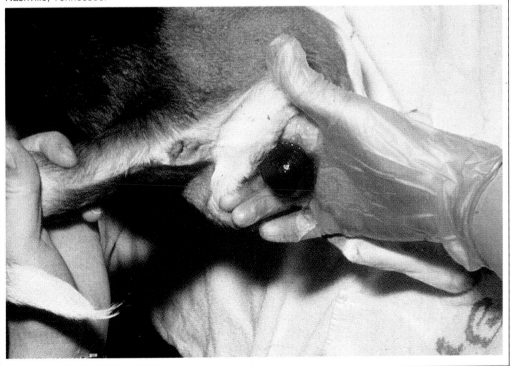

detectable by day 20 and the head and body can be discerned between days 34 and 37. Estimation of litter size is not accurate with ultrasonography, but the period between days 28 and 35 of gestation is believed to be the best time to attempt counting fetuses. Parts of the skeleton are unequivocally recognizable after days 38–40. Therefore, it is only after this time that radiographs will be able to correctly diagnose pregnancy.

The total body weight of the bitch increases 20–55% during the course of pregnancy. The mammary glands start to develop after days 38-40 and milk usually appears in the last week. The last few days of pregnancy are heralded by restlessness, a desire for seclusion, and poor appetite. These behaviors are intensified during the last 12–24 hours.

Stage I labor begins with uterine contractions and dilatation of the cervix, but not abdominal contractions. This lasts for 12–24 hours and often begins with a lowering of rectal temperature to 99°F (37°C). Therefore, taking the bitch's temperature morning and evening starting 58 days after the first breeding will allow the pet's owner to predict when labor should begin. Stage II is the propulsive stage, in which the chorioallantois ruptures (water breaks) and the pups begin to be delivered. This process should last for less than two hours. If the process is prolonged, there might be an abnormal delivery problem (dystocia) which requires intervention. Stage III labor occurs after

each pup is delivered and the chorioallantois is expelled from the uterus. The bitch may then rest for several minutes to a few hours before re-commencing Stage II with the next pup.

CESAREAN SECTION

Cesarean section is a surgical procedure that removes pups directly from the uterus (womb). There are many reasons why puppies are delivered by cesarean section. The most common are obstruction to the birth canal or medical reasons which prevent contractions being powerful enough to push the fetus through the birth canal.

An obstruction of the birth canal may occur because the fetus is too large to pass through the bony ring of the pelvis which surrounds the birth canal. This may occur simply because the fetus has grown too large in the womb or because it is in the wrong position to enter the canal. It should start into the canal head or tail first. If it tries to enter the canal sideways or bent double, it will likely become stuck and block its passage as well as that of its siblings. The female's pelvic ring may be too small due to fat that has been deposited within the pelvic canal of obese pets or because of previously sustained pelvic bone fractures that healed in the wrong position.

The second category of problems is physiological dysfunction. Basically this means some chemical imbalance that interferes with the body's messages to start parturition

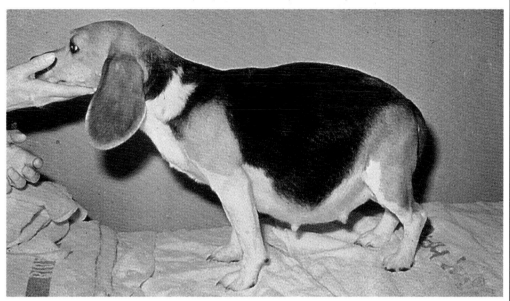

Full term female that required a cesarean section because of uterine inertia. Courtesy of Dr. Samuel L. Beckman, Tennessee Valley Veterinary Surgical Referral Center, Nashville, Tennessee.

(labor) or somehow prevents labor from continuing successfully. During labor the uterus and vagina function primarily as a sack made of muscle. As with other muscles, the proper balance of essential nutrients must be present so that they can contract hard enough and long enough to push the fetus out of the womb and through the birth canal.

Veterinary assistance should be sought for any female that is five days past the average 63-day gestation period or any female that strains in hard labor (hard contractions of the abdominal muscles) for more than two hours without delivering the first fetus or more than one hour since the last fetus was delivered.

A veterinarian will first determine that no problems exist, that no physical obstruction is causing the problem, and that the offspring are small enough to pass through the birth canal. If this is the case, medical therapy may be attempted to induce a vaginal delivery. This treatment consists of hormones to stimulate the uterine muscle to contract and glucose and minerals to furnish the nutrients that the muscle uses to contract. Stimulation of the birth canal with a sterile gloved finger may also be of some benefit.

The most common reason for a cesarean section is called uterine inertia. This term is used to describe a uterus that does not contract at all or has weak contractions that do not force the fetus out of the uterus. Uterine inertia may prohibit labor from starting or it may develop after prolonged straining with or without the delivery of part of the litter.

If medical therapy is not successful, then preparations should be made for a well-planned

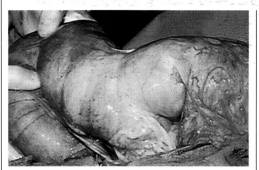

Full term uterus exposed during surgery. Courtesy of Dr. Samuel L. Beckman, Tennessee Valley Veterinary Surgical Referral Center, Nashville, Tennessee.

cesarean section. As with many surgical procedures, the success of a cesarean section depends to a large degree on attention to the details of patient care before and after surgery, not just during the surgical procedure.

Surgery

After the patient is safely anesthetized and placed on her back on the surgery table, a final antiseptic washing of her abdomen is done to kill any bacteria on the skin. An incision is made between the mammary glands from her umbilical scar (belly button) to the brim of her pelvis. A single incision is made into the body of the uterus and each puppy is "milked" out of the uterine incision. The umbilical cord of each newborn is sterilely clamped and the pup is then handed to an assistant. For each newborn delivered, a separate placenta (afterbirth) must also be removed from the uterus. If the owner elects, an ovariohysterectomy (spaying) can be performed after the deliveries have been completed. After the entire litter has been removed from the uterus, the uterine and abdominal incisions are sutured closed.

Puppy having just been removed from the uterus. Hemostatic clamps are present on the umbilical cord. Courtesy of Dr. Samuel L. Beckman, Tennessee Valley Veterinary Surgical Referral Center, Nashville, Tennessee.

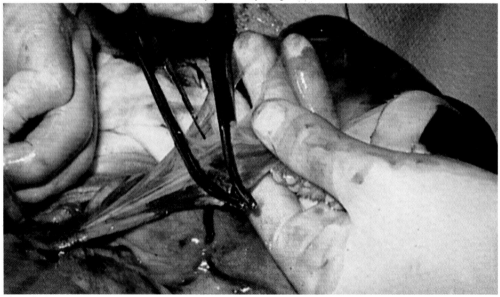

Each newborn is dried and rubbed briskly to stimulate it to breathe. The clamps are removed from the umbilical cord, but the cord may be tied with suture if it starts to bleed. The cord is also disinfected at this time to prevent infection. The pups should be placed in an incubator to keep them warm while the mother is recovering from anesthesia, which may take place in as little as 20–30 minutes. The pups can then be returned to the bitch so she can nurse them and keep them warm.

PSEUDOCYESIS (FALSE PREGNANCY)

Pseudocyesis results when bitches act like they are pregnant but really aren't. The reasons why pseudocyesis occurs in some bitches and not others is not known. Pseudocyesis tends to recur in bitches but not adversely affect the chances of conception.

Clinical Signs

Bitches with pseudocyesis show all the common manifestations of pregnancy, including mammary development, weight gain, and behavioral changes. Towards the end of diestrus (60–80 days following estrus), affected bitches display nesting behaviors, lactation (milk production), and may even "mother" inanimate objects.

Diagnosis

The diagnosis is easily made when ultrasound or radiographic studies fail to reveal developing fetuses. Palpation (feeling the abdomen) is not a reliable way to differentiate pseudocyesis from pregnancy.

Placenta being removed from the uterus. Courtesy of Dr. Samuel L. Beckman, Tennessee Valley Veterinary Surgical Referral Center, Nashville, Tennessee.

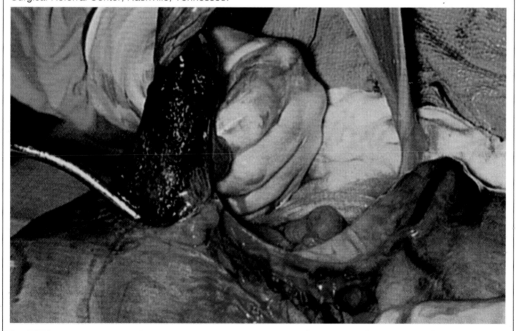

Therapy

Therapy is not needed in all cases as most bitches eventually revert to quiescent cycling. Drugs such as mibolerone are sometimes used daily for three to five days to speed the process. It is also advisable to decrease (slightly) the bitch's consumption of food and water to decrease milk production.

PYOMETRA

Pyometra is a common and serious condition in which the uterus becomes inflamed and fills with pus. The condition occurs only in intact females or those that have been incompletely ovario-hysterectomized (spayed). Most cases are reported within three months following estrus. Pyometra occurs during diestrus in the bitch, that stage of the estrous cycle in which progesterone is produced by the corpora luteum of the ovary.

The condition is most commonly seen in middle-aged to old intact bitches after one or more non-pregnant estrous cycles. The exact reason for the condition is still a matter of some debate but it is likely involved with cystic endometrial hyperplasia. Cystic endometrial hyperplasia is a condition of the uterus associated with uterine thickening and the accumulation of mucus within the uterus. As the condition progresses, the tissue becomes more inflamed. Cystic endometrial hyperplasia frequently but not always evolves into pyometra.

The effects of progesterone on the female reproductive system have also been blamed but this alone is insufficient to cause the condition. Also, pyometra can result in young bitches when they are administered estrogen compounds to prevent pregnancy or to induce estrus. However, there are other compounds that can accomplish this safely, and there is little justification for administering estrogens to breeding bitches.

Clinical Signs

Regardless of the underlying cause, pyometra results when the changes mentioned above interact with vaginal bacteria. The result is a bacterial overgrowth and accumulation of pus in the uterus. If the cervix is open, there will be drainage of pus from the vagina. If the cervix is closed, there is no visible discharge.

With the accumulation of pus in the uterus, bitches may be affected by the toxins produced. They may be lethargic, depressed, and inappetant but rarely have a fever. About 50% of affected bitches will have increased thirst and urination associated with kidney damage.

Diagnosis

If there is little vaginal discharge, it may be difficult to confirm pyometra clinically. Basic blood tests are very helpful in this case. Patients with pyometra typically have very high white blood cell counts but about 25% of cases will have counts in the normal range. Many affected bitches have mild anemia and most are dehydrated from the condition.

One of the most consistent blood test abnormalities in patients with pyometra is an elevation in one of the liver enzymes (serum alkaline phosphatase). This is seen in over 50% of cases and likely reflects kidney damage from the toxins in the uterus. Kidney function tests may also be abnormal because pyometra is known to be associated with kidney disease (tubulointerstitial nephritis). Blood tests can help identify this, but urine tests rarely show abnormalities.

The diagnosis can be confirmed by radiographic or ultrasonographic (ultrasound) examination of the abdomen. Ultrasound is preferred because an enlarged uterus is not always discernible on x-ray films. Ultrasound examination also permits early differentiation between pyometra and pregnancy.

Therapy

The treatment of choice for pyometra is surgical removal of the uterus and ovaries (ovariohysterectomy). It is wise to utilize intravenous fluids and antibiotics to stabilize patients prior to surgery, and antibiotics are usually required for at least a week following surgery.

When surgery is not an option, there are some medical ways to manage pyometra. A prostaglandin compound (Lutalyse: Upjohn) has been successfully used, but it is not licensed for use in the canine. It has been used experimentally with doses given once to twice daily for three to five days. Side effects such as restlessness, salivating, vomiting, and others are seen in most cases. Medical therapy is less satisfying than surgery because pyometra is likely to recur in treated bitches. Therefore, treatment is more likely to delay than to eliminate the need for surgery.

INFERTILITY IN THE STUD

Infertility in the stud is evaluated by looking at his history of siring and by semen evaluation. To be fertile, the male must first be able to maintain an erection, copulate, and ejaculate viable sperm into the bitch. The testes are responsible for producing normal motile sperm. These sperm can only be ejaculated if they have access to the urethra via the reproductive duct system. Finally, the sperm must be capable of capacitation (releasing important enzymes), penetrating the female's ovum (egg), and fertilizing it.

There are many reasons why a stud dog may not be capable of intromission (copulation) with the bitch. Some are behavioral (e.g., inexperience, poor libido) while others are conformational. Some conformational problems are congenital or acquired defects of the penis or breed-related conformations that make natural breeding difficult.

Azoospermia, a lack of sperm, can result from several different causes, some acquired and some congenital. The most common causes of acquired azoospermia are testicular tumors (e.g., Sertoli-cell tumor), immune-mediated diseases (lymphocytic orchitis), and infectious diseases (e.g., brucellosis). Congenital azoospermia can result from non-functional testicles or blockage of the ducts that carry sperm from the testicles to the urethra. Inbreeding may be involved in azoospermia because there is often a family history of reproductive dysfunction.

Most infertile dogs that have sperm present in their ejaculate either have too few sperm, abnormal sperm, or sperm without normal motility. Defects of sperm motility may occur with other congenital problems such as ciliary dyskinesia (immotile cilia or Kartagener's syndrome) which result in immotile sperm.

There are also a number of drugs that can interfere with sperm production. These include corticosteroids, anabolic steroids, testosterone, estrogens, cimetidine (Tagamet), and ketoconazole (Nizoral).

The diagnostic approach to these cases warrants a complete evaluation of health history, a physical examination, and semen evaluation. Radiography and ultrasonography (ultrasound) are useful in evaluating dogs with infertility associated with testicular or prostatic disease, including cancers. Laboratory evaluation of blood cells, organ function, brucellosis, and thyroid function are warranted in most instances. Specific hormone tests (e.g., testosterone, luteinizing hormone, follicle-stimulating hormone) may be helpful in some cases. When a genetic defect is suspected, chromosome analysis (karyotyping) may also be necessary.

Any treatment should be tailored to the exact cause of the problem. Using hormone therapies routinely is unlikely to be helpful and may have unwanted side effects.

INFERTILITY IN THE BITCH

Infertility is an inability to produce offspring. There are many reasons why this could occur in the bitch. Some cases occur because of breeding failures. Others are the result of abnormal estrous cycles. Finally, yet others are due to conception failures even though the estrous cycle appears normal. All bitches suspected of being infertile should have a thorough physical examination and routine evaluation of blood and urine samples. Underlying problems such as hypothyroidism, diabetes mellitus, and others could result in reproductive failure in the apparently healthy bitch. All breeding bitches should be screened for infectious diseases such as brucellosis and *Mycoplasma*, and a specific evaluation for uterine disease (e.g., cystic endometrial hyperplasia) may be warranted.

The most common cause for apparent infertility in the bitch is management. Breeding management is complicated by the fact that bitches have a confusing cycle and it is not always easy to predict ovulation periods. Owners often believe breeding should occur on predetermined dates relative to the day of the estrous cycle. Although proestrus typically lasts about nine days, there is considerable variation. Proestrus may last two days, then estrus commences, and then diestrus results by day 10. Alternatively, proestrus may last for 15 days. This makes breeding unpredictable when the onset of proestrus is used as a guideline for when ovulation is to occur. Therefore, breeding on days nine and 11 of the cycle cannot reliably pinpoint the best time for conception. If proestrus is either short or long, predetermined breeding dates may not correspond with behavioral estrus. Even a bitch with a typical, average cycle will usually display estrous behavior for longer than she is capable of conceiving. To complicate matters further, some bitches have a "split heat" in which a second fertile estrus occurs several weeks after the first. Therefore, just because she accepts a stud does not mean that conception will occur. Using ovulation-timing techniques during the next estrus is the best way to manage these causes of infertility in the bitch.

Certain anatomical problems can also complicate conception. Vaginal strictures (narrow compartments) are not rare in the bitch. However, since they may relax some during estrus, bitches should be evaluated at the time of breeding. Some bitches require surgical correction of these strictures if they are to breed and whelp naturally. Similarly, fibrous bands (septae)

may be present in the vagina and/ or cervix that can interfere with breeding. Septae that do not penetrate the cervix can be surgically removed.

MAMMARY CANCER

Mammary or breast cancer is as common in bitches as it is in women. These tumors can be benign or malignant. Benign is a descriptive characteristic of tumors that usually don't spread to other parts of the body. Malignant describes the potential of a tumor to invade other surrounding tissues or spread (metastasize) to other parts of the body. Cancer is the general term used frequently for the malignant neoplasms or tumors that have the capability for spreading throughout the body.

The incidence of mammary cancer is increasing as bitches are living longer than ever before (due to superior veterinary care and increased owner awareness). Mammary cancer is second only to skin malignancies in prevalence and is about twice as common in bitches as in women. Also, mammary cancers are more commonly seen in elderly animals. The incidence increases dramatically in bitches over ten years of age.

Fortunately, mammary cancers can be largely prevented by performing ovariohysterectomy (spay) in young bitches. In fact, it is very rare to diagnose breast cancer in a female dog who was spayed at or before about nine months of age, before the first heat (puberty). Dogs spayed after two-and-a-half years of age do not enjoy this cancer-sparing effect. Intact and neutered females over two years of age have a seven-fold increased risk of developing mammary gland tumors compared to females neutered prior to six months of age. In addition, no definitive study has shown a survival improvement by spaying a bitch at the time of the breast cancer diagnosis.

Clinical Signs

Mammary tumors are usually first noticed as a lump in the breast tissue. At least 50% of all dogs with mammary tumors will have more than one breast involved and usually they are found in the lowest glands. The dog usually has ten breasts with three pairs below the chest on the abdomen and two pairs of glands on the chest just slightly behind and parallel to the front legs.

A malignant mammary tumor most often spreads through the lymph nodes, primarily to the lungs. We do know that the cells can bypass the lymph nodes and travel through the bloodstream to the lung directly or to anyplace else they want to go.

Diagnosis

If a suspicious tumor (mass) is found associated in or on the breast, a thorough evaluation is warranted. Not only are the breasts themselves evaluated but the lymph nodes and draining lymph vessels as well. The abdomen is palpated (felt) and the chest lis-tened to with a stethoscope (auscultation) to help ascertain if there is any evidence of tumor spread.

It is important to note that it is impossible to determine if any lump is benign or malignant until the cells or tissues have been examined under a microscope. Sometimes, by sticking a needle into a tumor and withdrawing cells, microscopic examination of the collected cells may help with a preliminary diagnosis. This procedure (cytology) is not as exact as tissue biopsy and requires considerable experience in interpretation of cell types and activities. Tissue biopsies normally include part of the mass itself and sometimes tissue from the lymph nodes or vessels to see if there is any evidence of spread (metastasis).

Other tests that are useful include blood counts, biochemical profile, urinalysis, and radiographs of the chest. These tests help determine if there is any other internal involvement of the process. Radiographs are not absolute; microscopic growth of billions of cells must gather at least to 1 cm in size to be evident on radiographs. Therefore, even if radiographic evaluation does not suggest tumor, millions upon millions of cells could conceivably be present.

The same phenomenon holds true for the use of CAT (computed axial tomography) scans of the chest, abdomen, or bones. Though the CAT scan has a much more sensitive resolution to pick up smaller lesions, it too has its limitations by not picking up microscopic growth. Magnetic resonance imaging (MRI) can identify very small centers of cancer growth but its access and cost preclude its use in most pets.

Therapy

For most bitches diagnosed with a mammary malignancy, the recommendation is to remove the tumor(s) and the affected breast tissue with a wide surgical excision and submit the specimens to a pathologist for evaluation. If only one gland is involved, then usually only that area is removed. If more than one breast is involved, then all the tissue involved with each individual tumor is removed. In essence, a complete unilateral (one-sided) or bilateral (two-sided) mastectomy (breast removal) is only indicated if one or both sides are involved with multiple tumors. Because at least 50% of canine mammary tumors are benign, a radical procedure is not necessarily indicated before a confirmed diagnosis is available. Also, if the unfortunate patient has a very aggressive tumor which is diagnosed as being malignant, the cancer may have already spread internally, making mastectomy unwarranted.

For the patient with aggressive breast cancer, following surgery, most patients will live about 12-18 months with only perhaps 20% living two years beyond initial diagnosis. The cause of death is ultimately from the cancer itself.

With less aggressive cancer, without invasiveness or metastasis,

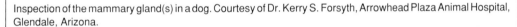

Inspection of the mammary gland(s) in a dog. Courtesy of Dr. Kerry S. Forsyth, Arrowhead Plaza Animal Hospital, Glendale, Arizona.

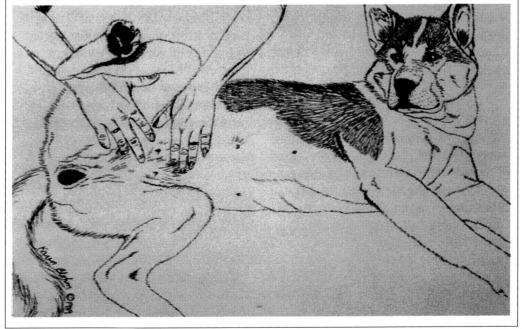

Benign prostatic hyperplasia refers to an increase in the number of prostate cells and it is not a cancer. Sometimes these result in cysts (cystic prostatic hyperplasia) or there can just be an increase in the size of the prostate gland. The increase in size of the gland is due to stimulation by male sex hormones or perhaps to an imbalance of male and female sex hormones.

Prostatitis is caused by an infection in the prostate; this is most commonly seen as a sequel to benign prostatic hyperplasia. Abscesses can also form on the prostate as a manifestation of infection.

Clinical Signs

In most cases, dogs do not suffer much from benign prostatic hyperplasia and the condition is noted during routine veterinary examinations. The enlarged prostate gland can cause problems as it occupies more space in the abdomen. Thus, it can result in constipation as the enlarged gland puts pressure on the rectum. Occasionally it can also cause perineal hernia or partial urinary-tract obstruction but this is rare in dogs.

Prostatitis can be more damaging and can result in recurrent urinary-tract infections, fever, depression, inappetance, and pain. If a prostatic abscess opens to the urinary tract, pus and hemorrhage may be noted in the urine. If the abscess ruptures into the abdomen, dogs will be systemically ill with fever and perhaps vomiting, diarrhea, and even shock.

Prostate cancers are usually malignant and cause many of the same signs as prostatic infections.

Diagnosis

Benign prostatic hyperplasia is usually recognized during a routine veterinary examination. Rectal evaluation detects an enlarged prostate gland, and sometimes even cysts or abscesses. This increase in size can be confirmed with radiographs or ultrasound evaluations.

When prostatitis is suspected, many other tests may be needed before therapy can be instituted. Basic blood work and urine analysis are needed to determine the extent of the infection and whether other body systems are involved.

A very useful test is known as the prostatic "wash." A catheter is inserted into the urethra and advanced toward the prostate. A gloved finger is inserted into the rectum and the prostate is "massaged." A sample of the fluid is then collected and sent for cellular analysis as well as culture.

In cases where a tumor is suspected, prostate biopsy is often needed. Newer techniques have allowed the biopsies to be done without surgery, by immobilizing the prostate or by using ultrasound to guide the biopsy instrument.

Therapy

Benign prostatic hyperplasia is the most common prostate disorder of dogs, and often requires no treatment whatsoever. If intervention is needed, castration (neutering) is the best option as it will cause a reduction in the size of the prostate without the need for drugs. Female sex hormones (estrogens) have been used in the past but often cause too many side effects to be recommended routinely (including squamous metaplasia, cysts, and possibly cancers). Androgen receptor antagonists have been used experimentally but are not yet licensed for routine use in dogs.

Progesterone administration is often effective in shrinking the prostate and often has fewer side effects than estrogens. Injections of medroxyprogesterone acetate usually cause shrinkage of the prostate gland within four to six weeks. In many cases, relapses are not seen for many months, sometimes as long as two years. A recent Japanese study showed that oral administration of chlormadinone acetate, an anti-androgen, was also effective when given for three to four weeks. Because of the anti-androgen effect, sperm counts and motility are decreased and more abnormal sperm are seen. Dogs usually remain in remission for six months or so before prostatic enlargement returns.

Neutering is also recommended for cases of bacterial prostatitis. This helps shrink the prostate tissue and resolve the condition, as well as helping to prevent future episodes. In acute prostatitis antibiotic therapy often needs to be given for three weeks, while chronic episodes usually require a minimum of two months of antibiotics. Prostatic abscesses sometimes respond to castration and antibiotics, but most cases require surgical drainage to resolve the situation.

Most cases of prostate cancer are malignant and treatment is usually unrewarding. Neutering may help shrink the prostate and associated tumor growth but will not cure the condition. Female sex hormones (estrogens) are also used for this purpose but have some severe side effects of their own, such as bone marrow suppression. Surgery and radiation therapy have had the most success to date. Most forms of chemotherapy have had disappointing results in managing prostate cancer.

BRUCELLOSIS

Brucella canis is a small bacterium that can cause infertility in dogs and abortions in bitches. Rarely, it can also be transmitted to people that handle the organism or an infected canine.

Most infections occur when organisms are inhaled or ingested. When brucellosis causes abortion in bitches, the aborted material and discharges may contain as many as 10 billion organisms per milliliter (one milliliter is one-fifth of a teaspoon). There are, however, yet other ways that brucellosis can be spread. Urine of acutely infected male dogs may contain up to one million organisms per milliliter of urine; fewer organisms are spread in the urine of females.

Brucellosis is considered a sexually transmitted disease in the

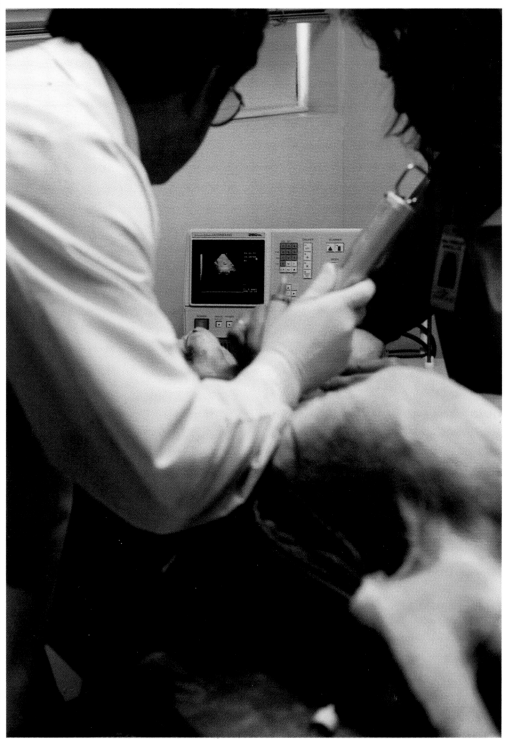

Dr. Kenneth Jeffrey of Mesa Veterinary Hospital, Mesa, Arizona performs a biopsy of the prostate, guided by an ultrasound image.

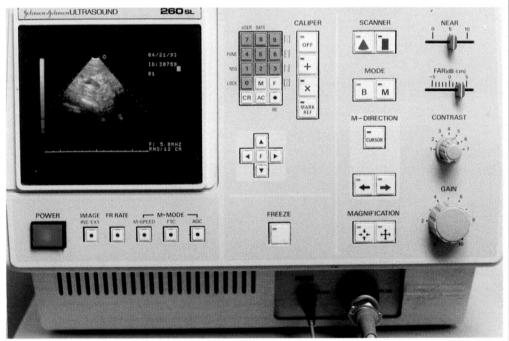

Closeup view of the ultrasound image of the prostate.

canine. Semen can serve as a source of infection because large numbers of organisms are shed in the semen of infected dogs. Most organisms are shed in the semen between three and 11 weeks after infection.

Brucellosis can be contracted by several different routes. It can be ingested or inhaled; the oral route is thought to be the most common. The organism can also penetrate abraded areas of skin. Brucellosis can also be present in semen samples used for artificial insemination; it has no problems surviving freezing or chilling.

Clinical Signs

There are several different syndromes caused by *Brucella* infection. When the bacteria enter the system, they are attacked by white blood cells, in which they continue to survive and reproduce. They can also replicate in the liver, spleen, and lymph nodes. Reproductive tissues that may be infected include the uterus of pregnant females and the testes and prostate of males.

Brucella canis infects the uterus of pregnant bitches where it localizes in the placenta. This results in the death of the fetus,

A canine brucellosis antibody test kit.

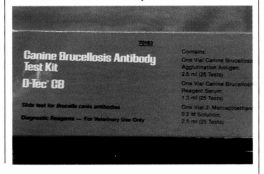

although occasionally some pups are born alive and fail to thrive. The classic picture is that of abortion occurring between 45 and 59 days of gestation in an otherwise healthy bitch. Non-pregnant bitches typically show no signs of disease, although they may be carriers and shedders of the infection. Infection does not appear to affect the estrous ("heat") cycle.

In males, the most commonly recognized sign of infection is infertility and abnormal semen quality. The infection is most pronounced in the epididymis, the cap-like structure on the base of the testes. Abnormal sperm are usually evident by five weeks after infection. Eight to 35 weeks after infection, scrotal swelling is found in some, but not all, infected dogs. Otherwise, these dogs do not have fever or any evidence of illness. In some cases, the testicles actually become involved in the inflammatory process (orchitis), but this is not common. The organism also involves the prostate gland without actually causing an inflammatory condition (prostatitis) there. The presence of *Brucella* organisms in the prostate likely accounts for the fact that male dogs shed more bacteria in their urine than do bitches.

There are some other manifestations of brucellosis. These include infections in the eye (anterior uveitis), brain (meningitis), kidney (glomerulonephritis), skin, and spine (diskospondylitis).

Diagnosis

Brucellosis is often suspected when an apparently healthy bitch has a spontaneous abortion in her last trimester of pregnancy or when an apparently healthy dog is infertile or has abnormal semen quality. Confirming these suspicions can be more difficult.

There are several blood tests used in the assessment of brucellosis suspects, but some of these tests are non-specific and therefore may give falsely positive results on occasion. This happens because most of these tests (rapid slide agglutination test) measure antibodies against cell wall anti-gens and these cell wall antigens may also be found in other bacteria, including staphylococci (common skin bacteria), *Bordetella bronchiseptica* (a cause of canine cough), and *Pseudomonas aeruginosa* (a common bacterial invader). Antibodies against *Brucella* can be detected eight to 12 weeks after infection and the levels (titers) usually remain high for several months. All positive results on the rapid slide agglutination tests should be confirmed with the more exacting tube agglutination tests, or agar gel immunodiffusion tests. The tube agglutination test is usually positive by three to six weeks after infection.

An agar gel immunodiffusion (AGID) test has been developed that measures internal (cytoplasmic) antigens unique to *Brucella*; this is the most specific diagnostic test available. The test may be positive by 12 weeks after infection and continue to be detectable for as long as 36 months after the organism is no longer circulating in the blood. The disadvantage of this test is that it may miss some infections because it is not as sensitive as the others, and that the test is technically difficult to perform.

A positive blood test should prompt more specific testing. The definitive way to confirm the diagnosis is to actually recover the organism from infected tissues. After an abortion, a vaginal culture is recommended; vulvar discharge is also a rich source of infectious organisms. For males, semen cultures are recommended especially between three and 11 weeks after infection. Within two to four weeks after infection, blood cultures are positive for *Brucella canis* and remain positive for at least 30 weeks. Most (about 80%) will still have evidence of bacteria in their blood one year after infection. The presence of bacteria in the bloodstream eventually subsides despite chronic infection. *Brucella* is shed in the urine, in variable concentrations, between eight and 30 weeks after infection.

Therapy

Antibiotics are typically not as effective in treating brucellosis because the organisms locate inside cells where it is hard for the drugs to penetrate. Since no treatments are 100% effective, some of these treated animals will therefore remain a source of infection for other animals and people.

Currently, minocycline, a derivative of tetracycline, is the antibiotic most often used in the treatment of brucellosis. Combinations of minocycline with drugs such as dihydrostreptomycin or gentamicin may be more effective, but the latter two drugs carry some significant side effects of their own. Therefore, the combination is usually only given for two weeks, followed by another two weeks of tetracycline only.

It is difficult to know when to discontinue antibiotic therapy in these cases. A dropping antibody titer and apparent return to health is no indication of success. Many animals become positive again within weeks or months of discontinuing antibiotic therapy. Also, it seems that *Brucella canis* is not eliminated from the prostate even with appropriate antibiotic therapy.

When a pet is infected with brucellosis, 100% control may not be needed since it is possible to isolate the animal and prevent contact with other dogs. In these cases, neutering tends to limit the amount of bacteria shed, and antibiotics may be sufficient to control, if not cure, the condition. This approach is usually not sufficient in breeding kennels in which many animals are present and reproductive status needs to be maintained. In this case, quarantine, identification, and elimination of infected animals is the best route. Antibiotic therapy alone is not sufficient because the infection will persist.

Prevention

It is important to prevent brucellosis because there are no vaccines available and because it can be devastating in a kennel situation. All new acquisitions should be quarantined for three months and tested monthly for brucellosis. Only animals negative on all tests should be admitted to the kennel environment. No animals previously exposed to brucellosis or completely recovered should be allowed into the kennel.

Brood bitches should be tested for *Brucella canis* before each breeding. All stud dogs should be certified to be negative for *B. canis* before being allowed onto the premises. Finally, any kennel animals that contact other canines should be considered "at risk" and treated as any new acquisition.

There is one other good reason to prevent brucellosis. It is potentially contagious to people. This poses considerable risk to individuals involved in breeding, those cleaning up after an abortion, and veterinarians involved in collecting specimens and treating infected animals.

HERPESVIRUS

Canine herpesvirus (CHV) primarily affects pups less than one week of age. It can result in a rapidly fatal disease. This virus has been found worldwide and has been isolated from clinically normal adult dogs. Pups acquire the infection while in the uterus or as they pass through the birth canal, or from contact with infected dogs or contaminated objects. Most dogs initially get infected via licking, shared bowls, or other contact items (fomites).

Clinical Signs

Dogs maintained as pets in households have a rate of infection of 10-15% compared to 80% for canines in kennel environments. However, canine herpesvirus causes mild or no problems in adult dogs so its presence is often difficult to detect. These animals function as carriers. The majority of infected dogs become immune and develop resistance to the disease themselves, but can still shed virus which is infectious to others.

The animals most susceptible to problems with canine herpesvirus are non-immune bitches and their puppies, from three weeks prior to three weeks after their birth. In the non-immune bitch, the virus can cause mild respiratory infection with flu-like symptoms and spare the pups, or it can affect the pups or the birth canal directly. It can also result in a vaginal rash which is not painful and usually not associated with any discharge. If the pups are infected in the uterus, abortion is likely or the pups will die shortly after birth. If the puppies become infected as they pass through the birth canal, some of the pups (about half) will fail to thrive and die within a few weeks.

Healthy pups can also be infected from other contact dogs or from owners who might carry the infection to them from other dogs. If they are exposed shortly after birth, most will become depressed, cry, and eventually die. Pups affected after three weeks of age may develop their own protective immune response.

Diagnosis

There are many causes of puppy mortality and the only way to confirm that herpesvirus caused the death of a pup is to have a postmortem examination (necropsy) performed by a veterinarian, prefer-ably a pathologist. Blood tests of the bitch only indicate exposure to the virus, not an indication that this particular virus was involved in the pup's condition.

Therapy

There is no specific treatment for canine herpesvirus infection. Hyperimmune serum has been used experimentally but is rarely effective. Surviving pups should be removed from the bitch and tube-fed with milk replacer. If they have any evidence of the disease, they are typically treated with antibiotics and electrolyte therapies. It is important that they be maintained in a warm environment.

Prevention

There is no vaccine available for canine herpesvirus. However, natural vaccination occurs when dogs contact other dogs, especially between three to six months of age. They can then pass the infection amongst themselves and develop their own immunity. Only bitches and young pups that have never been exposed to the virus before are susceptible to its detrimental effects.

Breeders should keep susceptible bitches quarantined from other dogs starting three weeks before whelping until three weeks afterward. Since the virus can survive outside the body for a week or so, good sanitation is critical. Chlorine bleach disinfectants (e.g., Clorox diluted 1:30) are suitable for killing the virus on hard surfaces.

NEOSPORA

Neospora caninum is a newly recognized parasite that can affect dogs, cats, cattle, sheep and horses. Unlike many other parasites, this one only crosses the placenta to infect the unborn from the mother.

Clinical Signs

Although dogs may be infected with *Neospora* at any age, congeni-tal disease is the most dramatic. If there is evidence that a breeding bitch is already infected, there is a great likelihood that her pups will be affected. As a rule, an infected bitch is a carrier of the parasite and shows no symptoms herself. The infected puppies usually first show clinical illness around three to six weeks of age. This includes progres-sive weakness, and paralysis and death can result. Diarrhea and pneumonia can also be part of the syndrome. There are several cases reported in which a bitch has given birth to more than one litter of infected pups. If the bitch acquires infection in the first month of pregnancy, it causes the death of the fetuses.

When adults are affected, ascending paralysis is not commonly seen. Other manifestations include encephalitis (inflammatory brain disease), myositis (inflammatory muscle disease), myocarditis (inflammatory disease of heart muscle), hepatitis (inflammatory liver disease), dermatitis (inflammatory skin disease), and generalized disease.

Diagnosis

The parasite can be recovered from affected animals by way of pathology samples. A blood test has been developed but is not widely available. These tests only measure exposure to the parasite, not that it is necessarily the cause of the problem. The parasite is similar to *Toxoplasma* but there are differences. This condition may be more common than appreciated because few people know what it is and therefore it is probably under-diagnosed.

Therapy

There is no known treatment for neosporosis. At present, the best approach seems to be a combination of trimethoprim and sulfa antibiotics. It is not known whether pups that survive carry the infection for life in a latent (hidden) form. Once a bitch has had one infected litter, there is a high probability that subsequent litters could be affected as well.

KIDNEY DISEASE AND KIDNEY FAILURE

The kidney has many important functions in the body; one of the most important is the removal of wastes and toxins. The body cannot survive long after kidney function has been lost. Animals are born with a specific number of filtering units (nephrons) which are not replaced after they are destroyed. When approximately two-thirds of the nephrons have been destroyed, the body has a difficult time conserving water and increased urination (polyuria) results. However, when three-quarters of the nephrons have been destroyed, toxins accumulate in the bloodstream and the situation becomes serious indeed. The body provides a great reserve of kidney function but when this is surpassed, there is none left.

There are many different causes of kidney (renal) disease. For purposes of discussion and therapy, kidney failure is usually divided into acute and chronic varieties. Acute renal failure results when there is an abrupt decline in kidney function. The most common causes are drugs, toxins and impaired blood flow. Some drugs that are specifically toxic to the kidneys include thiacetarsamide (used to treat heartworm), amphotericin B (an old remedy for systemic fungal infections), and several different antibiotics. Some of the more common toxins are ethylene glycol (antifreeze), heavy metals (e.g., lead), and rodent poisons that contain vitamin D (cholecalciferol). A variety of microbes (e.g., *Leptospira, E. coli*, infectious canine hepatitis) can also result in acute renal failure.

Every year thousands of pets die from exposure to ethylene glycol, the active ingredient in commercial automobile antifreeze. The sweet taste of the ethylene glycol encourages consumption by pets. Vitamin D (cholecalciferol) is an important component in a new class of rodent poisons. Dogs become poisoned by either ingesting the rodent poison itself or by feeding on poisoned rats. The poison works by increasing blood levels of calcium to excessive amounts, which in turn lodges in the kidneys and causes kidney failure and electrolyte disturbances.

The more common form is chronic renal failure, which results from disorders that slowly compromise the kidney over a period of time. For example, infections such as pyelonephritis and leptospirosis will destroy functional filtering units in the kidney over a period of months or years. Of course, as pets become older, they lose a certain percentage of their kidney filtering units (nephrons) as a consequence of aging. A variety of chronic diseases such as immune-mediated glomerulonephritis, amyloidosis, infarctions and cancers can also result in chronic renal failure.

Clinical Signs

For dogs with chronic renal failure, the clinical signs (symptoms) tend to vary with the extent and duration of the problem. Most dogs drink and urinate more than usual and may experience anorexia, lethargy, and weight loss. Because the kidneys produce a hormone (erythropoietin) that stimulates red-blood-cell production, dogs with chronic kidney disease usually have at least some degree of anemia. Because kidney disease interferes with the normal calcium/phosphorus regulation, affected dogs may experience bone pain and even spontaneous fractures.

Dogs with acute renal failure are noticeably ill. They may experience vomiting, diarrhea, depression, lethargy, and anorexia. Some dogs may be seen in a state of collapse. Rather than producing too much urine, these dogs tend to produce little or no urine; the toxins that are not excreted accumulate in the bloodstream. It is important that the severity of the condition is recognized and that veterinary attention is sought immediately.

When pets have been exposed to antifreeze (ethylene glycol), they may appear drunk and awkward initially, but coma and death are a common sequel if they are not attended to immediately. Some of the symptoms are caused by toxic effects on the liver, but the most dangerous are those effects on the kidney.

The signs of vitamin D poisoning depend on the total dose and usually occur 12-24 hours after ingestion. Most animals experience weakness, lethargy, vomiting, and constipation. With kidney failure, animals have increased thirst and increased urination. Neurological signs, including twitching and seizures, may occur as well, and coma and death can occur in a few days if damage is severe.

Diagnosis

Dogs with chronic renal failure deserve a full laboratory workup, including blood-cell counts, biochemical profiles, electrolytes, urinalysis, and radiography. Two measures of kidney function, creatinine and blood urea nitrogen (also known as BUN, urea), are typically elevated in the biochemical profiles. These animals often have an anemia and the urine remains dilute (as measured by specific gravity or osmolality) rather than being concentrated. If radiographs are taken, the kidneys are often smaller than normal and the bones of the skeleton may not be as dense as they should be.

When dogs have acute renal failure, evaluation of blood cells, organ profiles, and urinalysis should be performed immediately. Certain blood test results are usually elevated, including creatinine and urea. Other procedures, such as tests for specific toxins or drugs, are indicated; a kidney biopsy may be necessary if the cause can not be determined by other tests.

Therapy

Whenever possible, treatment should be directed at the specific cause of the problem. Supportive care is given to reduce stress, and fresh water and water-soluble vitamins are provided to compensate for urinary losses.

Dietary changes are made so that dogs are provided with high-quality protein (e.g., eggs, cottage cheese, liver), but in small amounts that won't further tax kidney function. Salt (sodium) is restricted to maintain normal blood pressure since kidney disease is one of the most common causes of hypertension in dogs. If anemia is profound, it may be warranted to stimulate red-blood-cell production with erythropoietin, nandrolone decanoate, or stanozolol (Winstrol).

Treatment for the dog with acute renal failure must be intensive and immediate if kidney function is to be preserved. If the cause of the problem is known, specific therapies should be directed to correct the problem. Fluid therapy is needed to correct fluid imbalances, electrolyte disorders, and alterations of pH. Specific drugs such as diuretics (water pills) are often needed, and dopamine is sometimes given to dilate renal blood vessels. Dialysis may be needed to help remove accumulated toxins if there are insufficient numbers of kidney-filtering units left viable. Other treatments are used to combat the clinical signs (vomiting) that often accompany acute renal failure.

It is important to recognize the signs of vitamin D (found in some rodent poisons) toxicity rapidly, as death can result. Patients should be kept inside, away from direct sunlight, since sun exposure stimulates vitamin D production by the skin. Most animals become dehydrated and require fluid therapy with saline. Diuretics are also sometimes given to help promote calcium excretion from the kidneys.

The standard treatment for ethylene glycol toxicosis has been ethanol, the common ingredient in drinking alcohol. It competes with enzymes and encourages the ethylene glycol to be excreted unmetabolized by the kidneys. There are several disadvantages and many side effects to this form of therapy. Recent studies suggest that 4-methylpyrazole is the most efficient and least toxic inhibitor of an enzyme (alcohol dehydrogenase) that normally turns antifreeze into its more toxic form within the body. There appears to be few side effects associated with this treatment and it may very well replace ethanol therapy in the very near future. Dog owners should also be aware of the availability of dog-safe antifreeze on the market—as always prevention is preferred over cure.

AMYLOIDOSIS

Amyloidosis refers to a group of diseases characterized by the accumulation of an abnormal protein (amyloid AA) in tissues. Amyloidosis in dogs has been reported in association with a number of different disorders, including systemic lupus erythematosus, blastomycosis, cyclic neutropenia, tumor of the spleen (hemangioma), chronic intravenous insulin therapy, and various inflammatory diseases. In many affected dogs, however, no underlying disease can be detected. An underlying inflammatory or cancerous disease process is found in perhaps 50% of dogs with renal amyloidosis, and, therefore, in animals the cause is thought to be "reactive."

Clinical Signs

Kidney deposits of amyloid protein usually develop in older dogs. Beagles, Chinese Shar-Pei, and Collies appear to be at higher risk than other breeds. The most common clinical signs in dogs with amyloidosis are anorexia, increased urination, increased thirst, weakness, lethargy, vomiting, dehydration, and weight loss.

Dogs affected with renal (kidney) amyloidosis eventually experience kidney failure as the amyloid deposits compromise kidney function and eventually result in significant scarring.

Diagnosis

Many routine tests can be conducted which suggest a problem in kidney function but not until relatively late in the course of the disease, when much of the kidney tissue has already been affected. Microscopic examination of actual kidney tissue is necessary to confirm the diagnosis. Occasionally, amyloid deposits will occur in other tissues, including the spleen, liver, adrenal glands, pancreas, and intestines.

Therapy

The prognosis for dogs with renal amyloidosis is poor, and kidney failure is the inevitable outcome. Renal amyloidosis is particularly resistant to medical treatment. The best chance is to uncover the underlying inflammatory or cancerous process, if it can be detected, and treat that specifically.

DMSO (dimethyl sulfoxide) and colchicine are products which have been used in people with amyloidosis, but experience in animals is limited.

CYSTITIS

Cystitis refers to an inflammatory process in the urinary bladder. There is usually some underlying cause for recurrent bladder infections. The most common microbes implicated in bladder infections are those that normally reside in the digestive tract and manage to invade the bladder. This is most easily accomplished if there is some process that interferes with the normal protective mechanisms. For example, crystal formation and urolithiasis (urinary tract "stones") are both a cause and effect of cystitis. Anything that causes the urine to pool in the bladder rather than be excreted quickly promotes infection. Also, conditions such as diabetes that dump glucose (sugar) into the urine make the bladder a good place for bacteria to flourish.

Clinical Signs

Most animals with cystitis are not physically ill. They may have difficulty urinating (straining, pain) but they usually don't have a fever and appear healthy otherwise. Sometimes affected dogs will pass urine that is cloudy or has blood in it.

Diagnosis

Most of the diagnostic testing done on dogs with suspected cystitis involves urinalysis, radiography, and perhaps microbial cultures. The urinalysis typically reveals blood, pus, and microbes in the urine but may also detect the presence of crystals. If a sterile procedure is used to collect urine, it can be sent off for a quantitative microbial count, identification, and sensitivity testing. Radiographs may help identify defects in the bladder, the presence of calculi (stones), or problems in the prostate.

Therapy

Whenever possible, it is important to identify and correct any underlying problems contributing to cystitis. Otherwise, the problem is bound to recur after the antibiotic has been discontinued. In most cases, antibiotics are needed for about three weeks in initial cases, and four to six weeks or longer for recurrent cases. Chronic cystitis recurs when the underlying problems have not been sufficiently addressed.

UROLITHIASIS

Urolithiasis is the disease caused when crystals combine to form "stones" in the urinary tract. These stones may also be referred to as calculi or uroliths. Uroliths can form in any part of the urinary tract, including the kidneys, ureters, bladder, or urethra.

Several types of uroliths have been identified and these may

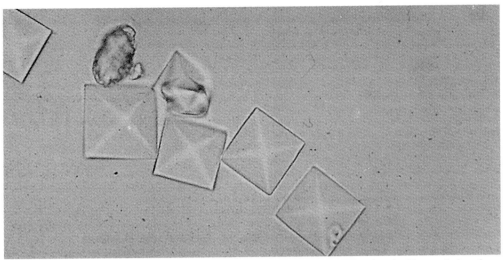

Urine sediment showing calcium oxalate crystals (magnified 160 times). Reprinted with permission, from Osborne CA and Stevens, JB: Handbook of canine and feline urinalysis, Ralston Purina, 1981.

contain magnesium ammonium phosphate hexahydrate (commonly called MAP stones, triple phosphate stones, or struvite stones), ammonium acid urate (also called urate stones), cystine uroliths, calcium oxalate, and others. The magnesium ammonium phosphate uroliths are by far the most common, accounting for about 60% of uroliths.

Calculi can and do occur in all breeds of dogs but the most commonly affected breeds include Schnauzers, Poodles, Dachshunds, Shih Tzu, Dalmatians, Cocker Spaniels, Pugs, many terriers, Basset Hounds, Corgis, Bulldogs, and Yorkshire Terriers. However, there is some breed variation when it comes to individual types of uroliths. For instance, MAP (struvite) uroliths are most commonly seen in Miniature Schnauzers, Welsh Corgis, Dachshunds, Poodles, English Cocker Spaniels, Beagles, and Scottish Terriers. Calcium oxalate crystals (the most common type in people) are most commonly seen in Miniature Schnauzers, Miniature Poodles, Yorkshire Terriers, Lhasa Apsos, and Shih Tzus. Approximately 60% of urate uroliths are seen in Dalmatians. Most cystine uroliths are seen in Dachshunds, Mastiffs, Australian Cattle Dogs, Bulldogs, Chihuahuas, Bullmastiffs, Newfoundlands, Basenjis, Australian Shepherds, Scottish Deerhounds, Staffordshire Terriers, Miniature Pinschers, Pit Bull Terriers, Welsh Corgis, Silky Terriers, and Bichons Frises. Most silicate uroliths are seen in German Shepherd Dogs.

Over 90% of canine uroliths occur in the bladder or urethra and not in the kidneys. In the female urinary tract, most small stones pass through the urethra because it is shorter, straighter, and wider than that of the male. In the male

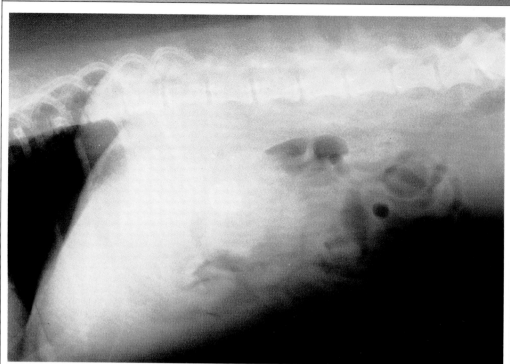

Radiograph of the abdomen showing a white spot that corresponds to a urolith lodged in the kidney.

Urine sediment showing MAP (triple phosphate) crystals.

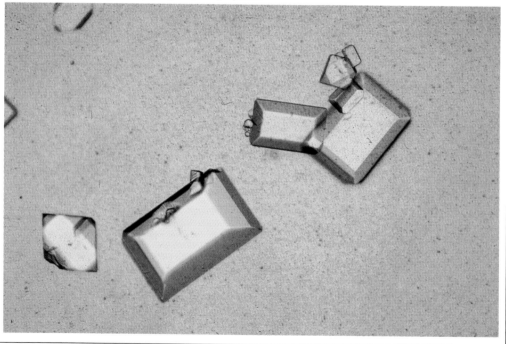

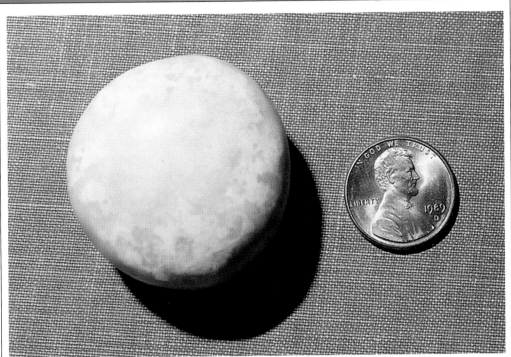

A typical urolith surgically removed from the bladder of a dog. The penny is shown for size comparison. Courtesy of Dr. Randy Walker, Sun Lakes Animal Clinic, Sun Lakes, Arizona.

Uroliths composed of 60% calcium apatite and 40% magnesium ammonium phosphate hexahydrate, which were surgically removed by Dr. Jack Henry of Mesa Veterinary Hospital, Mesa, Arizona. Analysis and photo by the Urolithiasis Laboratory, Baylor College of Medicine, Houston, Texas.

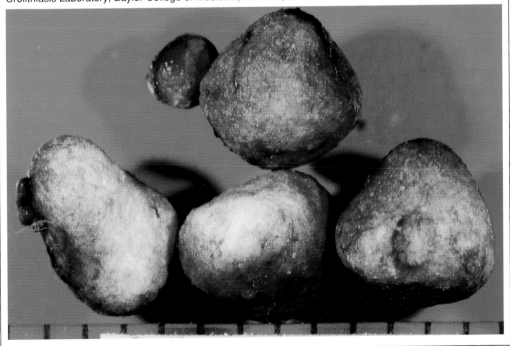

urinary tract, it is common for the stones to occlude or "plug up" the urethra, thereby causing a situation in which the dog cannot urinate until the stones are removed.

Although the exact cause of urolith formation cannot always be determined, some contributing factors to stone formation have been identified. These include: urinary tract infection with urea-splitting bacteria; genetic metabolic abnormalities producing crystals; infrequent urination so that urine accumulates in the bladder allowing time for stones to form; and acquired disorders resulting in the excretion of abnormal amounts of certain compounds into the urinary tract.

Clinical Signs

In most dogs, there are no problems from crystal formation in the urine. There is only a problem when the crystals form "stones" or when they abrade or damage portions of the urinary tract.

Some clinical signs that may be evident in dogs with urolithiasis are: blood in the urine, difficulty urinating (dysuria), inappropriate urination, and reduced size and force of the urine stream. Abdominal discomfort may result from straining, and signs of kidney failure (vomiting, loss of appetite, lethargy) may occur if calculi obstruct the flow of urine from the body.

Diagnosis

Urolithiasis can usually be easily diagnosed by examining urine and by taking appropriate radiographs.

Sometimes, large stones can even be felt in the bladder by careful palpation.

Urine analysis (urinalysis) can be easily performed on samples and often helps to detect the crystals which form uroliths. It can also aid in detecting such conditions as bacterial infections, tumors, diabetes, etc. Since bacterial infections are commonly associated with urolithiasis, culture and sensitivity testing of urinary tract microbes may also be helpful. Together with other tests, blood counts and organ profiles are often performed to produce a more complete picture of overall patient health.

Radiography and ultrasonography (ultrasound) are very helpful in detecting the presence of "stones." Radiographs of the abdomen are often taken in suspect cases because most stones are more dense than the surrounding tissues and will show up on a radiograph. Some stones (most notably urate uroliths) are the same density as the surrounding tissues and will not show up on a plain radiograph. Other methods must be used to diagnose these stones, such as contrast studies. Ultrasound examinations are very helpful in detecting urinary tract stones but are not commonly available in all veterinary clinics.

If a urolith is found in the urine or is "passed," it can be analyzed to determine its chemical composition. This is important because it can help predict the cause of the problem and the best ways to avoid future episodes. This can also be

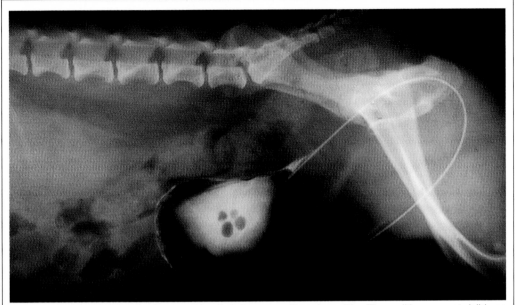

Radiograph of the bladder of a six-year-old male Schnauzer with urate uroliths. The uroliths were not visible on standard radiographs but can be distinguished when liquid contrast media is injected into the bladder, as in this case. Courtesy of Dr. Randy Walker, Sun Lakes Animal Clinic, Sun Lakes, Arizona.

accomplished by using a special technique to collect bladder stones with the aid of a urinary catheter. Special laboratories can determine the actual makeup of stones by sophisticated tests such as optical crystallography, x-ray diffraction, or infrared spectroscopy. Knowing the chemical composition of the urolith helps determine how and why it occurred and the best methods of treatment and preventing relapses. Approximately 60% of uroliths are MAP (struvite), 15% are calcium oxalate, 6% purines (e.g., uric acid), 2% are cystine, and most of the others are mixtures.

Therapy

The treatment for canine urolithiasis can involve either surgical removal of the stones or attempting to dissolve them so they can pass out in the urine. Surgery is usually preferred when a quick remedy is needed, such as when animals are in pain or when a stone is blocking the kidney or ureter. In these cases, uroliths should be sent to a laboratory in order to determine the type and the most appropriate way to prevent further occurrences.

Medical approaches to the problem center on causing the stones to dissolve in the urine so that they can be more easily passed. Often the solubility can be increased by changing the pH of the urine; some uroliths are more prevalent in alkaline urine, and some in acidic urine. Reducing the amount of stone-forming crystals in the urine usually means that fewer stones are likely to form. Increasing the volume of urine produced is more likely to dilute the crystal concentration.

Adjusting the pH of the urine is a good way to encourage uroliths to dissolve. MAP (struvite) crystals tend to form in alkaline urine and are best dissolved if the urine can be made more acidic. Other stones may be more prevalent in acidic urine and so can be dissolved if the urine can be made more alkaline. Changing the pH of the urine can be done with medications, certain nutritional supplements, or with special diets. These special diets tend to limit the specific mineral found in the urolith and reduce the urine concentration of urea in addition to changing the pH of the urine. These diets often produce more urine so that crystals become diluted and dogs urinate more frequently. This frequent urination is important so that crystals can be excreted before they become large enough to cause problems.

Treating bladder infections with antibiotics is often needed because bacterial infections are commonly associated with these conditions. Antibiotics are often continued during the entire time that the uroliths are being dissolved because, as the stones form, bacteria are trapped within the stone and will become released and start new infections as the various layers of the stone dissolve. A urease inhibitor, acetohydroxamic acid, is sometimes used to dissolve those struvite uroliths that are resistant to antibiotic and dietary treatment.

When medical management is used rather than surgery, periodic radiographs and urinalyses should be performed to check progress. If successful, medical management is usually continued for at least one month after the stones are no longer visible on the radiograph to make sure that they have been completely dissolved. It sometimes takes several months to dissolve uroliths completely.

ADDITIONAL READING

Bamberg-Thallen, B; Linde-Forsberg, C: Treatment of canine benign prostatic hyperplasia with medroxyprogesteron acetate. *Journal of the American Animal Hospital Association*, 1993; 29(3): 221-226.

Bartges, JW; Osborne, CA; Polzin, DJ: Recurrent sterile struvite urocystolithiasis in three related English Cocker Spaniels. *Journal of the American Animal Hos-pital Association*, 1992; 28: 459-469.

Beckman, S: Cesarean section. *Pet Focus*, 1990; 2(2): 7-8.

Bull, RW; Gerlach, JA: Paternity testing in small animals. *Compendium for Continuing Education of the Practicing Veterinarian*, 1992; 14(1): 44-50.

Case, LC; Ling, GV; Franti, CE; *et al*: Cystine-containing urinary calculi in dogs: 102 cases (1981-1989). *Journal of the American Veterinary Medical Association*, 1992; 201(1): 129-133.

Chastain, CB; Ganjam, VK: *Clinical Endocrinology of Companion Animals*. Lea & Febiger, Philadelphia, 1986, 439-548.

Cook, SM; Dean, DF; Golden, DL; et al: Renal failure attributable to atrophic glomerulopathy in four related Rottweilers. *Journal of the American Veterinary Medical Association*, 1993; 202(1): 107-109.

Forsyth, K: Mammary Cancer. *Pet Focus*, 1990; 2(2): 18-20.

Gilbert, RO: Diagnosis and treatment of pyometra in bitches and queens. *Compendium for Continuing Education of the Practicing Veterinarian*, 1992; 14(6): 777-783.

Hahn, KA; Richardson, RC; Knapp, DW: Canine malignant mammary neoplasia: Biological behavior, diagnosis, and treatment alternatives. *Journal of the American Animal Hospital Association*, 1992; 28: 251-256.

Johnson, CA; Walker, RD: Clinical signs and diagnosis of *Brucella canis* infection. *Compendium for Continuing Education of the Practicing Veterinarian*, 1992; 14(6): 763-772.

Kawakami, E; Tsutsui, T; Shimizu, M; et al: Effects of oral administration of chlormadinone Acetate on canine prostatic hypertrophy. *Journal of Veterinary Medical Science*, 1993: 55(4): 631-635.

Kerwin, SC; Lewis, DD; Hribernik, TN; et al: Diskospondylitis associated with *Brucella canis* infection in dogs: 14 cases (1980-1991). *Journal of the American Veterinary Medical Association*, 1992; 201(8): 1253-1257.

Krawiec, DR; Heflin, D: Study of prostatic disease in dogs: 177 cases. *Journal of the American Veterinary Medical Association*, 1992; 200(8): 1119-1122.

Lulich, JP; Osborne, CA: Catheter-assisted retrieval of urocystoliths from dogs and cats. *Journal of the American Veterinary Medical Association*, 1992; 201(1): 111-113.

Odin, M: Dubey, JP: Sudden death associated with *Neopspora caninum myocarditis* in a dog. *Journal of the American Veterinary Medical Association*, 1993; 203(6): 831-833.

Olson, PN; Schultheiss, P; Seim, HB: Clinical and laboratory findings associated with actual or suspected azoospermia in dogs: 18 cases (1979-1990). *Journal of the American Veterinary Medical Association*, 1992; 3(1): 478-482.

Peter, AT; Jakovljevic, S: Real-time ultrasonography of the small animal reproductive organs. *Compendium for Continuing Education of the Practicing Veterinarian*, 1992; 14(6): 739-746.

Reberg, SR; Peter, AT; Blevins, WE: Subinvolution of placental sites in dogs. *Compendium for Continuing Education of the Practicing Veterinarian*, 1992; 14(6): 789-796.

Walker, R: Canine urolithiasis. *Pet Focus*, 1990; 2(1): 16-19.

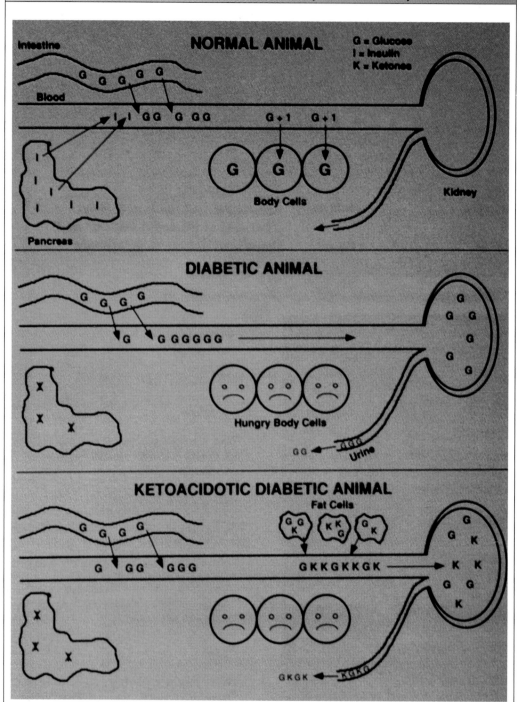

Relationship of glucose, insulin, and ketones in the body of a normal, diabetic and ketoacidotic dog. Courtesy of Dr. Katherine Rogalle, East Maryland Animal Hospital, Scottsdale, Arizona.

Endocrine (Hormonal) Disorders

The endocrine system is a complex collection of glands that produce hormones and secrete them directly into the bloodstream. Some diseases are caused when hormone levels get too low (e.g., hypothyroidism), some are caused when levels are too high (e.g., Cushing's disease) and others may be an indirect reflection of disease (e.g., growth hormone-responsive dermatosis).

Most hormone systems function by a negative feedback mechanism, like the furnace in a house. When hormone levels in the blood get too high, the system turns off; when those levels get too low, the system turns back on. In this way, the hormone levels fluctuate throughout the day between their high and low values. This happens as an active process every minute of every day for all hormones and this is what complicates evaluation of these hormone levels.

Because hormone levels in the blood fluctuate so widely throughout the day, taking one blood sample and hoping for a diagnosis is often wishful thinking. Very often it is necessary to "stimulate" the system or "suppress" it to see how high or low the levels actually go, or to perform more exacting tests.

DIABETES MELLITUS

Diabetes mellitus in dogs is not rare. It is primarily caused by processes that damage the pancreas, killing those specific cells that produce insulin. Genetics is only rarely implicated; a line of Keeshonden is believed to have a genetically determined form, and a familial form of the disease has been reported in Golden Retrievers. Regardless of the cause, diabetes mellitus is characterized by a relative deficiency of the hormone insulin. Insulin is responsible for directing the tissue uptake, utilization, and storage of glucose (blood sugar). Therefore, with insulin deficiency, blood levels of glucose rise. This is also facilitated by another pancreatic hormone, glucagon, that tends to increase in secretion as insulin levels fall.

Insulin is produced in the pancreas by specialized endocrine cells (B cells) which empty their product directly into the bloodstream. It is the role of insulin to allow all of the cells of the body to absorb glucose for energy. This glucose, in turn, is derived from the food we feed our pets, which is absorbed from the intestines into the bloodstream. Without insulin, glucose cannot be absorbed by body cells, regardless of the amount of glucose present in the bloodstream. Without glucose, the

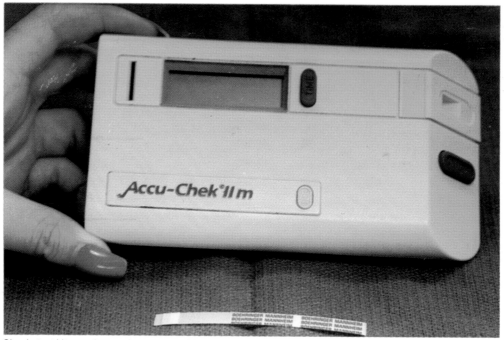

Simple test kits can be used to measure blood glucose levels in the clinic or at home.

cells have no energy to function and the animal feels hungry despite the fact that the animal continues to eat and has abundant levels of glucose in the blood. When the body cells become extremely starved for energy, they will break down body stores of fat which releases glucose and ketones. The bloodstream can only hold so much glucose, and when the amount becomes excessive (approximately 180 mg/dl where normal is 60-100 mg/dl), the excess spills over into the urine.

Diabetes in people is usually subdivided into three types: insulin-dependent diabetes mellitus (IDDM), noninsulin–dependent diabetes mellitus (NIDDM), and secondary diabetes mellitus. Insulin-dependent diabetes mellitus (IDDM) is the most common form of diabetes seen in the dog. However, unlike the situation in people, this is more commonly seen in middle-aged and older dogs.

Secondary diabetes mellitus is also common in the dog. Blood-sugar levels can be elevated in several other conditions, such as hyperadrenocorticism (Cushing's syndrome), acromegaly, and pancreatitis. It can even develop in association with estrus ("heat") in bitches and with chronic administration of corticosteroids or progesterone-like drugs. Finally, there is at least compelling circumstantial evidence that diets high in processed carbohydrates (especially sugars) might precipitate diabetes mellitus in dogs as well as in people.

Clinical Signs

When glucose can't get to body cells, it can't be used for energy. Therefore, dogs with diabetes mellitus tend to feel hungry even though they're eating well. Because these same dogs lose glucose in their urine, they urinate more. In turn, this makes them thirsty, even though they're drinking plenty. These are the cardinal signs of diabetes—dogs eat more, drink more, and urinate more than usual.

Even though dogs with diabetes mellitus tend to eat and drink more than usual, they urinate more than usual and tend to progressively lose weight. This is because they can't absorb the glucose they derived from their food.

If diabetes is left untreated, the animal will begin to break down body fat into glucose and ketones to feed the starving cells. This additional glucose causes higher blood-sugar levels, and ketones make the blood acidic. Abnormal acid levels in the blood can be very dangerous. Ketones also "spill over" into the urine. Diabetes, in its uncontrolled state, also increases the risk of infections and cataracts.

Diagnosis

The diagnosis of diabetes is usually not difficult since blood and urine profiles often reveal significantly elevated levels of glucose and/or ketones. Animals should be fasted prior to assessing blood-glucose levels since glucose levels rise following feeding. Normal dogs have fasting glucose levels below 110 mg/dl while fasting levels greater than 200 mg/dl are generally considered diagnostic for diabetes mellitus. Glucose tolerance tests are rarely indicated in dogs but may be useful in cases of high blood-glucose levels without glucose loss into the urine.

Non-insulin-dependent diabetes mellitus occurs in some dogs, as it does in people. These dogs tend to be overweight and they may go into spontaneous remission from time to time without insulin. In these cases, it is appropriate to measure

Urine levels of glucose and ketones can be tested by comparing the color of the dipstick (once dipped into the urine) with the color codes on the bottle.

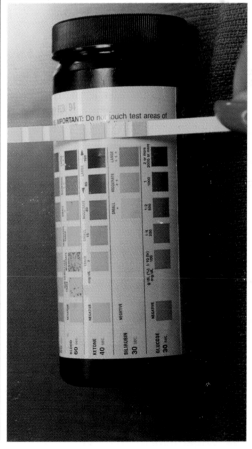

insulin levels which tend to be inappropriately high for the amount of glucose in the blood. This indicates that the diabetes is a secondary phenomenon.

A suspect diabetic is often a good candidate for full blood and urine diagnostic screening tests, not only to pinpoint the correct diagnosis but also to assess other organ function including that of the liver, pancreas, and kidney. Diabetes often results in fat deposition in the liver, elevated cholesterol, and altered electrolytes.

Based on laboratory findings, diabetics are often categorized depending on the extent of their problem. Animals with uncomplicated diabetes mellitus have all the characteristics of diabetes without the potentially life-threatening complications of acidosis or coma. Diabetic ketoacidosis is a sequel to untreated diabetes mellitus, in which there are ketones present in the blood which makes the system more acidic. Nonketotic hyperosmolar syndrome is a rare form of diabetes seen in animals with heart or kidney failure. These dogs also have sodium imbalances and may be found unconscious or severely depressed.

Therapy

Animals diagnosed with diabetes require daily insulin injections. Insulin cannot be given orally because it is digested and broken down into ineffective by-products. Also, oral hypoglycemic drugs used in people are not useful in most

dogs although they have been effective in a small percentage of obese animals.

When diabetes mellitus is first diagnosed, it is advisable to hospitalize the dog for careful scrutiny and repeated blood and urine testing. During this time, the dog will be stabilized with the correct insulin dose. Although there are guidelines for dosing based on body weight, each dog is an individual and the optimal dose will be determined after several days of testing. Most dogs with diabetes are treated with beef/pork insulin unless problems of resistance develop. Eli Lilly and Company planned to discontinue its Ultralente Iletin (Extended beef/pork insulin zinc suspension) as of September 1, 1993. Other insulin sources include pork, beef, and recombinant human insulin. Dog insulin is identical to pork insulin. However, because its effects are shorter lived than the beef/pork combination, it is not the first choice for therapy. Regular insulin is most often used to treat ketoacidosis initially. This type of insulin works quickly but doesn't last very long (five to eight hours) in the body.

Before a pet is released from the hospital, you must learn how to give insulin injections and to collect and test a pet's urine for glucose. A regimented diet (type, quantity, schedule) will be prescribed. It is important to keep accurate records. Urine test results, insulin dose, appetite and water consumption, as well as weekly body weight, should all be recorded. A wall calendar works well for this purpose.

Dogs with diabetes mellitus need to lead regulated lives. They need to be fed the same food, in the same amounts, and at the same time each day. This is because the insulin requirement depends on diet and exercise (which affect glucose levels). Irregularities in schedule make it more likely that dogs could receive an insulin overdose, which is potentially fatal.

The insulin injections can be painlessly given into the subcutaneous fat, after the morning urine has been analyzed for glucose and ketones. This is accomplished with test strips available from pharmacies. The procedure is repeated prior to the evening meal. The dose can be altered as per a veterinarian's instructions. Once stabilized and well managed at home, the symptoms of diabetes will disappear and an animal can have a good quality life for many years. In most cases, twice-daily injections of insulin get better control than injections given only once daily.

For animals receiving insulin, it is important to check blood levels of glucose often. This has been simplified in people with the use of at-home tests. A new alternative for pets is an implanted capillary filtrate collector (CFC). It allows blood samples to be collected frequently without the need for multiple needle punctures. A device can be simply implanted beneath the skin surface in about ten minutes with local anesthesia only, and the animal fitted with a jacket that has a zippered pocket to hold the external portion. The device pulls fluid painlessly from small vessels located in the subcutaneous fat and makes it available for laboratory analysis of glucose levels as well as other tests. The animals could then be maintained the same way people are, with glucose level checks as often as three times daily. This reduces stress, allows appropriate dosing of insulin, and should lessen the complications which may be associated with diabetes.

Diabetes exists when the blood-glucose levels get too high (hyperglycemia). However, with insulin treatment, occasionally the blood-sugar level can get too low (hypoglycemia). This can occur for many reasons, such as injecting too much insulin, a dog not eating all its food, or too much exercise or stress for the amount of insulin given. Signs of low blood sugar include weakness, confusion, dizziness, staggering, convulsions or "fits," and occasionally even collapse. If any of these symptoms occur, the pet needs sugar immediately. In this emergency situation, place two to three tablespoons of Karo syrup in the animal's mouth. The sugar only needs to contact the animal's gums where it will be absorbed; it does not need to be swallowed. Be careful not to use too much syrup as there is danger of the pet choking. If the pet does not recover or improve within ten to 15 minutes, a veterinarian should be

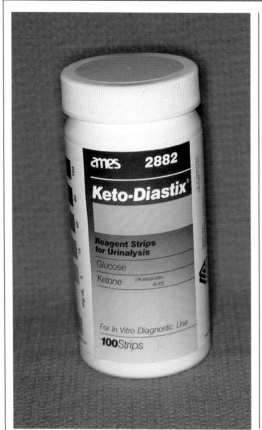

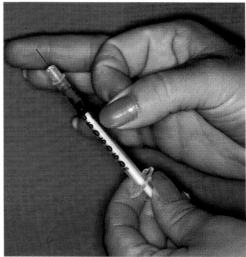

Above: Insulin is administered with special syringes that are measured in units and have a very fine needle. Courtesy of Dr. Katherine Rogalle, East Maryland Animal Hospital, Scottsdale, Arizona.

Left: Dipstick tests for glucose and ketones can be purchased at a pharmacy for use at home. Courtesy of Dr. Katherine Rogalle, East Maryland Animal Hospital, Scottsdale, Arizona.

Below: In-home use of the capillary filtrate collector (CFC), for diabetic animals. Courtesy of Ash Medical System, Inc, W. Lafayette, Indiana.

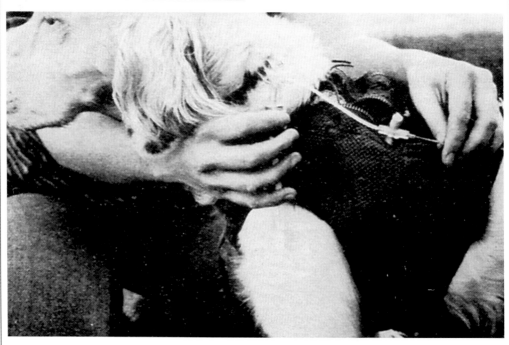

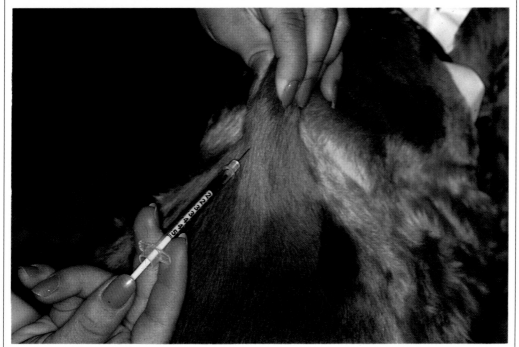

Insulin can be administered as a painless subcutaneous injection. Courtesy of Dr. Katherine Rogalle, East Maryland Animal Hospital, Scottsdale, Arizona.

The most commonly used insulin products for home maintenance of the diabetic dog.

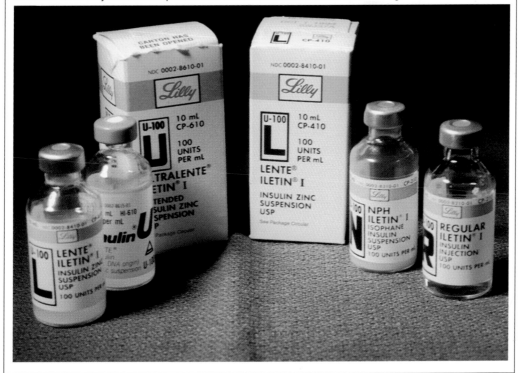

contacted immediately. It does not hurt a pet to have high blood-glucose levels temporarily but low blood glucose is life-threatening and constitutes an emergency.

Both the quality and quantity of food given to a diabetic pet are important. Usually a veterinarian will have determined the amount of food required and the specific times of day to feed the animal. It is essential to stick to this amount and schedule precisely as variation will affect the pet's insulin requirement. The type of food (dry, semi-moist or canned), the brand, and even the flavor (beef, chicken, liver, etc.) may affect the energy content of the food as well as digestibility. This affects the amount of glucose a pet absorbs from each meal. Since the same amount of insulin is injected every day, a pet's meals should consist of the same amount, same type of food, and be given at the same times each day. Remember, *no* table scraps or treats between meals. Water should be available at all times. It is essential to adhere to the standardized diet.

For diabetic dogs that are overweight, a safe weight-loss program should be considered. Obesity is associated with insulin resistance and decreased glucose tolerance. In fact, appropriate weight loss may be sufficient to control secondary diabetes without any insulin at all. Restricting the caloric intake to 60% of that required for an animal of normal weight will accomplish safe weight loss of about 3% of body weight per week. Most of the commercially available reducing diets are relatively high in fiber. This allows dogs to eat a usual amount but actually ingest fewer calories. Also, fiber has been found to be an important regulator of blood-glucose levels in diabetics. Diets with a fiber content of about 15% on a drymatter basis are recommended. There are several of these diets available from veterinarians and specialty outlets. Finally, semi-moist diets should be avoided because of their high sugar content.

Just like people, pets can also experience insulin resistance. Insulin resistance is a condition in which a normal amount of insulin produces an inadequate response; the anticipated dose fails to regulate the blood sugar level. The phenomenon may result from a decreased sensitivity to insulin, a decreased maximum response to insulin, or a combination of the two.

There are many reasons why some animals develop insulin resistance. Some are relatively simple to deal with and some are not. The female progesterone sex hormones, often referred to as progestagens, affect blood-glucose levels and therefore problems are anticipated in cycling bitches or those animals receiving these compounds used to treat other conditions. Other causes include: problems in insulin administration; inactive or outdated insulin; hyperadrenocorticism (Cushing's syndrome); acromegaly; infection;

anti-insulin antibodies; obesity; impaired absorption and pancreatic tumors. If insulin resistance is suspected, further diagnostic testing is always warranted.

Current research is examining other options for managing the 14 million human diabetics in the United States, and some of the benefits are likely to be applied to animals as well. Studies at the Johns Hopkins School of Public Health in Baltimore are experimenting with insulin inhalers. Patients using the device actually inhaled five to ten times the amount of insulin in normal injections in order to simulate the same effect. The insulin reaches the lungs and is then absorbed into nearby capillaries. The inhaler is not only more convenient but it may actually control glucose levels better than injections.

HYPOTHYROIDISM

Hypothyroidism is the most commonly diagnosed endocrine disorder in dogs. That said, it is also one of the most difficult endocrine diseases to diagnose accurately. For purposes of definition, hypothyroidism describes a condition in which there are low levels of thyroid hormones in the blood.

Like most endocrine glands, the thyroid gland produces hormones in response to stimulation by other hormones. Thyrotropin-releasing hormone (TRH) is produced in the hypothalamus of the brain. This then stimulates the pituitary gland, located at the base of the brain, to secrete another hormone, thyroid-stimulating hormone (TSH). Finally, TSH stimulates the thyroid gland to produce two hormones, thyroxine (T-4) and 3,5,3-triiodothyronine (T-3). Although hypothyroidism may be attributable to low levels of either T-4 or T-3, decidedly T-4 is the more important hormone and the one most likely to cause problems in hypothyroidism. This is true, even though T-3 is three to four times more potent than T-4.

The most common cause of hypothyroidism in dogs is lymphocytic thyroiditis, known in people as Hashimoto's thyroiditis. The second most common cause is idiopathic follicular atrophy, which is degeneration of the thyroid tissue for no apparent reason. Iodine deficiency is almost never a cause of hypothyroidism in dogs fed commercial diets.

There is now much evidence that many cases of hypothyroidism have a genetic basis, and many breeds are prone to developing hypothyroidism. Thyroiditis usually starts between one and three years of age and progresses throughout middle age and may only be clinically detectable later in life.

One of the reasons that hypothyroidism is so difficult to diagnose accurately is that many drugs and different illness can profoundly affect the levels of thyroid hormones in the blood. These dogs have conditions that are variably referred to as "borderline hypothyroidism," "nonthyroidal illness" or "euthyroid sick syndrome." Usually, their

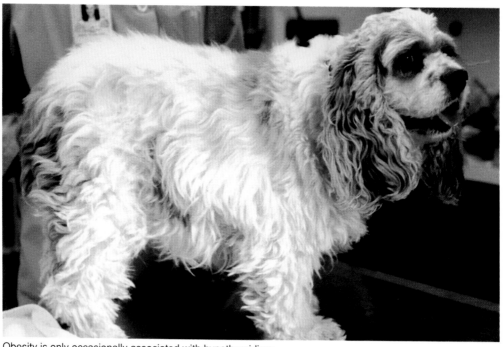

Obesity is only occasionally associated with hypothyroidism.

problem is not related to thyroid function at all. Many drugs, especially corticosteroids, sulfonamides, phenylbutazone, diphenylhydantoin (Dilantin), phenobarbital, diazepam (Valium), and salicylates (e.g., aspirin) profoundly influence the levels of thyroid hormones in circulation. Also, any problem that causes animals not to eat properly for more than two days can dramatically affect thyroid-hormone levels. Several diseases are also known to affect thyroid-hormone levels, including diabetes mellitus, Cushing's disease, kidney disease, liver disease, congestive heart failure and others. Also, since sex hormones can also profoundly affect testing, thyroid profiles are difficult to interpret in intact females within two months following estrus (heat).

The following breeds are prone to hypothyroidism:

Afghan Hound
Akita
Alaskan Malamute
Boxer
Brittany
Chinese Shar-Pei
Chow Chow
Cocker Spaniel
Dachshund
Doberman Pinscher
English Bulldog
Golden Retriever
Great Dane
Irish Setter
Irish Wolfhound
Newfoundland
Pomeranian
Poodles
Schnauzers
Vizsla.

Clinical Signs

There are many misconceptions about the clinical signs seen with hypothyroidism in dogs and how it is best diagnosed. Despite the attention it receives, obesity is only rarely associated with hypothyroidism. Dogs will often appear entirely normal until they have completely used up their reserve of thyroid hormone, which may take several years. The most common clinical signs of hypothyroidism in dogs are lethargy and recurrent infections. Dogs may develop skin problems such as hair loss with hypothyroidism but this is not seen in all (or even most) dogs.

When dogs do have skin problems associated with hypothyroidism, hair loss and cutaneous infections are most commonly seen. The hair loss is not associated with inflammation.

Also, the hair loss is not itchy in the vast majority of cases. Affected dogs have smooth patches of hair loss for no apparent reason, and it is equally divided on both sides of the body. This is referred to as bilaterally symmetrical alopecia.

Diagnosis

The accurate diagnosis of hypothyroidism is difficult because many conditions that have nothing to do with thyroid function can affect test results. Because of this, it is likely that many dogs are diagnosed as hypothyroid but actually have some other problem. There is no single test (other than thyroid biopsy) that will be accurate in all cases. Thyroid biopsy is not routinely done because it poses several surgical and anesthetic risks.

The most common approach to diagnosing hypothyroidism is to

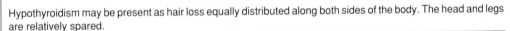

Hypothyroidism may be present as hair loss equally distributed along both sides of the body. The head and legs are relatively spared.

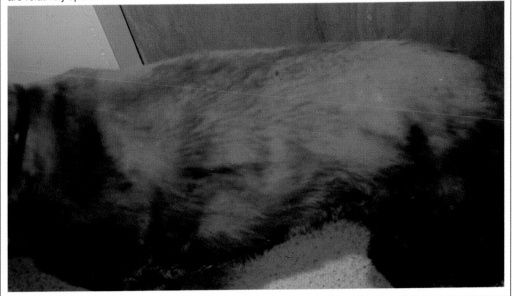

run blood cell tests, biochemical profiles, and thyroid hormone levels to help discern true hypothyroidism from other conditions that might confuse the picture. Over 50% of hypothyroid dogs have high blood cholesterol and often increased triglycerides and lipoproteins as well. A small percentage of affected dogs is also anemic.

Total T-4 and T-3 tests are easy to perform and inexpensive but unreliable on their own because we know that thyroid hormone levels fluctuate greatly throughout the day. At any one time, thyroid levels may be normal in 30-60% of hypothyroid dogs and abnormal in 20% of normal dogs.

There is also some variation in normal thyroid levels related to age, breed, and sex. Puppies have total thyroxine (T-4) concentrations two to five times the normal adult concentrations until about four months of age. After that time, levels continuously decrease with age. There is also some breed variability and the Greyhound has been shown to have lower T-4 levels and higher T-3 levels than mixed-breed dogs. As a general rule (with exceptions), small-breed dogs have higher concentrations of T-4 than do larger breeds. Finally, concentrations of T-4 and T-3 are consistently higher in bitches that are pregnant or in diestrus.

To try and be more specific, other special tests are employed to help confirm the diagnosis. Some laboratories can measure "free" levels of thyroid hormones, the levels which are available to tissues. In general, these have been very helpful. However, recent studies bring into question whether free levels of thyroid hormones provide additional information about thyroid gland function than total levels alone.

TSH stimulation is regarded as the classic diagnostic test for hypothyroidism because it measures the maximum output of thyroid hormones after stimulation of the thyroid gland. Blood samples are collected before and four to six hours after an intravenous injection of TSH. This measures the ability of the thyroid gland to respond to maximal stimulation and is a useful test, though TSH is expensive and difficult to obtain. A similar test, TRH stimulation, is sometimes used when TSH is in short supply, which happens from time to time. The TRH stimulates the pituitary gland to release TSH which in turn stimulates the thyroid gland to release its T-4 and T-3.

In people, a test that measures TSH is regularly used as a reliable measure of thyroid function. A canine version of this test is not yet available and, unfortunately, human test kits cannot reliably measure canine TSH and therefore have not proved useful.

When veterinarians realized that an accurate blood test for hypothyroidism was an elusive goal, predictive formulas (K values) were proposed to help sort out the problem cases. These formulas combine the results of two or more tests (e.g., TSH stimulation, cholesterol, free T-4) to provide a more balanced assessment. It is unlikely that they provide any greater insight into thyroid function than other appropriate individual tests, but the jury is still out on their usefulness.

Thyroid autoantibodies are specific antibodies in the bloodstream that target the thyroid gland, the thyroid hormones, or the protein thyroglobulin. They can be useful predictors of "risk" but do not confirm a diagnosis on their own. Great Danes, Irish Setters, and Old English Sheepdogs have an increased occurrence of autoantibodies. High levels of autoantibody only indicate risk; they do not confirm a diagnosis. Roughly 50-60% of hypothyroid dogs have antithyroglobulin antibodies. The presence of anti-thyroglobulin antibodies (ATA) alone is not an indicator of hypothyroidism; it merely suggests the presence of lymphocytic thyroiditis.

Autoantibody levels alone do not confirm a diagnosis but can be useful as part of a genetic screening program. Together with other thyroid profiles, the presence of anti-thyroid antibodies might suggest a breeding prospect be reconsidered. It can also be used to screen animals at risk of developing the disease. Those animals with normal thyroid function tests but antithyroid antibodies should be further screened every six months for onset of disease. Dogs can also have circulating autoantibody that targets the thyroid hormones, especially T-3. It is important to remember, however, that anti-thyroid hormone antibodies alone do not cause hypothyroidism.

Treatment

Fortunately, treatment of hypothyroidism is simple, inexpensive and very successful. It involves supplementing the hormone (T-4) that is lacking, and doses can be calculated based on body weight or body-surface area. For dogs that are very small or very large, body-surface area is actually a better way to determine dosage than weight. Dogs are typically medicated twice a day, and they will require therapy for the rest of their lives.

Typically, patients are reevaluated after six weeks on therapy and thyroid levels measured four to eight hours after the morning pill is given. This represents the highest level the thyroid hormones are going to reach. If levels are well into normal range, once-daily dosing may be considered, but most dogs are maintained on twice-daily treatment for life. After this, levels should be repeated annually to ensure that the pet is still being maintained in normal range and that the dosage does not require alteration.

It must be remembered that not every dog that appears to benefit from thyroid-hormone replacement actually has hypothyroidism. That would be like saying that if an antibiotic cleared up an infection that it proved the dog had an antibiotic deficiency. Thyroid hormones have many effects, even in dogs with normal thyroid function. This is because of the effects of thyroid hormones on other circulating hormones. Also thyroid hormones may be involved in the regulation of fatty-acid activity in serum as well as in the skin. In these dogs, the improvement seen with replacement therapy is usually temporary.

HYPERPARATHYROIDISM

The parathyroids are small glands that nest in tissues next to the thyroid glands in the neck. They produce the important compound parathyroid hormone (PTH) that regulates calcium balance in the body. When PTH is secreted, it instructs the body to add more calcium to the bloodstream. It accomplishes this by several mechanisms. It causes the kidneys to conserve more calcium, it causes bone to give up some of its calcium, and it indirectly increases calcium absorption in the intestines. The other end of the balancing act is performed by the thyroid hormone calcitonin. It is the job of calcitonin to help lower the blood-calcium levels when they get too high.

Primary hyperparathyroidism occurs when there is a tumor in the parathyroid gland that produces excessive amounts of PTH. This is quite rare in the dog. There is also a rare inherited (familial) form of this disorder which has been reported in the German Shepherd Dog. Once again, this is very rare. More common than this (but still rare) is pseudohyperparathyroidism, in which other cancers produce hormones that act like PTH and cause blood levels of calcium to rise abnormally.

The most common form of hyperparathyroidism is known as secondary hyperparathyroidism. It is called secondary because the problem is not centered in the parathyroid glands themselves. The parathyroid glands only respond to abnormal conditions elsewhere. The most common reasons for this are: chronic kidney disease, intestinal disease with poor absorption, and dietary imbalances.

There are two major reasons why kidney disease can result in secondary hyperparathyroidism. The first is that phosphorus levels in the blood increase in kidney disease and, in general, when phosphorus levels go up, calcium levels go down. This then causes a situation in which the parathyroid glands secrete PTH to try to increase the level of calcium in the blood. The second reason is that vitamin D is important in regulating calcium levels, and vitamin D requires the kidney to become its "activated form." The more kidney damage, the less activated vitamin D, and the blood calcium starts to drop. This once again sends a message to the parathyroid glands and they secrete more PTH.

Hyperparathyroidism due to intestinal disease can occur with any problem that affects the absorption of vitamin D, calcium, or phosphorus from the gut for the reasons listed above. This is usually easy to identify because the "malabsorption" will result in diarrhea that is hard to miss.

One of the most common forms of hyperparathyroidism, and the form that is entirely preventable is secondary nutritional hyperparathyroidism. This occurs when the diet contains too little calcium or too much phosphorus for the amount of calcium in the diet. The ratio of calcium to phosphorus in the diet is critical because too much phosphorus has a negative impact on calcium, as described above. The ideal ratio of calcium to phosphorus in the diet is about 1.3 parts calcium to every one part phosphorus. High-phosphorus diets are usually those inexpensive diets based largely on cereal products. Owners can contribute to the problem by feeding low-calcium foods such as meat, liver, rice, potatoes, and eggs. Another dietary cause of the condition is diets with too low a level of vitamin D and limited exposure to sunlight. This can cause rickets in young animals, but is quite rare.

Clinical Signs

Primary hyperparathyroidism, that caused by a parathyroid tumor, and pseudohyperpara-thyroidism are usually seen in older animals. These dogs secrete excessive amounts of PTH, which causes their blood-calcium levels to climb to abnormal ranges. Since the calcium has to come from somewhere, and diets provide a limited source, most of the calcium dumped into the bloodstream comes from bone. Of course, when the calcium is removed from bone it loses much of its strength. Bony facial swellings, loose teeth, and weakened jaws ("rubber jaw") may all be manifestations. Bones may even break on their own as their mineral content is substantially depleted.

Secondary hyperparathyroidism due to kidney disease is seen at the final stages of kidney failure, when phosphorus levels climb excessively in the bloodstream. Most of these dogs are old but there are exceptions. Congenital and inherited kidney disease has been reported in Norwegian Elkhounds, Cocker Spaniels, Lhasa Apsos, Shih Tzus, Beagles, German Shepherd Dogs, Dachshunds, Miniature Schnauzers, Samoyeds, and Alaskan Malamutes. This congenital form results in rickets (osteomalacia). Teeth may become loose and jaws become moveable (rubber jaw) as the bones of the head lose their supportive strength.

Secondary hyperparathyroidism due to intestinal disease is associated with malabsorption and displays itself as chronic diarrhea. The diarrhea results because some disease has rendered the intestines unable to absorb nutrients found in the diet. Along with loss of other nutrients, the lack of calcium, phosphorus, and vitamin D leads to hyperparathyroidism.

Secondary hyperparathryoidism due to dietary problems can be insidious because most owners don't realize they're doing anything wrong. These dogs don't have symptoms of kidney disease and they don't develop diarrhea. In many cases they seem like they're in good health, have a shiny coat, and may even be obese. Therefore, these dogs may be in trouble before anything abnormal is ever noticed. The problem may start out as a "shifting-leg lameness" or a reluctance to move or play. They may have difficulty eating and eventually they may lose teeth. In young dogs, they may not grow as well as expected and some may develop bowing of the legs (rickets). At this point they are in big trouble and at risk of breaking bones because their bones are severely weakened.

Diagnosis

The diagnosis of the different forms of hyperparathyroidism are based on routine laboratory tests and, if needed, specific measures of parathyroid hormones.

When blood levels of calcium are very high (hypercalcemia), primary hyperparathyroidism and pseudohyperparathyroidism are the most likely diagnoses. A careful physical examination and routine laboratory tests are essential since lymphosarcoma (a tissue cancer of lymphocytes, a type of white blood cell) and malignant cancers of anal sac glands are actually more common than primary cancers of the parathyroid glands. If necessary, measurements of actual parathyroid hormone (PTH) can be performed and elevated levels would suggest a primary parathyroid cancer.

Routine blood tests are also handy when diagnosing secondary hyperparathyroidism. These conditions differ from primary hyperparathyroidism and pseudohyperparathyroidism in that blood-calcium levels are usually decreased, not elevated. Animals with kidney disease will have abnormalities in their blood and urine profiles to suggest the cause of the problem. Animals with chronic diarrhea will have the diagnosis of malabsorption made on the basis of blood and stool evaluations. Laboratory findings in the dog with dietary causes for the disease will include low levels of calcium or high levels of phosphorus in the blood, but these are rarely conclusive.

One diagnostic test that may shed light on the situation is using radiography (x-rays). When the mineral content of bone is decreased, this can usually be depicted on radiographs as thinning bone. Dental radiographs may show loss of bone in the jaws and loosened teeth. A search for reasons may turn up hyperparathyroidism as the cause.

Therapy

Obviously, the treatment for hyperparathyroidism differs radically depending on the ultimate cause. Animals with cancers of the parathyroids or other tissue will require cancer therapy which may involve surgery or chemotherapy. Animals with kidney disease or bowel disease will need their specific maladies addressed and corrected if possible.

Most attention on treatment should be directed at secondary hyperparathyroidism of dietary origin. This can be done simply and safely by placing dogs on a balanced diet with appropriate levels of calcium, phosphorus, and vitamin D. If no fractures have occurred, skeletal strength can return to normal in about three months. Dogs should have their activity restricted for the first four to eight weeks so that they don't cause fractures while skeletal strength is still weak.

HYPERADRENOCORTICISM (CUSHING'S DISEASE)

Hyperadrenocorticism, commonly called Cushing's disease or Cushing's syndrome, describes a condition in which the body produces too much cortisol, its own form of cortisone. Cortisol is produced in the adrenal glands, which are located at the top poles of the kidneys. Other hormones are also produced by these glands, including small amounts of sex hormones.

The adrenals work on a negative feedback loop similar to the thyroid gland. When blood levels of cortisol get below normal, CRF (corticotropin-releasing factor) is released from the hypothalamus in the brain. This causes ACTH (adrenocorticotropic hormone) to be released from the pituitary gland at the base of the brain. This, in turn, causes the adrenals to release cortisol into the blood.

Because of the way the loop works, hyperadrenocorticism can result from several different mechanisms. Most (approximately 85%) result from pituitary brain tumors that secrete large amounts of ACTH. This, in turn, stimulates the adrenal glands to produce excessive cortisol. In a smaller percentage of cases (15%), the disorder is caused by a tumor on one of the adrenal glands. This tumor then secretes large amounts of cortisol directly. The tumors that cause hyperadrenocorticism do not need to be malignant to cause problems. Most tumors of the pituitary are benign but result in the secretion of ACTH which, in turn, causes high levels of cortisol. About half of the adrenal tumors are actually malignant. The Boxer, Boston Terrier, Poodle, and Dachshund are prone to hyperadrenocorticism.

There is one other common way that dogs can develop a form of Cushing's syndrome—if they are treated with corticosteroids, a family of cortisone compounds. These drugs are used commonly in veterinary medicine, especially to treat allergies, immune-mediated diseases, and other inflammatory conditions. We refer to this variant as iatrogenic (doctor-caused) Cushing's syndrome. This syndrome can result from the use

One of the most common blood abnormalities seen in dogs with Addison's disease is electrolyte imbalances. Sodium levels have a tendency to be lower than normal and potassium levels have a tendency to be higher than normal. This is because the adrenal hormone aldosterone is responsible for electrolyte regulation. If potassium levels get high enough, they can be toxic to the heart, which might be evident on electrocardiograms (EKG) and radiographs (x-rays). The ratio of sodium to potassium is therefore an important indicator of electrolyte balance, and indirectly reflects adrenal gland function. This is a helpful clue but not absolute in all cases.

The diagnosis of Addison's disease is made by utilizing the ACTH stimulation test, the same one used in the diagnosis of Cushing's syndrome. With Cushing's disease, the cortisol level in the blood tends to markedly increase after an injection of ACTH. On the other hand, with Addison's disease, the cortisol level fails to stimulate after the ACTH injection. This is because the adrenal glands can't make enough cortisol to respond to the injection in dogs with Addison's disease.

Since Addison's disease is potentially fatal, it is sometimes necessary to start therapy before the results of the ACTH stimulation test are available. If this is necessary, a rough guide to the likelihood of the diagnosis being correct can be made by looking at white blood cell counts before and after the injection. Normal dogs tend to increase their eosinophil counts and decrease their neutrophil-to-lymphocyte ratio after the injection. Evaluating these changes and any important electrolyte imbalances may allow for a presumptive diagnosis while awaiting confirmation.

Therapy

When Addison's disease has not been promptly diagnosed, the consequences may be dire and emergency measures necessary. These dogs may have significantly decreased blood pressure (hypotension), abnormal electrolyte levels, and their blood may be too acidic. All of these abnormalities can result in death if not effectively dealt with. These will therefore need to be addressed with prompt fluid therapy before specifically dealing with the adrenal disorder.

The treatment for dogs with Addison's disease is to replace the hormones the dogs are unable to make themselves. Replacing cortisone is not difficult because prednisone is inexpensive and readily available. Also the dose of prednisone used is quite low so it causes few if any side effects.

The difficult part of therapy has always been the replacement of mineralcorticoids, the hormones responsible for regulating electrolyte levels in the body. The treatment may involve daily administration of fludrocortisone acetate (e.g., Florinef: Squibb) but now there are some other alternatives. Recently, an injectable form, desoxycorticosterone pivalate (DOCP), has been found to suitably control the condition in dogs. It can be given as intramuscular injections every 21-25 days, making it more convenient in some cases than the daily oral form. A final option is the surgical implantation of DOCA pellets beneath the skin. These may provide controlling medication for up to ten months. However, implants are often the most expensive and least reliable form of therapy. Day-to-day levels may fluctuate greatly, and overdosage is a major concern. Whichever form of therapy is selected, blood tests will need to be collected periodically to monitor response to treatment and to allow dosage changes as needed.

GROWTH HORMONE-RESPONSIVE/ADRENAL SEX HORMONE-RELATED CONDITIONS

By the title of this condition it should be obvious that there are a lot of questions unanswered that lead to much confusion in this area. The condition was originally called growth hormone-responsive dermatosis because it was thought that the hair loss in these dogs was due to a relative deficiency of growth hormone. If growth hormone is deficient in young animals, they become dwarfs; it was thought that a growth-hormone deficiency later in life might cause hair loss. This is a fine theory with very little real evidence to back it up. In fact, there is mounting evidence that the cause of the problem is actually an imbalance of sex hormones that come from the adrenal gland. Therefore, this condition may actually be a variant of Cushing's syndrome. The defect, in Pomeranians at least, appears to be similar to late-onset 21-hydroxylase deficiency in human beings.

Clinical Signs

Males are much more commonly affected than females, and most affected animals are quite young, often one to three years of age. Various breeds are affected, but those predisposed include the Chow Chow, Pomeranian, Poodle, Airedale, Samoyed, American Water Spaniel and Keeshond. Affected animals start to lose hair on their trunks but the legs and head remain relatively spared. In time, the skin often becomes quite dark in the areas of hair loss. These animals have no "disease"; they are perfectly healthy except for the hair loss and darkening of the skin.

Diagnosis

Because the exact cause of the condition is still a matter of debate, it should not be surprising that diagnostic testing is also controversial. The first test used when this condition was originally described was growth-hormone-stimulation testing. Drugs are given that stimulate maximal secretion of growth hormone and the diagnosis confirmed in those animals that do not stimulate adequately.

The most exciting breakthrough in diagnosis of this perplexing condition is the use of adrenal sex hormone levels. It is thought that sex hormones produced by the adrenal gland may be at the root of the problem. These include dehydroepiandrosterone sulfate (DHEAS) and androstenedione, which are increased in many cases. Unfortunately, these hormone tests are only available from a very few specialized laboratories.

Treatment

Therapy for this perplexing condition can be directed at correcting either growth-hormone or sex-hormone levels. Since the condition does not affect the health of the animal, treatment is only indicated for cosmetic reasons. Neutering is always an excellent recommendation, especially in Chow Chows and Samoyeds, which respond especially well to this form of therapy.

Growth hormone can be used in therapy but it is scarce and quite expensive. Although many regimens exist, it is usually administered twice weekly for six weeks, or every other day for three weeks. Hair growth is expected within about three months. Treatment with growth hormone is not without risk, and diabetes mellitus may result because of the effect on insulin levels. Therefore, blood-glucose levels should be monitored throughout treatment.

Ketoconazole has been shown to affect sex-hormone levels and has successfully managed cases of growth-hormone-responsive dermatosis. Undoubtedly, its effect on adrenal hormones is the reason for its success. This drug is more commonly used to treat deep (systemic) fungal infections.

Mitotane (o,p'DDD; Lysodren) is a treatment for pituitary-dependent hyperadrenocorticism (Cushing's syndrome) but is receiving attention for its success in treating some of these disorders. It has been particularly helpful in Pomeranians, in which an adrenal enzyme deficiency has been documented. Of course, this treatment is not without risk so monitoring is a critical aspect of therapy.

SEX-HORMONE DISORDERS

The common sex hormones of females (e.g., progesterone, estrogen) and males (testosterone) can sometimes cause problems in dogs, but much less often than most people think. Because more and more dogs are being neutered at a young age, hormonal abnormalities are becoming even less common.

Hyperestrogenism results when levels of the female sex hormone estrogen get too high in the bloodstream. This can occur for several different reasons. Although some bitches may produce abnormal amounts of estrogen from cysts or tumors on their ovaries, many more are affected by drugs that contain this hormone. Drugs such as diethylstilbesterol (DES) contain estrogen and are

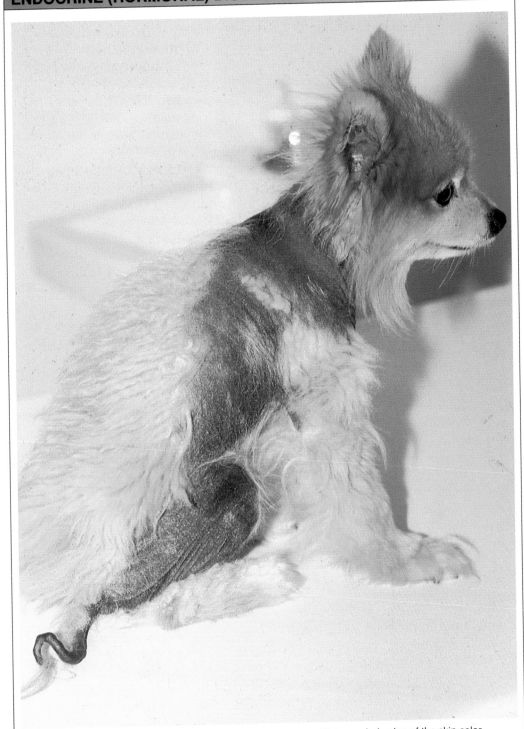

Growth-hormone-responsive dermatosis usually has hair loss and intense darkening of the skin color.

used to treat conditions such as incontinence.

Estrogen-responsive dermatosis occurs when blood levels of estrogen are too low. It has never been documented, however, that these animals are really deficient in estrogen. It is presumed that the cause is low levels of estrogen because it is most commonly seen in bitches that were ovariohysterectomized (spayed) at a young age. The followup argument is that these bitches often improve if treated with estrogen compounds such as DES. However, many researchers are currently re-investigating this condition in search of real answers.

Testicular tumors can sometimes secrete female sex hormones and result in hyperestrogenism in male dogs. The incidence is much higher in cryptorchid dogs, those dogs in which one or both of the testicles have not descended entirely into the scrotum. It is presumed that the increased temperature of the testicle within the body makes it more prone to developing cancers. Some of these cancers, especially Sertoli-cell tumor, produce estrogen that can reach toxic levels in the bloodstream.

Hormonal hypersensitivity is a rare hormonal problem in which dogs develop allergic reactions to the hormones they produce. As might be anticipated, this is an exceptionally rare condition. It is most commonly seen in females, especially those with a history of pseudopregnancy, cystic ovaries or irregular "heat" cycles.

Clinical Signs

With hyperestrogenism, there is hair loss around the genitals, on the underside, and extending down the hind legs. Often the vulva and nipples are swollen because of the high circulating levels of female sex hormones. Itchiness, waxy ears, and a greasy, scaly haircoat are frequent secondary features of the disorder and heat cycles are irregular, prolonged, or suppressed. There may also be a history of previous endometritis or pyometra. In time, the gums may be pale because estrogen is toxic for the bone marrow.

Bitches with estrogen-responsive disorders usually have dribbling of urine (urinary incontinence). There may be hair loss around the genital areas and down the backs of the hind legs. When there is hair growth in these regions, it is soft and downy. The vulva and nipples remain infantile in appearance because of lack of stimulation from sex hormones.

For dogs with testicular tumors, the cancerous testicle is not always obvious, especially if it has remained within the body (cryptorchidism). These dogs often develop what is referred to as "feminizing syndrome." Because of the female sex hormones the cancerous testicle is producing, they may develop hair loss around the genitals, grow breasts (gynecomastia), and have a drooping prepuce. In time, they may also develop prostate problems and estrogen-induced bone-marrow suppression.

Most canines with hormonal hypersensitivity are females. They tend to develop most of their itchiness around the genitals and hind end. In time, they may develop waxy ear conditions (ceruminous otitis), which are also common with other allergies.

Diagnosis

The diagnosis of sex-hormone-related conditions is complicated by the fact that there may be many different forms of hormones involved and that most veterinary laboratories do not have the capability of running these tests.

For hyperestrogenism, blood counts are evaluated since chronically high circulating estrogen levels cause bone-marrow suppression. Blood samples for estradiol and estrone levels may be helpful sometimes, but not consistently. The preferred diagnostic test is ovariohysterectomy (spaying) since it represents diagnosis and treatment in one step. Obviously this is not a desirable option for breeding bitches.

For estrogen responsive conditions, most diagnostic tests are not helpful. Once bitches have been spayed, measuring sex hormones in the blood is a futile task. The condition is described as "estrogen-responsive" rather than "estrogen deficiency" because these animals respond to treatment with estrogens even if they don't have an actual deficiency. At this point, we really don't know the exact cause. However, estrogens should be used cautiously because of possible suppression of the bone marrow.

Dogs with testicular tumors may have detectable lumps on a testicle but these are not always evident. If this diagnosis is suspected, blood counts are usually performed since the high estrogen levels may suppress bone marrow activity. Surgical removal of the testicles and their assessment by a pathologist will provide a diagnosis in most cases. Since about 10% of these tumors are malignant and may spread (metastasize), chest radiographs (x-rays) are advised if the tumor turns out to be malignant.

Hormonal hypersensitivity is very rare and somewhat difficult to diagnose. A modified allergy test can be performed using the classic sex hormones (estrogen, progesterone, testosterone) but the diagnostic accuracy of this test is presently unknown. The best option is neutering. If the cause of the itchiness is hormonal hypersensitivity, there will be a dramatic reduction of the problem within ten days of neutering.

Treatment

The treatment of choice for naturally occurring hyperestrogenism is ovariohysterectomy (spaying). This removes the cysts or tumors that are producing abnormal levels of estrogen. After surgery, improvement is noted within three to six months. When the condition is the result of treatment utilizing estrogen-containing drugs, treatment options should be carefully evaluated, and the estrogen discontinued if possible. The long-term toxic effects of estrogen therapy include bone-marrow suppression, which can be fatal if not properly managed.

By definition, the condition estrogen-responsive dermatosis responds to estrogen. However, estrogen has many side effects, the most important of which is bone-marrow suppression. Otherwise, these bitches do not have a medical condition that would do them any harm. Sometimes the incontinence can be managed by very low doses of estrogens given infrequently, and sometimes other medications will suffice.

The only treatment of choice for testicular tumors is surgical removal of the testicles. Actually, castration is suggested for any dog with retained testicles. Since these animals can't be used for show purposes anyway, there is little reason for them not to be neutered

Canines with sex-hormone imbalances usually display hair loss down the back of the thighs and around the genital area.

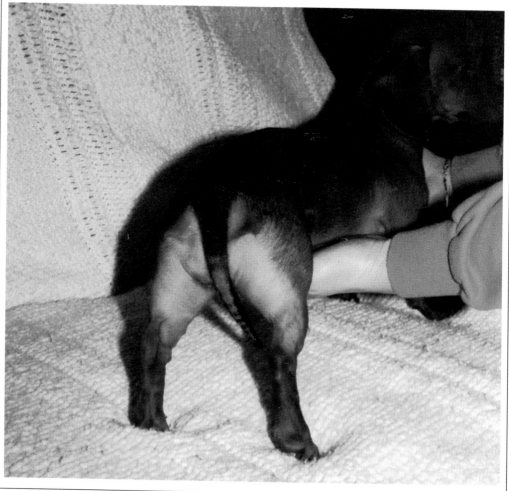

while young. This not only prevents any risk of testicular tumors but also makes prostate problems later in life an unlikely prospect. If a malignancy has been confirmed by biopsy, it is important that radiographs of the chest be taken to look for evidence of spread. This would warrant specific cancer therapy.

Hormonal hypersensitivity is rare and so few treatment options have been explored. Neutering is the preferred approach and results in resolution of the itching within a week or so. If the itching does not resolve, it is likely that the diagnosis was incorrect to begin with. Hormonal hypersensitivity does not respond well to antihistamines or corticosteroids the way allergies might.

ADDITIONAL READING

Ackerman, L: *Practical Canine Dermatology*. American Veterinary Publications. Goleta, CA. 1989, 369 pp.

Beale, KM; Keisling, K; Forster-Blouin, S: Serum thyroid hormone concentrations and thyrotropin responsiveness in dogs with generalized dermatologic disease. *Journal of the American Veterinary Medical Association*, 1992; 201(11): 1715-1719.

Beale, KM; Halliwell, REW; Chen, CL: Prevalence of antithyroglobulin antibodies detected by enzyme-linked immunosorbent assay of canine serum. *Journal of the American Veterinary Medical Association*, 1990; 196(5): 745-748.

Campbell, L; Davis, CA: Effects of thyroid hormones on serum and cutaneous fatty acid concentrations in dogs. *American Journal of Veterinary Research*, 1990; 51(5): 752-756.

Chalmers, SA; Medleau, L: Identifying and treating sex-hormone dermatoses in dogs. *Veterinary Medicine*, 1990; 1317-1330.

Feldman, EC; Mack, RE: Urine cortisol: creatinine ratio as a screening test for hyperadrenocorticism in dogs. *Journal of the American Veterinary Medical Association*, 1992; 200 (11): 1637-1641.

Fiorito, DA: Hyperestrogenism in bitches. *Compendium for Continuing Education of the Practicing Veterinarian*, 1992; 14(6): 727-729.

Jensen, RB; DuFort, RM: Hyperadrenocorticism in dogs. *Compendium for Continuing Education of the Practicing Veterinarian*, 1991; 13(4): 615-620.

Lynn, RC; Feldman, EC; Nelson, RW: Efficacy of microcrystalline desoxycorticosterone pivalate for treatment of hypoadrenocorticism in dogs. *Journal of the American Veterinary Medical Association*, 1993; 202(3): 392-396.

Nelson, RW: Dietary therapy for diabetes mellitus. *Compendium for Continuing Education of the*

Practicing Veterinarian, 1988; 10(12): 1387-1392.

Nelson, RW; Feldman, EC; Ford, SL: Topics in the diagnosis and treatment of canine hyperadrenocorticism. *Compendium for Continuing Education of the Practicing Veterinarian,* 1991; 13(12): 1797-1805.

Nelson, RW; Ihle, SL; Feldman, EC; Bottoms, GD: Serum-free thyroxine concentration in healthy dogs, dogs with hypothyroidism, and euthyroid dogs with concurrent illness. *Journal of the American Veterinary Medical Association,* 1991; 198(8): 1401-1407.

Nichols, R: Recognizing and treating canine and feline diabetes mellitus. *Veterinary Medicine,* 1992; March: 211-222.

Panciera, DL: Canine hypothyroidism. Part I. Clinical findings and control of thyroid

hormone secretion and metabolism. *Compendium for Continuing Education of the Practicing Veterinarian,* 1990; 12(5): 689-701.

Panciera, DL: Canine hypothyroidism. Part II. Thyroid function tests and treatment. *Compendium for Continuing Education of the Practicing Veterinarian,* 1990; 12(6): 843-857.

Reimers, TJ; Lawler, DF; Sutaria, PM; *et al:* Effects of age, sex, and body size on serum concentration of thyroid and adrenocortical hormones in dogs. *American Journal of Veterinary Research,* 1990; 51(3): 454-457.

Rogalle, K: Diabetes mellitus. *Pet Focus,* 1990; 2(3): 44-46.

Wilson, SM; Feldman, EC: Diagnostic value of the steroid-induced isoenzyme of alkaline phosphatase in the dog. *Journal of the American Animal Hospital Association,* 1992; 28(3): 245-250.

Vaccines and Vaccination

To properly understand vaccination, it is first important to understand the immune system and how it attempts to protect the body naturally. Only then can it be fully appreciated what a vaccine can hope to do.

The immune system is a remarkable system that helps keep animals and people safe from a variety of invaders and diseases. The immune system does not consist of one organ, such as the liver or thyroid, but is a complex array of interrelated cells and organs that function in a balanced and integrated fashion.

The immune system was heralded long before its processes were understood. Vaccination was practiced before viruses were even known to exist and long before we understood the role of antibodies. Somehow it was comprehended that we could inoculate a person or animal with a mild strain of an infectious microbe and the body would develop "immunity" and be protected from that infection in the future. We have used this knowledge to all but completely eradicate smallpox and polio from the human population and greatly reduce the incidence of a variety of infectious diseases in our pets.

IMMUNITY

Immunity refers to all the mechanisms used by the body as protection against environmental agents that are foreign to the body. These foreign substances include drugs, microbes, foods, chemicals, and various inhalants (e.g., pollens).

Although an individual is born with the capacity to mount the defenses provided by the immune system, immunity is only acquired after exposure to the foreign agent. Therefore, pets are not born with protection from rabies. We must introduce it to their system so that they can mount an appropriate, and hopefully protective, response. The substance that triggers the response is known as an antigen, and the protective protein produced by the immune system is called an antibody.

Animals do receive some "passive" immunity from their mothers during nursing. The most important period is the first 24 hours in which colostrum, a antibody-rich portion of the milk, is produced. We call this immunity "passive" rather than "active" because the immunity was actively produced by the mother and then passively transferred to the young; the offspring therefore received some short-lived protection from their mother but have yet to produce antibodies themselves. This provides some residual protection of the newborn for the first few months of life. Vaccination schedules are established to augment this passive immunity by stimulating antibody production by the young at a time when maternally provided antibody levels are waning. As the antibody protection derived from the mother begins to dwindle, we vaccinate so that the young start to produce their own antibodies.

THE IMMUNE SYSTEM

In a very simplified version of the immune system, one can imagine two different but balanced arms, with special white blood cells, the lymphocytes, controlling both. One arm of the system, manned by B-lymphocytes, is known as the B-cell system and functions to produce antibodies. The other arm of the system, manned by T-lymphocytes, is known as the T-cell system and patrols the body perimeter. They are aided in their function by a variety of other cells and cell products.

The B-cell system is most responsive to vaccination because these B-cells evolve into antibody-producing cells known as plasma cells. They produce antibodies which are a response to specific agents. If an animal contracts rabies, specific anti-rabies antibodies are produced by the body in an attempt to control the infection. Unfortunately, with natural infection, most animals die before they can create a sufficient immune response.

Antibody and foreign agent (antigen) fit together like a lock and key so that the collection can be removed by other scavenging cells of the immune system. Sometimes our antibody response is sufficient

Pictorial representation of various different viruses and bacteria. Courtesy of Kenvet.

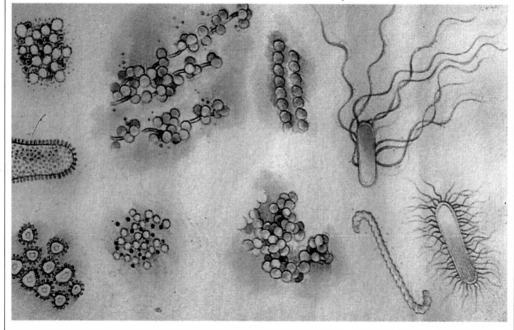

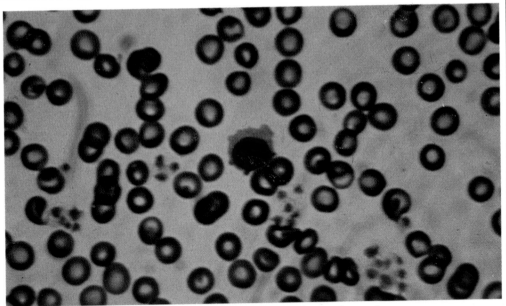

A single lymphocyte found among many red blood cells in a blood smear from a dog.

to control disease and other times it is not. These antibodies are special proteins, also known as immunoglobulins, and in general they can be subdivided into different types.

Immunoglobulin M (or more simply IgM) is the first antibody produced when a foreign substance is introduced to the system. It is a large antibody, perhaps five times larger than the others, and capable of removing many foreign invaders such as viruses and bacteria.

As the immune system becomes more refined, and the infection persists, another antibody (IgG) is produced which is the most common immunoglobulin found in the bloodstream of animals and people. When we vaccinate our pets, it is this antibody (IgG) which is most often produced, and the antibody is specific for the particular disease agent (eg. rabies,

distemper, etc.). These antibodies latch onto the agent when it is encountered and allow it to be cleared from the body by the rest of the immune system.

Another immunoglobulin, IgA, is responsible for resistance to disease in those parts of the body directly communicating with the environment such as the respiratory, digestive, integumentary (skin), and urinary/ reproductive systems. It is a surface-acting antibody that helps control infections at these important boundaries to the outside world. Vaccines that are given into the nose (intranasally) as a spray, such as the ones for tracheobronchitis (canine cough), try to take advantage of producing specific IgA rather than IgG to catch the infection in the respiratory passages before it gets into the bloodstream. Also, IgG does not reach as high levels in the respiratory secretions as does IgA. Several breeds of dog have been recognized with IgA deficiency, the most common of which is the Chinese Shar-Pei.

Finally, IgE is a specific antibody that is involved in the development of allergy. In an evolutionary sense, we believe this antibody was originally important as a response to parasites, but with current hygiene and medical treatment, this has proved unnecessary and even problematic.

It can therefore be seen that there are many different classes of immunoglobulins available to produce antibodies and a limitless number of specific antibodies that can be produced in response to disease-causing agents.

The T-cell system of T-lymphocytes helps moderate the immune response, and some may have helper or suppressor effects on B-lymphocytes. They perform a variety of functions, including helping B-cells make antibodies (T-helper cells), suppressing the production of antibodies (T-suppressor cells), directly attacking target cells, and mediating delayed hypersensitivity reactions (e.g., contact allergy). They also have direct effect by producing special substances (lymphokines) rather than antibodies. The T-cells themselves are not directly responsible for making antibodies but they do help the B-cells recognize when they have to make antibodies in response to infection or vaccination.

THE CONCEPT OF VACCINATION

The purpose of a vaccination program is to prevent the development of disease caused by a variety of infectious agents. It was recognized for centuries, prior to even a fundamental understanding of immunology, that milk maids exposed to cowpox rarely developed smallpox; if they did, it was invariably milder than those in the general population. Edward Jenner, in the late 18th century, experimentally induced immunity to smallpox by inoculating a young boy with pus from a lesion of a dairy maid who had cowpox. The boy was then protected against smallpox. From this protective phenomenon came the term vaccination, from the Latin *vacca*, for cow.

The concept of vaccination was expanded by Louis Pasteur and Paul Ehrlich almost 100 years later. It was only at this time that it became apparent to scientists and doctors that microbes were the cause of those diseases. It was inconceivable to the scientific minds of the day that humans and animals could be harmed by organisms too small to be seen without a microscope.

We now know that by injecting organisms into an animal or person, we stimulate them to produce protective antibodies against those organisms. These antibodies circulate in the bloodstream and engage microbes if they encounter them, removing them from our system before they can do harm. In general, the more identical the vaccine microbe is to the infectious organism, the higher the degree of protection afforded. This is a point of controversy.

As veterinarians, we are proud to be able to provide pets with protective immunity to a number of diseases that were once devastating. Most dogs are protected from rabies, distemper, parvovirus, coronavirus, adenovirus, parainfluenza and others by appropriate vaccination. An initiating series of vaccinations is often necessary to confer immunity, which can then be maintained by periodic "boosters."

An ideal vaccine should include organisms that stimulate an immune response to disease-causing agents, yet not cause any problems of its own. Thus, there are two types of vaccine available: modified-live and inactivated ("killed").

MODIFIED LIVE VACCINES

Modified live vaccines contain a living but relatively harmless strain of a particular microbe. Because the microbes are still alive, they persist well in the animal and stimulate an excellent immune response. The organisms have been modified or "attenuated" so that they do not result in disease when injected. When Jenner injected his young patient with pus containing cowpox virus, he created protection against the related and deadly smallpox virus with an organism causing much milder symptoms.

Unfortunately, although effective for immune stimulation, modified live vaccines are not without problems. Their main problems are that the living organisms can become altered, they can affect the overall immune status, they can be shed and spread to other animals, and they are not safe for use in pregnant animals. Problems can occur if the once-safe organism used in the vaccine reverts in the body to a more dangerous form. This is similar to the occasional outbreak of polio in children when the vaccine was first introduced. This does not happen often but the potential always exists for modified live vaccines. A similar problem occurred in pet ferrets vaccinated with modified live canine distemper vaccine; this can result in actual distemper in the vaccinated animal.

The second problem, one of altered immune status, is potentially more insidious. This problem is compounded by the fact that most vaccines are polyvalent, which means they contain several different microbes. For example, there are many five-way and six-way vaccines on the market, in which one vaccine contains parvovirus, parainfluenza, hepatitis, distemper, and leptospirosis. Could one of the microbes in the vaccine suppress the immune system sufficiently to make it more susceptible to one of the others modified by still-living vaccine organisms? There is at least some early evidence that this is in fact possible. The combination of organisms appear to suppress the immune system to a much greater degree than when the organisms are injected individually. Interactions appears to be most profound when distemper virus is combined with the adenoviruses (adenovirus 1 causes canine hepatitis).

Virus shedding by vaccinated animals does occur and can be beneficial or dangerous depending on the organism. It is known that live canine adenovirus 1 strains can be shed in the urine of vaccinated dogs, and this is one reason there has been a shift to using adenovirus 2 vaccines. Dogs vaccinated with live parvovirus vaccine shed the virus in their feces beginning three to eight days after vaccination. This shedding generally terminates by day 14 but in the interim, contact dogs can acquire the virus and may show some signs of disease.

The main advantages of modified live vaccines are that the weakened virus reproduces in the body and promotes a very high level of protection against infection. Modified live vaccines have been instrumental over the years in greatly reducing the incidence of viral diseases in animals.

"KILLED" VACCINES

Inactivated, non-infectious, or "killed" vaccines are generally safer since the organisms injected are not alive, cannot reproduce in the body, and can never become infectious. They are also not as good at stimulating an immune response because they are less similar than live organisms to the actual agents capable of causing disease. They must often be combined with adjuvants, which are compounds capable of increasing the immune response. These compounds are often irritating and may cause reactions when injected.

Subunit vaccines are different still in that they try to include in the vaccine the important compounds of the microbe that stimulate an immune response without including the whole organism. As we learn more and more about immunology and what it takes to initiate protective immunity, subunit vaccines will undoubtedly become more important. Currently, subunit vaccines are used in the protective vaccination of cats for feline leukemia virus infection.

The principal disadvantage of "killed" vaccines is also its main advantage: the virus does not persist and reproduce in the body. This results in a shorter period of protection, and less actual protection, but the organism can never revert to an infective form and is safer for pregnant and immunosuppressed animals. A further disadvantage posed is that "killed" vaccines may help prevent animals from actually showing disease, but may not be effective enough to actually stop them from being infected. They might thus harbor an infection and pass it along to contacts.

A BALANCED PERSPECTIVE?

There is little doubt that modified live vaccines are more effective.

There is also little doubt that they are indeed safe for the general population of pets. In fact, most vaccines in human medicine come from live viruses, including measles, mumps, and rubella. "Killed" vaccines are safer to use but in most cases are not as effective at conferring protection and often must be given more frequently. Which is the most critical issue, safety or effectiveness? The question is a relative one because clearly both modified live and "killed" vaccines are safe (although "killed" vaccines are safer), and in general both are effective (although modified live vaccines are more effective).

The future will definitely tend away from modified live vaccines in favor of "killed" vaccines, subunit vaccines, and even recombinant DNA vaccines. For instance, the human hepatitis B vaccine introduces a virus that reproduces only particles, not complete organisms. Until technology has advanced significantly, the vaccines we have used for years are both safe and effective and have continued to protect our pets from a variety of devastating diseases while rarely causing problems.

ADVERSE EFFECTS OF VACCINATION

Aren't vaccines always good? Don't we give them because they protect our pets, not hurt them? This is a lofty ideal but, unfortunately, there is no such thing as a drug that is always beneficial. When we use vaccines, we accept the risk of taking the potential bad along with the potential good.

Facial swelling in a dog resulting from vaccination.

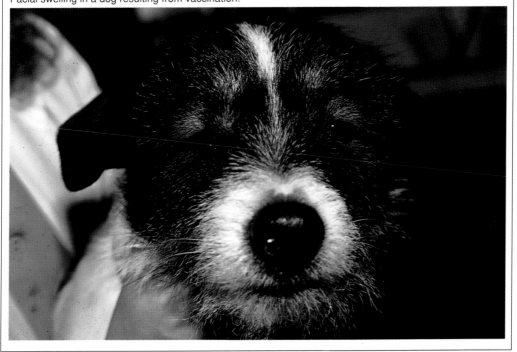

Most experienced veterinarians will tell you that vaccine risks are minimal. But these risks do exist. We are injecting a foreign substance, and often a living microbe into our pets with the hopes of conferring protection. This protection is achieved in the majority of cases if the vaccine was properly handled and administered. It is only reasonable to assume that there must be some risks in return.

Some vaccine reactions may be mild and include soreness at the injection site, mild lethargy, and occasionally hives or swelling of the face. These clinical signs usually disappear a day or two after vaccination. Occasionally life-threatening (anaphylactic) reactions are noted which might include vomiting, diarrhea, seizures, and inability to breathe. These are usually evident within 30 minutes of vaccination and should be treated as veterinary emergencies.

Studies in the dog have clearly demonstrated that polyvalent (more than one microbe) vaccines significantly suppress the lymphocyte count in the blood and the ability of lymphocytes to be stimulated. There is also a decrease in the platelets, the clotting cells of the blood, that lasts for three to ten days following vaccination. These changes do not occur when the vaccine constituents are given individually. The most profound effect occurs when canine distemper virus is combined with canine adenovirus 1 or canine adenovirus 2 in a polyvalent vaccine. And yet, polyvalent vaccines are preferred by pet owners because they are more convenient. Because of these changes, dogs should not be stressed or have surgery for at least ten days after vaccination.

Some components of vaccines can cause adverse reactions on their own. *Leptospira*, the organism that causes leptospirosis, can cause irritation and an adverse reaction in dogs. Since this is mainly a threat to rural dogs only, it would seem sensible that urban and suburban dogs not routinely require vaccination with this microbe.

In recent years, subcutaneous rabies vaccines have become available. Previously, rabies vaccines were given by deep injection into the muscle. The newer vaccines are quicker to administer and cause less pain, but there are some tradeoffs. Over the last several years, these vaccines have caused vaccine-site reactions in several dogs. The breed most susceptible to these reactions appears to be the Poodle. There is hair loss and scarring in a round-to-oval region in the site of the vaccination.

There is also evidence that modified live distemper vaccine given to young dogs can result in disease. Although animals most at risk are under four weeks of age, even in six- to eight-week-old puppies the distemper vaccine may occasionally induce disease.

Several other vaccine-induced reactions have been reported and are only now being thoroughly evaluated. These reactions tend to occur one to three days or ten to 21 days after vaccination, depending on the level of protection the pet already has. Typical signs are fever, stiffness, sore joints, and abdominal tenderness. More severe reactions, such as liver dysfunction and seizures, have also been noted occasionally.

Recently, pathologists have reported a worrisome trend in feline medicine. It seems that particular malignant cancers (sarcomas) have been associated with vaccination sites in cats. The numbers are not epidemic in proportions but troubling nonetheless. It is thought that the reaction may be to aluminum, which is included in some feline vaccines, but this is only conjecture. The real reason for these vaccine-site cancers in cats is not yet apparent, but the same trends have not been noted in dogs.

VACCINE SCHEDULES

Just as initial vaccinations are given to match the waning level of protection pups get from their mother, booster vaccines are given to match waning protection from previous vaccinations. There is no benefit in vaccinating pups four weeks of age or younger. Overvaccination is no better than undervaccination. When vaccines are given too often or spaced improperly (less than ten days apart), the immune system can actually be suppressed, which is counterproductive. This not only hinders the ability of the immune

system to make protective antibodies in response to the vaccination but may also increase the risk of disease. Ideally, vaccinations should be spaced three to four weeks apart to allow the immune system to fully process the vaccines before they are repeated.

The initial vaccination schedule is meant to increase your pet's protection just as the temporary protection it received from its mother is waning. If you vaccinate too early, you just interfere with maternal protection. If you vaccinate too late, you leave a period of time when your pet is defenseless. A compromise is therefore reached, and vaccinations generally commence at six to eight weeks of age and continue every three to four weeks until 16–20 weeks of age. These last vaccines are the most important because they are given at a time when there should be no interference from maternal antibodies the pup received while nursing. You may see quite a variation in vaccination schedules between different veterinarians depending on the types of vaccine used, local risk factors, and personal preferences.

A vaccination schedule may include various immunizations so it's best follow your own veterinarian's advice because schedules will reflect local conditions and risks. Vaccine schedules are not static because we learn more each year about vaccination than we did the year before. It now seems apparent that one vaccina-

A Sample Vaccination Schedule

AGE	VACCINE
6 weeks	Parvovirus Coronavirus (depending on risk)
8 weeks	Distemper Hepatitis Parainfluenza Parvovirus Coronavirus
12 weeks	Distemper Hepatitis Parainfluenza Rabies Parvovirus Coronavirus
16 weeks	Parvovirus Distemper Hepatitis Parainfluenza
20 weeks	Parvovirus (depending on risk)
12–16 months	Parvovirus Distemper Hepatitis Parainfluenza Rabies
Annually	Rabies (every one to three years) Parvovirus (every three to 12 months) Distemper Parainfluenza
Others	Bordetella Lyme disease Leptospirosis

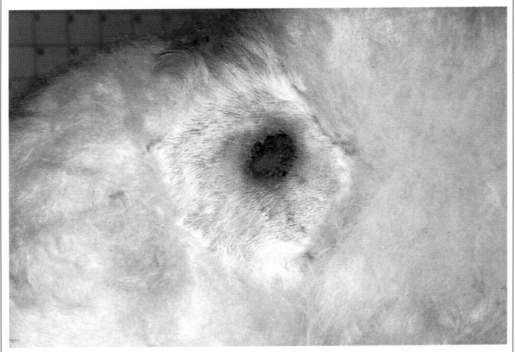

Injection site reaction from vaccination.

Rabies is a public health threat. Make sure your dog is vaccinated and not a danger to others. Courtesy of Toronto Academy of Veterinary Medicine, Toronto, Canada.

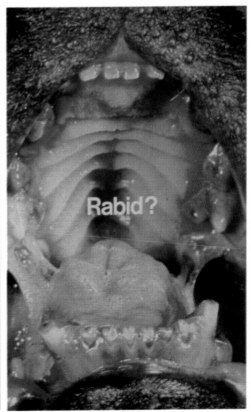

tion with adenovirus, the hepatitis virus, may confer immunity for life. However, until this is definitively proven, annual vaccination will likely still continue. Parvovirus vaccination was once thought to last a year; it is now likely that dogs at risk of exposure should be vaccinated twice yearly to assure that protective levels stay high.

There are some guidelines that do affect vaccine schedules. No animal that is ill should receive vaccinations. This only serves to compromise their immune system further. Similarly, pups stressed with other diseases (e.g., diarrhea, canine cough, internal parasites) should not be vaccinated until they are suitably recovered. Modified live virus vaccines should not be given to pregnant bitches. Whenever possible, vaccines should not be given at the same time as corticosteroids (cortisone), anti-inflammatory agents (e.g., phenylbutazone), estrogens (e.g., diethylstilbesterol), or organophosphate insecticides. The combination can severely suppress the pet's immune system.

There is also some likelihood that the amount of vaccine administered might be altered, depending on the individual animal. At present, the same dose is administered regardless of whether the patient is a five-pound Chihuahua or a 150-pound Great Dane. Recent studies with the hepatitis B vaccine in human children have shown adequate and safe protection with one-fifth of the adult dose. Shouldn't we follow suit in veterinary medicine? This will need further research but the benefits may be worth the effort.

There is one final concern when it comes to vaccination schedules and dosages. Modified live vaccines are formulated and tested by manufacturers with the assumption that they are being given to animals with normal immune systems. Since we have no way of determining in advance which normal-appearing animals do not have normal immune systems, there will always be unknowns with regard to vaccination. This probably explains, to some degree, why some animals that have been properly vaccinated still contract diseases for which they have been "protected." Vaccines must be cautiously administered to pets with known immunodeficiencies.

HOME VACCINATION

Recently, some vaccines have become available, over the counter, from retail outlets and even by mail order. For the most part, the quality of these vaccines seems acceptable. As to their effectiveness and safety, it is more difficult to say since handling and administration are critical issues.

To be effective, vaccines must be administered to healthy pets so that the pet is capable of mounting an appropriate immune response. The vaccine must be kept refrigerated until administered, properly loaded into a syringe, and injected into the proper location. If the pet is actually ill, even though it may appear fine, vaccination may do more harm than good, because it taxes the immune system to some extent. When the vaccine is purchased on a shopping trip, does it sit in the car for several hours while the rest of the shopping is being done? Both heat and freezing affect the vaccine.

There is also a concern for public health when it comes to home vaccination. Needle sticks can be a serious concern for owners and discarded supplies are potential risks for all family members. All medical supplies are intended to be disposed of hygienically so as not to endanger people or the environment. That means that they should not be discarded in the family garbage.

Vaccinations must also be given into the correct location to be effective. Injection around a nerve can result in paralysis. Injection into a small blood vessel can result in potentially fatal reactions. Injection into the skin (intradermal injections) can cause lumps and adverse immunologic reactions. And, if there is an adverse reaction to the injection (it's rare but it does happen), you are in no position to deal with the situation effectively at home. It is hard to justify the cost savings with so many risks.

If you are extremely money-conscious, it may seem reasonable to buy and administer your own vaccines, but it hardly makes sense where your pet's health and well-being are concerned.

RABIES

Rabies was first described as early as 2300 B.C. and is a potentially fatal disease in pets; and, of course, it poses risks to people as well. In nature, rabies survives from year to year in several wildlife species. Although the rabies virus can potentially infect any warm-blooded animal, there are three species that are responsible for most cases in the United States and Canada. These are the skunk, fox, and raccoon. Although bats carry rabies as well, rabies in bat populations is not on the rise. Also, preliminary evidence does not suggest that bats play an important role in transmitting disease to wildlife such as skunks, foxes, and raccoons.

Approximately 90% of all cases of rabies in the United States are found in wildlife. And these numbers are on the rise. For example, from 1990 to 1991, there was a 46.8% increase in rabies cases. Raccoons represent 44.1% of all cases, followed by skunks (29.7%), bats (9.9%), foxes (4.6%), and others. This incidence is very geographic. For instance, during the same period of time, 81.6% of rabies cases in Mexico were in dogs. In Canada, 45.9% of rabies cases involved foxes, 23.7% were in skunks, and 15% were in cattle. It can be concluded that, in the United States and Canada, rabies in dogs and cats is well controlled by vaccination. However, rabies is on the rise, especially in cats, and this is likely due to the fact that owners are letting their pets roam and not vaccinating them as diligently as before.

The fact that many pets remain unvaccinated and many animals run at large makes the situation difficult to contain. Without a large vaccinated pet population, there is little to buffer the advance of the disease. Without pet control ordinances, pets run at large or remain ownerless and serve as carriers of the deadly disease.

Clinical Signs

The virus that causes rabies exists in wildlife, especially skunks, raccoons, foxes and bats. When they meet up with wandering pets, bites can be fatal. The typical "mad dog" scenario of movies is rarely like the real thing. The stages of rabies can usually be classified as prodromal, furious, or paralytic, although there is much individual variability.

The prodromal stage is characterized by apprehension, anxiety, and personality changes. This typically lasts two to three days in dogs. During the second stage, the furious stage, dogs may be irritable, overly sensitive, and aggressive. Rabid dogs are more likely to exhibit symptoms of paralysis, awkwardness, excessive salivation, and difficulty eating than being aggressive and foaming at the mouth. This stage tends to last from one to seven days.

The paralytic or dumb stage may develop one to ten days after the first clinical signs begin. Paralysis progresses from the site of injury towards the brain and then the rest of the nervous system. It is at this stage that dogs have difficulty drinking water because of paralysis of their facial and throat nerves. This has been described as hydrophobia, or "fear of water," although this is obviously a poor descriptive term. This stage typically lasts two to four days and affected dogs die within ten days after onset of illness.

Diagnosis

Because of the risk to humans, suspected cases of rabies in dogs must be carefully evaluated. There are several tests that have been developed for use in living dogs, but a negative result can not conclusively prove that the dog doesn't have rabies. Tests can be performed on biopsies taken from the whisker areas of the face, scrapings from the corneal surface of the eye, and the cerebrospinal fluid. However, if a dog has not been vaccinated, public health officials would prefer the dog be euthanized and that the diagnosis be made safely from postmortem samples.

Therapy

If a vaccinated dog is exposed to rabies, it is typically revaccinated and confined and observed for 90 days. On the other hand, it is too dangerous to manage dogs that have not been previously vaccinated. The recommendation in these cases is euthanasia. Alternatively, postexposure vaccination and the administration of immune globulin, such as done

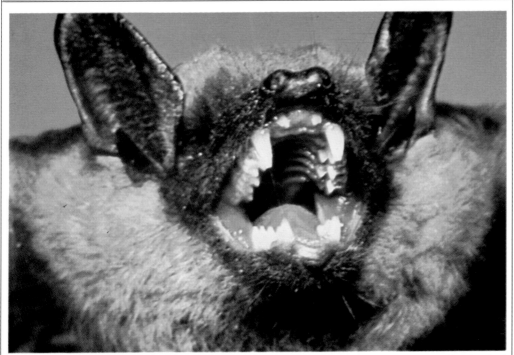

Bats can spread rabies but are not the major cause of rabies in wildlife. Courtesy of Toronto Academy of Veterinary Medicine, Toronto, Canada.

in people, can be attempted, but this poses considerable risk to owners and other in-contact individuals. These animals would need to be quarantined for six months and vaccinated one month before release.

Prevention

Since both animals and people can die from rabies and it is entirely preventable, *all* dogs should be vaccinated for rabies, starting from about three months (12 weeks) of age. The vaccination needs to be repeated as boosters one year later and then at intervals of one to three years, depending on the type of vaccine and the incidence of rabies in each geographic area. In the United States and Canada, rabies vaccination of dogs is mandatory. Unfortunately, in several states there is still no legislation making rabies vaccination mandatory for cats.

Rabies in dogs has been dramatically lessened as a result of vaccination and stray-dog-control programs. Vaccination for rabies can only be performed by veterinarians, and there is no excuse for pets not being protected.

Rabies is a potentially fatal disease in pets, and of course it poses risks to people as well. Sadly, over 20,000 human deaths occur yearly from rabies throughout the world. Many pets remain unvaccinated and many animals run at large (especially cats), despite the widespread warnings in the published word and media. In

New Jersey, for instance, a report estimated that about 50% of dogs and only about 20% of cats were vaccinated.

Strangely enough, lack of legislation is central to the issue of vaccination. In many areas where there are no cat-licensing ordinances, most cats remain unvaccinated as well as unlicensed. In Connecticut, where a strong public awareness program has been instituted, it was estimated that 90% of dogs and 60% of cats statewide were vaccinated. Still, in 1991 there were 200 cases of rabies in Connecticut, compared with 300 in 1990. Without a large vaccinated pet population, there is little to buffer the advance of the disease. Without pet-control ordinances, pets run at large or remain ownerless and serve as carriers of the deadly disease.

In the wild, rabies is carried mainly by raccoons, skunks, and foxes. Raccoons are the most important wildlife vector in the mid-Atlantic region. Research is currently underway to test a wildlife vaccine which has been added to bait in an attempt to create a barrier of immune animals to stop the advance of the disease. It has been proven safe; now it just has to work. If it is successful, it will undoubtedly be used in areas in which rabies is already rampant.

DISTEMPER

Distemper was introduced from Asia about 200 years ago and has nothing to do with a dog's temper. It is caused by a virus which is related to the human measles virus. Severe, fatal distemper can occur in dogs of any age but most commonly affects unvaccinated, exposed puppies three to six months of age. Infected dogs shed large amounts of virus in all their secretions and excretions for 60-90 days after they become infected and pose much danger to other dogs.

Distemper is spread principally by respiratory secretions and aerosols, and it colonizes the cells of the upper respiratory tract. It then spreads in the blood to all the tissues of the body and localizes in the epithelial and nervous-system tissues.

Clinical Signs

Dogs that are exposed to distemper virus but have a well-functioning immune system may only develop mild or inapparent disease. On the other hand, young or immunocompromised dogs often develop brain disease (encephalomyelitis) from infection. Older dogs tend to develop a progressive demyelinating disease with symptoms similar to multiple sclerosis in people. At one time it was feared that distemper in dogs might be linked to multiple sclerosis in people, but this has never been substantiated. It is far more likely that multiple sclerosis is related to measles than distemper.

During mild disease, pups may be listless and have decreased appetite. Often they have discharge from the eyes and nose. Most will also develop a fever. These clinical signs can advance to include vomiting, diarrhea, dehydration, digestive upsets, and a cough.

The most damaging aspect of severe infection is that brain involvement may be evident one to three weeks after apparent recovery. These dogs may suffer from seizures, awkwardness, weakness, and rigidity. Often associated with these neurological signs is thickening of the footpads and scaling of the nose, referred to as nasodigital hyperkeratosis ("hard pad").

Many other clinical signs may be noticed, depending on when infection took place. Infection in the pregnant bitch results in abortions, stillbirths, and the birth of weak puppies. Surviving dogs may have mottled teeth, immune dysfunction, heart ailments (cardiomyopathy), and eye problems. Better than 50% of adult dogs that contract the disease will die. Among puppies, the death rate often reaches 80%.

Diagnosis

Distemper is often suspected in young dogs when there is a history of non-vaccination coupled with respiratory and neurological disease. Basic laboratory work is usually nonspecific. These dogs often have low-blood-lymphocyte counts but this is common in many different diseases.

In animals with neurologic problems, a cerebrospinal fluid (CSF) examination is usually performed. A needle is inserted into the area around the spinal cord and some fluid is removed for analysis. Dogs with distemper tend to have increased protein and cells in their cerebrospinal fluid. Electroencephalography (EEG) may also be performed in dogs with neurological disease and may detect abnormalities more than 90% of the time. A careful ophthalmic examination may detect eye changes (retinochoroiditis) in about 40% of cases of distemper-induced brain disease.

Absolute diagnosis of distemper can be made by tests detecting virus particles or by measuring the change in distemper antibody levels in the blood. Antigen tests can be used to detect distemper in cellular smears from the mucous membranes of the tonsils, nose, or eyes from five to 21 days following infection. They can also detect distemper antigen in footpad biopsies during the first two months of infection.

Single antibody tests will not confirm diagnosis because vaccinated dogs as well as dogs that were previously exposed to distemper will have positive blood tests (titers). In fact, very high titers probably indicate relative immune protection. Therefore tests are performed and repeated ten to 14 days later to see if the titer rises. This would signify active infection. The same testing can be performed on cerebrospinal fluid samples, if needed.

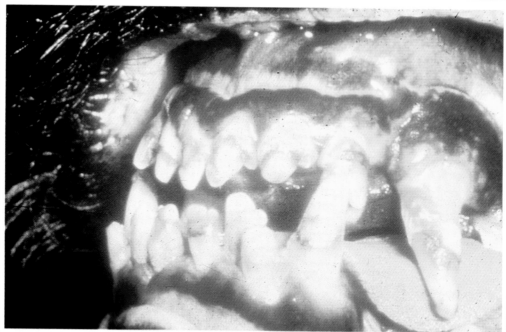

Mottled teeth in a dog with distemper. Courtesy of Dr. Anthony Shipp, Dr. Shipp's Animal Hospital, Beverly Hills, California.

Therapy

There are no specific treatments for distemper. All are symptomatic and supportive. Animals are kept in a clean, warm, and draft-free environment and their clinical signs (symptoms) are treated. Antibiotics are often prescribed, even though they don't directly affect the distemper virus, because affected dogs are susceptible to bacterial infections. High doses of the B vitamins and vitamin C may be helpful because these dogs tend to lose most of the vitamins that they ingest. Intravenous administration is the most direct route for supplementation.

For more severely affected dogs, intravenous therapy will be necessary to correct fluid and electrolyte disturbances. Seizure medications and corticosteroids (cortisone) are sometimes needed to battle the neurological signs that may accompany the disease. Progressive neurological dysfunction is an indication that the disease process has not been halted and warrants a poor prognosis.

For dogs that do recover, it is important to remember that they can continue to shed the virus. Neighbors should be alerted to the diagnosis so they can ensure that their dogs have had booster vaccinations for distemper within the past six months.

Prevention

Distemper is not always easy to diagnose and treatment is symptomatic at best, so prevention is very important. Bitches should be vaccinated before breeding (with a "killed" product) to increase the level of protection they pass on to the pups. The extent of the protection depends on whether the pups nurse immediately and ingest colostrum. In pups that received colostrum from their mothers, protective antibodies will protect them for the first nine to 12 weeks of life. Pups that nurse but didn't get colostrum only have enough protection to last them one to four weeks.

Vaccination should begin in pups six to eight weeks of age with boosters at ten to 12 weeks and again at 14–16 weeks. Some researchers suggest that distemper vaccination should not be given at the same time as parvovirus because there may be interference. Many other researchers appear convinced that there is no legitimate reason for this conclusion.

Dogs older than 16 weeks of age and previously unvaccinated should receive at least two vaccinations at three- to four-week intervals. Occasionally, the first vaccinations given to pups less than 12 weeks of age may be a combination distemper-measles product. Dogs are protected beginning two to three days after vaccination and boosters are given every one to two years. There is also some evidence that vaccination may be effective in preventing an outbreak of distemper if it is administered within four days of exposure, using a modified live virus vaccine.

PARVOVIRUS

Parvovirus ("parvo") is a potentially fatal disease of dogs first

A ten-week-old Rottweiler with severe parvovirus infection. Intravenous fluids were placed in the rear leg due to vein collapse in the forelimbs. Courtesy of Dr. Nita Gulbas, Desert Sage Veterinary Clinic, Phoenix, Arizona.

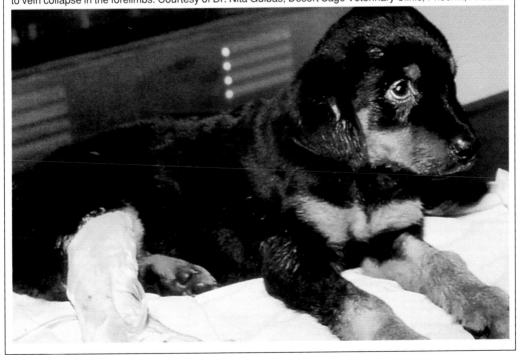

recognized in 1978. By 1980, the disease was being reported worldwide. It is highly contagious and a major cause of diarrhea in dogs, especially young dogs.

Dogs can pass the virus even when they don't seem sick. They can be spreading virus in their stool within three days of exposure, even though they don't usually appear ill until four to seven days following exposure. Although virus shedding in the feces begins to slow down after seven to eight days, the virus will persist in the environment for up to six months under proper conditions.

Clinical Signs

Canine parvovirus is a highly contagious viral infection, causing lethargy, loss of appetite, vomiting and diarrhea, that can be severe and fatal in all ages of dogs. It occurs more commonly in young dogs than in adults.

Dogs get infected when they ingest the virus. The virus then spreads throughout the body, especially to the intestines, bone marrow and, in the young dog, the heart. Approximately three days after exposure and even before displaying overt clinical disease, an exposed animal can begin to shed the virus in normal-appearing stool. Virus shedding decreases after seven to eight days and is rarely present in the stool longer than 12 days following exposure. Even though a dog may stop shedding virus within a week or so, parvovirus will persist in the environment for up to six months.

Many dogs get infected with parvovirus, but not all actually get sick from it. These normal-appearing dogs, however, can shed the virus and spread it to others.

The most common manifestation of parvovirus is severe diarrhea. Dogs developing clinical illness will begin to display signs four to seven days following exposure to the virus. Initially, dogs will be lethargic and depressed. Lack of appetite is accompanied by vomiting and diarrhea, which may contain blood.

The parvovirus targets the small intestine, especially the jejunum and ileum, while the stomach, large intestine, and upper small intestine (duodenum) are usually spared. This part of the small intestine performs some critical functions. It is an important site for absorption of nutrients and also an important region for antibody production by the immune system. Both of these functions are compromised by parvoviral infection. The intestines are no longer capable of fully absorbing nutrients, and the immune system is suppressed. The result can be death if appropriate therapy is not quickly instituted.

Parvovirus can also affect the heart in young puppies, usually when the infection occurs in the first four weeks of life when the heart muscle is rapidly developing. These affected pups usually die by 12 weeks of age, although there have been reports of puppies' surviving and developing heart failure months to years after infection. When the heart is affected, young puppies may display difficulty in breathing, crying, retching, and foaming at the mouth and nostrils. Treatment is often heroic, and rarely successful.

Diagnosis

Parvoviral infection is usually tentatively diagnosed when a dog develops severe diarrhea and vomiting with no known exposure to poisons. Often there is blood present in the stool, and these dogs tend to be dehydrated. Preliminary blood work does not confirm a diagnosis, but the white blood cell counts are often depressed in dogs with parvoviral enteritis (intestinal infection).

An examination of stool for viral particles will confirm parvovirus infection because it actually detects the presence of the virus. There are two testing kits available using fecal hemagglutination (HA) and enzyme-linked immunosorbent assay (ELISA), and both tests have a high rate of accuracy. It must be remembered, however, that if an animal is tested after being ill for greater than one week, virus particles may no longer be present in the stool in high numbers, and the test may therefore be negative even though parvovirus is the actual cause.

Blood tests do not test for the presence of the virus, but rather the unique antibody response to the infection (protective titers). Unfortunately, these tests cannot indicate active infection; they only signify exposure to the virus and the production of antibodies.

Blood tests are convenient when dealing with breeding bitches and trying to determine the level of protection she will confer upon her pups during pregnancy and while nursing. Approximately 80% of the protection is acquired through the milk, and 20% through the placenta when the puppies are still in the mother's uterus. This is important in determining a puppy's vaccination schedule as the antibody protection derived from the mother interferes with vaccination.

Therapy

Rigorous and immediate therapy is needed for the patient affected with parvovirus, or permanent (and potentially fatal) damage can result. Intravenous fluids are critical, because these dogs tend to quickly dehydrate from the vomiting and diarrhea and they suffer from electrolyte imbalances. Medications can also be given intravenously since it is difficult to give oral medications to a dog with vomiting and diarrhea. In mild cases, subcutaneous fluid therapy may be adequate. However, necrosis (tissue death) and sloughing of the skin from subcutaneous administration of fluids has been reported.

Antibiotics are often administered, even though they have no direct effect on parvovirus itself. The viral infection tends to suppress the immune system, which predisposes the animal to secondary bacterial infections, especially bronchopneumonia and

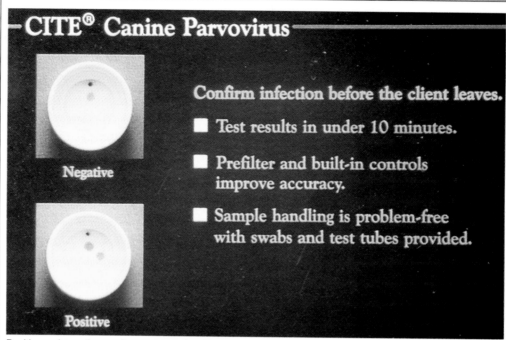

CITE® Canine Parvovirus

Negative

Positive

Confirm infection before the client leaves.

■ Test results in under 10 minutes.

■ Prefilter and built-in controls improve accuracy.

■ Sample handling is problem-free with swabs and test tubes provided.

Positive and negative results on a parvovirus ELISA test (CITE®) performed on stool samples. Courtesy of IDEXX Corporation.

bacterial-associated shock (septic shock). Injectable antibiotic therapy is indicated in these cases.

Prevention

The prevention of parvoviral infection is far more rewarding than therapy. This can be readily accomplished by vaccination and environmental decontamination.

Vaccination against canine parvovirus (CPV) remains the most important tool in protecting the canine population. When parvovirus in dogs was first discovered, there were no canine vaccines and we were forced to rely on feline parvovirus and mink enteritis vaccines, which are caused by similar viruses. These vaccines were not very good and have now been almost completely replaced by vaccines of canine origin.

Both modified live and "killed" parvovirus vaccines are available. As usual, the modified live virus (MLV) vaccines tend to provide the best protection and the "killed" products are thought to be safer. Dogs immunized with canine origin MLV will shed low numbers of living virus in their stool and can thereby "vaccinate" other susceptible animals without causing major disease. As with most vaccines, MLV products should not be used in the pregnant bitch.

Killed vaccines may provide only short-lived protection but are the only safe vaccines for use in the pregnant bitch. It is beneficial to vaccinate a bitch prior to breeding so that she may provide maximum protection to her unborn pups. The vaccination does not interfere with conception or litter size.

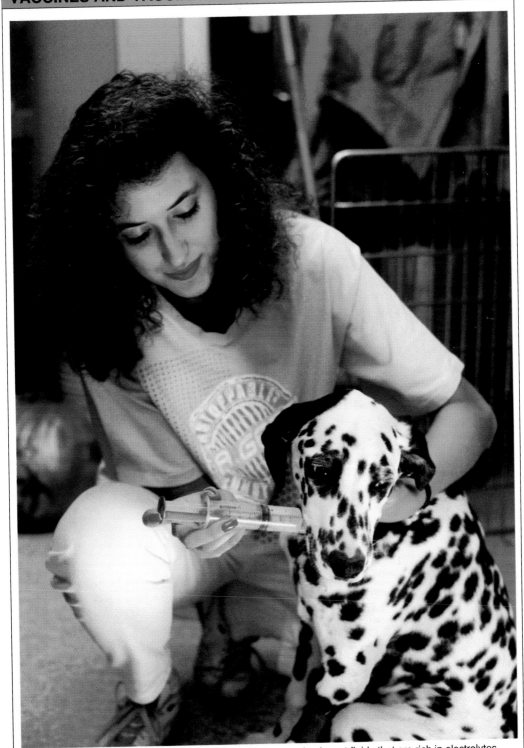

When pups with parvovirus are feeling better, they are coaxed to ingest fluids that are rich in electrolytes.

Viral shedding may still occur in dogs vaccinated with killed vaccines. It is not the vaccine virus that is being shed but infectious parvovirus the dog contracted elsewhere. Therefore killed vaccines prevent active infection if parvovirus is encountered, but the dogs might still acquire and shed that natural virus, even if it doesn't make them ill. This may have significant implications in the kennel environment.

Vaccination should begin at six to eight weeks of age and continue every three to four weeks until the puppy is 16–20 weeks of age. Alternatively, the optimal times to start vaccination can be determined by evaluating antibody levels in the bitch. This will allow an estimate of when the maternal antibodies will likely drop to a point where they won't interfere with vaccination. After this time, the vaccines are continued on schedule, every three to four weeks until 16–20 weeks of age. It is imperative not to stop the vaccinations at too young of an age or young puppies may remain unprotected. Boosters are given every three to 12 months, depending on risk. MLV vaccines should not be given to puppies less than six weeks of age, but killed vaccines are suitable if needed. Since parvovirus may last six months in the environment, bitches that are at risk are often vaccinated (with a killed product) one week before breeding.

Environmental control is another important aspect of parvoviral prevention. Infected dogs shed large amounts of virus in the stool, and this can quickly contaminate an environment for up to six months. It is unlikely that the virus can be totally eliminated in kennel environments, but precautions can be taken to aid in decreasing contamination. Isolation of infected animals is critical. If possible, infected animals should be placed in an area that can be thoroughly cleaned and disinfected. A 1:30 dilution of chlorine bleach (e.g., Clorox) is effective in deactivating the virus on hard surfaces. Daily cleaning and disinfection of animal premises are important in decreasing viral contamination. Feeding animals inside and keeping food supplies well protected so as to avoid contamination of food by flies, roaches, and other insects will aid in decreasing the spread of disease.

CORONAVIRUS

Canine coronavirus is a cause of digestive upset (gastroenteritis) in dogs which is similar to (but usually milder than) parvovirus infection. The virus is similar to one causing gastroenteritis in pigs and to the feline infectious peritonitis virus of cats. People are not likely susceptible to infection. The disease is usually mild, but stress and other infections can increase the severity of the disease. For some reason, outbreaks are more common during the winter months.

Clinical Signs

Canine coronavirus affects only dogs, and the virus is shed in the feces. When acquired by a susceptible dog, the virus spreads throughout the small intestine within four days. Fortunately, coronavirus does not penetrate as deeply into the small intestinal tissue as parvovirus and so less permanent damage is done.

Most dogs affected with coronavirus have a disease similar to parvovirus enteritis, but usually milder. However, poor appetite and lethargy can progress to vomiting, diarrhea, and dehydration, which can be fatal. The digestive upset then persists or is intermittent for the next three to four weeks. Most dogs then recover within seven to ten days.

Diagnosis

The diagnosis is usually rendered based on clinical signs and preliminary laboratory testing. A test for parvovirus on stool samples should yield negative results. If confirmation is needed, blood tests for coronavirus antibodies can be taken initially and repeated in ten to 14 days. Rising levels (titers) suggest active infection with coronavirus.

Therapy

Rigorous and immediate therapy is needed for the patient affected with coronavirus. Intravenous fluids are critical with vomiting and diarrhea because these dogs tend to quickly dehydrate and suffer from electrolyte imbalances. Medications can also be given intravenously since it is difficult to give oral medications to a dog with vomiting and diarrhea. Antibiotics may also be needed.

Prevention

The vaccine currently available for dogs is safer than the one which was originally produced: this had some side effects and was taken off of the market. Typically, the new vaccine is given at six, nine, and 12 weeks of age and offers safe protection from this very contagious and potentially devastating infection.

Environmental control is another important aspect of coronaviral prevention. Infected dogs shed large numbers of viruses in the stool, and this can quickly contaminate an environment. Isolation of infected animals is critical. If possible, infected animals should be placed in an area that can be thoroughly cleaned and disinfected. A 1:30 dilution of chlorine bleach (e.g., Clorox) is effective in deactivating the virus on hard surfaces. Daily cleaning and disinfection of animal premises are important in decreasing viral contamination. Feeding animals inside and keeping food supplies well protected so as to avoid contamination of food by flies, roaches, and other insects will aid in decreasing the spread of disease.

HEPATITIS

Infectious canine hepatitis (ICH) is a viral disease that primarily affects the liver. It was first described in 1947 and is caused by a virus called canine adenovirus type I (CAV-1). Dogs and foxes serve as reservoirs for this virus and can shed virus in their urine for up to nine months. The virus is highly contagious and is transmitted by contact with infected animals, parasites, and items that have been in contact with infected animals.

Clinical Signs

The disease is most commonly seen in dogs less than one year of age, particularly in pups nine to 12 weeks of age. Most dogs are infected by breathing in infectious viral particles. The virus localizes in the tonsils and then disperses the virus to all body tissues, including the liver, kidney, and eyes. The bodies of most healthy dogs recognize the virus and make protective antibodies. This clears the virus from the system and the dog recovers. Even in unvaccinated dogs, almost half will become resistant to hepatitis infection.

When dogs produce insufficient amounts of antibodies, they develop the syndrome recognized as infectious canine hepatitis. They often look like they've been poisoned. They have fever, abdominal pain, bruising on the gums and other mucous membranes, and convulsions and coma may also occur. Severely affected pups may be dead within a few hours.

Less severely affected dogs will be depressed, weak, and disoriented. They have little interest in eating, may have a fever, and often have vomiting and/or diarrhea. Their lymph nodes (often referred to incorrectly as "glands") may be enlarged.

Whereas a high antibody level results in cure, and a low antibody levels results in hepatitis, intermediate levels of antibody may cause yet another syndrome—immune complex disease. These dogs may have mild disease symptoms but their immune response is insufficient to clear the virus. What happens then is that clumps of virus and antibody circulate in the bloodstream; some lodge in the eye and cause uveitis, which clinically is referred to as "blue eye." This blue-eye phenomenon was more common when the first vaccines for hepatitis were introduced. Since then, the virus present in the vaccine has been changed so that this doesn't occur, or at least very rarely.

Dogs with chronic disease caused by this virus develop liver disease (hepatitis), as well as complications from the clumps of virus and antibodies circulating in the bloodstream. This can result in glaucoma, pyelonephritis (kidney infection), and disseminated intravascular coagulation.

Diagnosis

Infectious canine hepatitis is often suspected based on clinical signs and preliminary laboratory findings. It should not be surprising that blood tests indicate liver disease. In addition, blood sugar (glucose) and lymphocyte counts are usually lower than normal.

The virus can be isolated if samples are collected from throat swabs, or from urine or feces. This helps differentiate this disease from leptospirosis, which may share similar clinical signs and laboratory results. Antibody levels can also be helpful. They can be measured initially and then ten to 14 days later to see if the level (titer) increases. This would indicate active infection.

Therapy

Treatment is only supportive in dogs surviving acute infection as there are no specific drugs that will cure viral hepatitis. Affected dogs are treated symptomatically for their liver impairment as well as other problems.

Prevention

Puppies acquire protective antibodies from their mothers in colostrum, the first milk. These levels decrease significantly by nine to 12 weeks of age (sometimes five to seven weeks) at which time the pups are susceptible to infection. Therefore, vaccination should begin in pups eight to ten weeks of age and be repeated at least once three to four weeks later, then annually.

LEPTOSPIROSIS

Leptospirosis is caused by a bacterium that can cause severe disease in people and pets. It is somewhat regional in its distribution and is often spread by rodents. Blood-testing surveys indicate that about 5% of household dogs have been exposed to leptospirosis; up to 37% of stray dogs have been exposed.

Leptospira organisms enter through mucous membranes (e.g., mouth, nose, conjunctiva of eyes) or through abraded skin. After four to ten days, the microbe spreads via the bloodstream and invades the internal organs. The kidney is most often infected. The dog then sheds the bacteria in the urine, where it is communicable to other animals and people. The liver can also be involved, resulting in clinical signs similar to infectious canine hepatitis.

Clinical Signs

There is quite a bit of variability as to the clinical manifestations of leptospirosis. This depends somewhat on the age and immune status of the dog, and the infective strain of the bacteria. Peracute infections can result in fever, muscle pain, vomiting, dehydration, shock, and sudden death. Other animals may be infected yet show mild or no clinical signs.

More moderate infections result in fever, inappetence, vomiting, dehydration, hemorrhage, and evidence of kidney and/or eye (anterior uveitis) disease. The kidney disease can be progressive and irreversible and active hepatitis can also develop.

Diagnosis

A basic diagnostic workup usually includes blood counts, biochemical profiles, and urine analysis. This type of workup is warranted in any dog with evidence of internal disease. Biochemical changes usually reflect damage to the kidneys and/or liver. Electrolyte abnormalities are also common. With kidney damage, there is usually evidence to be found in the urine analysis although the changes are not specific for leptospirosis. Severely affected dogs may have bleeding disorders evident on coagulation profiles.

Leptospire bacteria can be detected by special dark field microscopic examination of urine samples, but cultures are less often helpful. There have been several blood tests developed to help confirm the diagnosis as well. Some are done on single blood samples, but others require comparison between initial samples and those taken two to four weeks later.

Therapy

Unlike the viruses discussed previously, there are antibiotics that can kill the leptospire bacteria. The most common choices are procaine penicillin, tetracycline, the cephalosporins, and the fluoroquinolones. This usually kills the organism and prevents shedding of infectious microbes.

Supportive therapy is also necessary for the other internal disorders present in these dogs. The most challenging aspects of management are treating potential kidney, liver, and coagulation disorders associated with leptospirosis.

Prevention

Not all pets need to be vaccinated for leptospirosis unless your veterinarian feels they are at risk. Current vaccines do not protect against the carrier state and do not invoke a very high level of immunity. Also, they are the components in multivalent (multiple) vaccines that have the highest incidence of hypersensitivity reactions. It is best to concentrate on vaccinating dogs at risk and administering the product every four to eight months, as warranted.

When vaccinations are necessary, they are normally given as three to four injections, two to three weeks apart. Protection is not significant until one to two weeks after the second injection and lasts perhaps six to eight months. Since bacteria are shed in the urine and are infectious to people, hygiene is a critical issue when dealing with infected dogs.

PARAINFLUENZA AND BORDETELLA (CANINE COUGH)

Canine infectious tracheobronchitis (also known as canine cough or kennel cough) is a contagious respiratory infection that causes a persistent hacking cough in dogs. The disorder is more a nuisance than a disease and is very common wherever dogs contact infected dogs, such as boarding kennels, groomers, dog shows, and veterinary clinics.

Canine cough is a complex of respiratory infections involving at least one type of virus and one type of bacteria. The most common virus implicated is parainfluenza and several others are also commonly recovered. These viruses are spread rapidly among susceptible animals. The most prominent bacterium present is *Bordetella bronchiseptica*. Thus, canine cough is actually a mixed infection, starting with a virus and being complicated by bacteria.

Clinical Signs

Canine cough is a mild condition in which dogs develop a hacking cough. The cough may sound bad, but most dogs remain relatively healthy throughout the course of the condition. Occasionally there might be associated discharge from the nose and mouth, and bronchitis and pneumonia can develop as a consequence of the disorder. This is only encountered in 10–20% of cases. The majority resolve spontaneously over a period of five to 25 days.

Diagnosis

The diagnosis is usually rendered when dogs have a history of exposure (e.g., pet shop, groomer, kennel, dog show), a hacking cough, and no other clinical abnormalities. Often the dog can be made to cough by gently squeezing the trachea (windpipe).

Basic blood profiles and radiographs are warranted if it appears that bronchitis or pneumonia is developing. In these cases, it is also worth trying to identify the causative organism(s).

This can be done by culturing throat swabs and by measuring specific antibody levels initially, then again ten to 14 days later. A rise in titers signifies active infection for the organism being tested.

Therapy

Antibiotics may be warranted if bronchitis or pneumonia is developing, but otherwise they probably have little or no benefit. More important is providing good supportive care and perhaps using a nebulizer or mild non-prescription cough medications.

Prevention

Parainfluenza virus is included in most polyvalent (multiple) vaccine combinations. Although it will not protect entirely against canine cough, it does protect somewhat against the most common virus that initiates the condition.

If animals are going to be boarded or be otherwise at risk, they should be vaccinated for bordetella. Vaccination for this organism can be accomplished by injection or by spraying a product into the nostrils. This should be given at least ten days before anticipated exposure, and the protection is anticipated to last six to 12 months. Natural infection also appears to confer resistance to reinfection for about six months.

Many vaccines for this respiratory infection are given intranasally by actually squirting the aerosolized vaccine into the

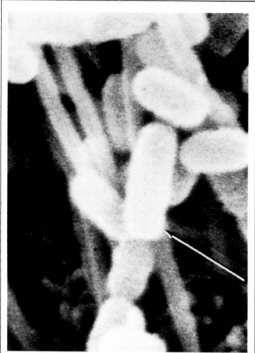

Bordetella attached to canine cilia. Courtesy of Schering Animal Health.

nose. It is estimated that the vaccine affords approximately 80% protection. For intranasal vaccination, protection starts within four to five days.

The intranasal bordetella vaccination is designed to stimulate local immunity in the nasal passages. In this way it traps viruses that may be trying to enter the animal's body. However, giving an intranasal vaccination to a patient that is already harboring the organism offers little benefit. In this case, the dog already has the infectious organism in the throat, so placing a road block in the nasal passages isn't much of a deterrent.

Injections of bordetella vaccine into a muscle stimulate good protection within the bloodstream but less protection within the nasal passages. The intranasal vaccine provides good local protection but less systemic protection. There is some thought that there might be advantages to combining the two approaches. Perhaps the intramuscular injection should be given initially and repeated annually, and the intranasal "booster" be given immediately prior to anticipated exposure. This hypothesis needs to be more thoroughly explored.

LYME DISEASE (BORRELIOSIS)

Lyme disease, or borreliosis, is a disease which we have recognized since the turn of the century, but only in 1975 did we discover and isolate the causative agent, *Borrelia burgdorferi*. The first case in dogs was reported in 1984. The disease

The bordetella vaccine is best given directly into the nostrils. Courtesy of Schering-Plough Animal Health.

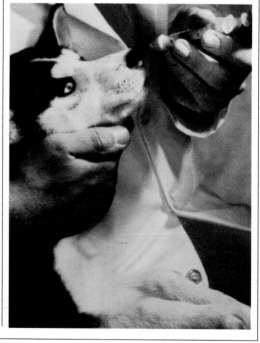

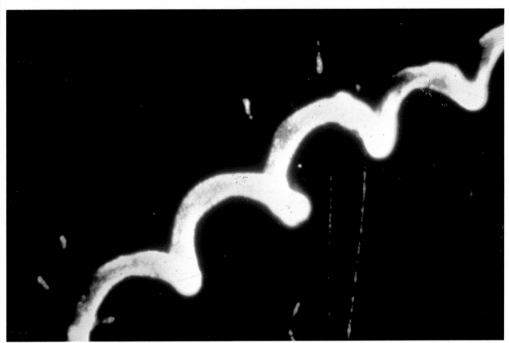

Closeup of the spirochete bacterium that causes Lyme disease. Courtesy of Fort Dodge Laboratories, Fort Dodge, Iowa.

Example of the rash that Lyme disease can cause in people. This is often referred to by physicians as Erythema chronicum migrans (EMC). Courtesy of Fort Dodge Laboratories, Fort Dodge, Iowa.

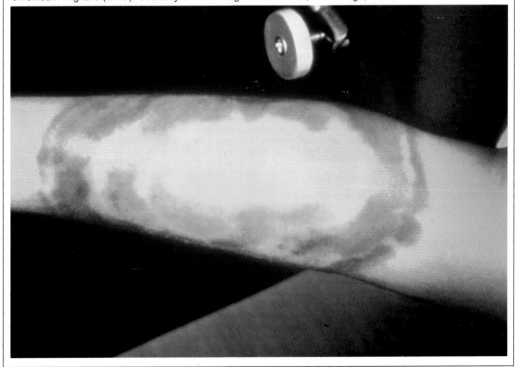

is seen in dogs, cats, horses, cattle, and people, but most cases are seen in people. Although reported in many states, the condition is still most prevalent in the northeastern and midwestern United States, as well as the West Coast. The majority of all cases reported in people has been from New York, New Jersey, Connecticut, Pennsylvania, Massachusetts, Rhode Island, California, Minnesota, and Wisconsin. More and more cases are starting to be reported in the southeastern United States and in Texas. Nearly 50,000 cases of Lyme disease have been reported in the late 1980s and early 1990s (in people), including 9,677 in 1992. In some areas, over 50% of dogs may be infected, with only about 10% actually showing signs. Current studies do not suggest that Lyme disease is transmissible between pets and people, only by contact with ticks.

Although Lyme disease was first reported in 1975 to describe a syndrome seen in patients in Lyme, Connecticut, researchers have found the organism (*Borrelia burgdorferi*) in Long Island ticks from as far back as the 1940s and it is likely that the origins of the organism span back several thousand years. Why the epidemic now?

It appears that the microbe is carried by white-footed mice, spread by two species of ticks, and reproduces profusely in white-tailed deer. It took these three factors to produce the epidemic we're seeing today.

Recent factors such as habitat manipulation, hunting regulations, depletion of natural predators, and reforestation have allowed deer populations to rise dramatically. There were fewer than 30 deer in Connecticut at the turn of the century, but over 30,000 today. Reforestation has helped increase deer and ticks to significant numbers.

The only ticks that transmit Lyme disease are those that are members of the *Ixodes ricinus* complex. The deer tick, previously named *Ixodes dammini,* is the most important, and has recently been renamed *Ixodes scapularis.* The tick primarily responsible for transmitting the microbe, *Ixodes scapularis* (deer tick), dates back to the 1920s and '30s but its numbers have increased greatly in recent times as the deer population has increased. One of the other ticks that carries the microbe, *Ixodes pacificus* (western black-legged tick), is less of a problem because it targets lizards as the principal host (which don't carry the disease) rather than deer. In Europe, *Ixodes ricinus* is the most common vector of Lyme disease in people and pets. Recent research by the U.S. Public Health Rocky Mountain Laboratory and the Department of Entomological Science at the University of California at Berkeley has revealed that the Lyme disease-causing bacterium can also be carried by the Lone Star tick, the American dog tick, and the Pacific Coast tick.

Thus, Lyme disease came about suddenly because of changes to the

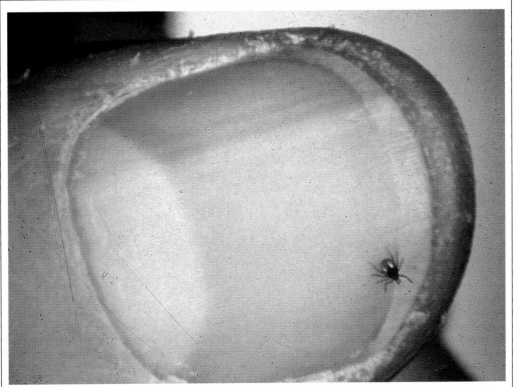

Relative size of the deer tick, the most common carrier of Lyme disease. Courtesy of Fort Dodge Laboratories, Fort Dodge, Iowa.

environment, which allowed it to change from a local phenomenon to a widespread concern.

Clinical Signs

Lyme disease in dogs can cause fever, lethargy, lameness, joint swelling, and a decrease in appetite. Lameness is the most common manifestation. Most clinical signs occur about a month after exposure. A rash, which is so common in people, rarely ever occurs in dogs.

In the United States, 80% of the cases occur from May through August, with peak incidence in July. A resurgence of the disease occurs in mid-September through November. In some areas, Lyme disease is a year-round threat, depending on feeding patterns of the tick vectors. Lyme disease has become the most common tick-borne disease of people in the United States. Currently, only human cases of Lyme disease must be reported to the Centers for Disease Control, so the full impact on the dog population is not yet known. Some experts estimate that the incidence in dogs may be six to ten times higher than in humans.

Diagnosis

Diagnosis of the disease in animals is often challenging for the veterinarian, because blood tests have drawbacks. Finding ticks on a dog is suggestive, but there is no

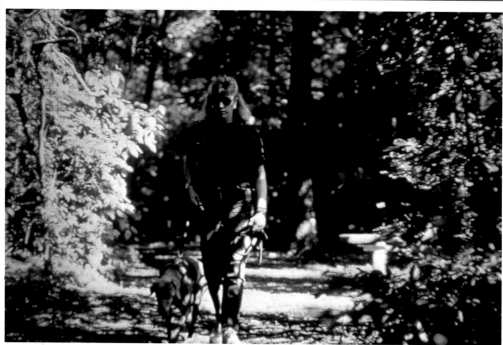

Walking in the woods increases exposure to ticks, especially the varieties that cause Lyme disease. Courtesy of Fort Dodge Laboratories, Fort Dodge, Iowa.

way of knowing whether those particular ticks were carrying the disease organism.

The development of antibodies to the bacteria (which is what is measured in the test) may take up to six months after tick transmission. However, there are serious questions as to how reliable this test is. In a recent study, there was no significant difference between infection rates in dogs with positive tests and in those which tested negative. Also, it has been suggested that dogs with periodontal disease may test positive for Lyme disease with current test kits. It is suspected that spirochetes in the mouth, such as *Treponema*, might be responsible for the false-positive test results. Therefore, blood tests are a poor predictor for determining which animals will eventually develop Lyme disease. However, blood tests can be performed and repeated in two to four weeks to see if the titer is climbing. This is suggestive that active infection with *Borrelia* is present. More specific forms of the test are currently being developed.

Therapy

Since it takes from 24–72 hours for the tick to transmit the bacteria, prompt removal of ticks from pets greatly lessens the chances for them to become infected.

The infection is treated with antibiotics and is most effectively managed early in the course of the disease. Anti-inflammatory agents like aspirin may be used to help alleviate joint pain.

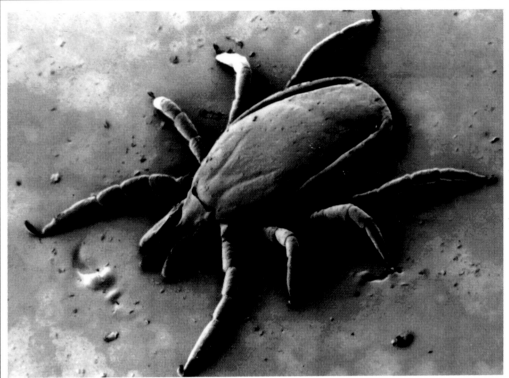

An electron micrograph (approximately 250 times the actual size) of a deer tick nymph. Lyme disease is most often transmitted by a deer tick during this stage of life. Its barbed mouthpart makes removal difficult. M. Fergione photo provided by Boehringer Ingelheim Animal Health, Inc.

Lyme-disease bacterin. Courtesy of Fort Dodge Laboratories, Fort Dodge, Iowa.

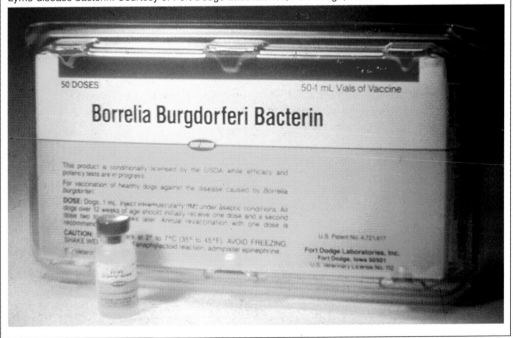

Prevention

A commercial Lyme disease vaccine containing killed organisms is currently available, and the manufacturer claims that the product has been shown to protect against experimentally induced borreliosis. This would seem to have some value in pets at risk in high-incidence areas. Ask your veterinarian for details because there is some question as to whether the vaccine will protect against all of the 200 strains of *Borrelia burgdorferi* that ticks might be carrying. The initial series consists of two vaccinations given two to three weeks apart and an annual revaccination.

A subunit vaccine of *Borrelia burgdorferi* has recently been formulated. The outer membrane protein of the bacterium has been extracted and utilized experimentally as a vaccine. This is not yet commercially available but it is eagerly awaited for use as a Lyme-disease vaccine.

In addition to vaccination, it is important to keep ticks and pets as far away from one another as possible. Rodent control is also critical.

ADDITIONAL READING

Bemis, DA: Bordetella and mycoplasma respiratory infections in dogs and cats. Veterinary Clinics of North America, *Small Animal Practice*, 1992; 22(5): 1173-1186.

Chu, H-J; Chavez, Jr., LG; Blumer, BM; et al: Immunogenicity and efficacy study of a commercial *Borrelia burgdorferi* bacterin. *Journal of the American Veterinary Medical Association*, 1992; 201(3): 403-418.

Esplin, DG; McGill, LD; Meininger, AC; Wilson, SR: Post-vaccination sarcomas in cats. *Journal of the American Veterinary Medical Association*, 1993; 202(8): 1245-1247.

Gulbas, NK: Canine parvovirus infection. *Pet Focus*, 1989; 1(1): 15-17.

Hendrick, MJ; Dunagan, CA: Focal necrotizing granulomatous panniculitis associated with subcutaneous injection of rabies vaccine in cats and dogs: 10 cases (1988-1989). *Journal of the American Veterinary Medical Association*, 1991; 198(2): 304-305.

Kazmierczak, JJ; Sorhage, FE: Current understanding of *Borrelia burgdorferi* infection, with emphasis on its prevention in dogs. *Journal of the American Veterinary Medical Association*, 1993; 203(11): 1524-1528.

Krebs, JW; Strine, TW; Childs, JE: Rabies surveillance in the United States during 1992. *Journal of the American Veterinary Medical Association*, 1993; 203(12): 1718-1731.

Levy, SA; Magnarelli, LA: Relationship between the development of antibodies to

Borrelia burgdorferi in dogs and subsequent development of limb/joint borreliosis. *Journal of the American Veterinary Medical Association*, 1992; 200: 344-347.

McDonald, LJ: Factors that can undermine the success of routine vaccination protocols. *Veterinary Medicine*, 1992; March: 223-230.

Ohlers, C: Tracing the roots of *Borrelia burgdorferi. Journal of the American Veterinary Medical Association*, 1991; 199(10): 1249-1250.

Phillips, TR; Jensen, JL; Rubino, MJ; *et al*: Effects of vaccines on the canine immune system. *Canadian Journal of Veterinary Research*, 1989; 53: 154-160.

Pollack, RVH: The parvovirus Part II. Canine parvovirus.

Compendium for Continuing Education of Practicing Veterinarians, 1984; 6:653-664.

Robinson, LE; Fishbein, DB: Rabies. *Seminars in Veterinary Medicine and Surgery*, 1991; 6(3): 203-211.

Sela, M; Arnon, R: Synthetic approaches to vaccines for infectious and autoimmune diseases. *Vaccine*, 1992; 10(14): 991-999.

Tizard, I: Risks associated with use of live vaccines. *Journal of the American Veterinary Medical Association*, 1990; 196(11): 1851-1858.

Walker, PD: Bacterial vaccines: old and new, veterinary and medical. *Vaccine*, 1992; 10(14): 977-990.

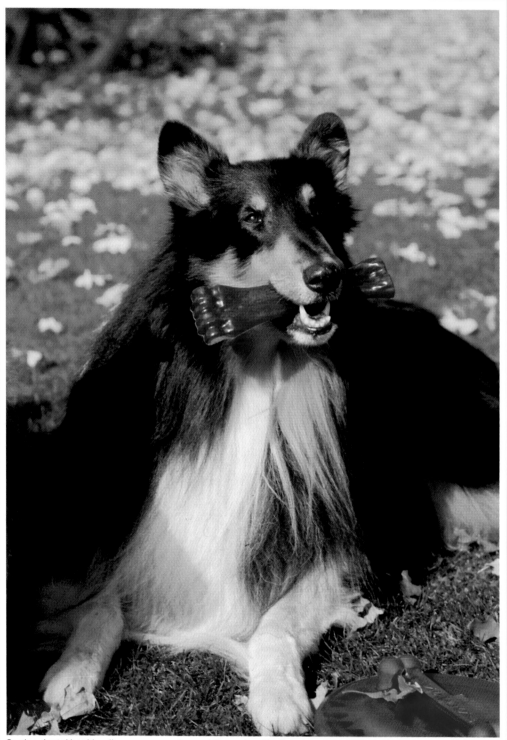

Canine dental health relies upon owner's providing safe, effective chew toys. This Collie is content with his new Gumabone®.

Dental Disorders

We all know that pets have teeth but few owners have spent the time to really familiarize themselves with their pet's teeth and how to keep those teeth healthy. Some mistakenly believe that animals don't need dental care because they wouldn't receive any in the wild—this is foolish; we wouldn't receive any dental care in the wild either, so what does this mean? The fact that these animals are in our care and no longer in the wild is further argument that we should endeavor to meet our pet's dental needs, as we do our own. The first step to understanding those needs is to appreciate how the teeth develop and where problems are likely to occur.

BASIC GUIDE TO YOUR DOG'S TEETH

Eruption of Teeth

Puppies are born without teeth, and the first teeth start to erupt when the pups are a few weeks old. Puppies, like their owners, get two sets of teeth, the deciduous or puppy teeth and the permanent teeth. The puppy incisors erupt around two to four weeks of age on average and all puppy teeth are usually present by eight weeks of age. There are a total of 28 deciduous or puppy teeth in dogs. Because the puppy teeth provide the pathway for the permanent teeth to follow, puppies should have their teeth checked by eight weeks of age to make sure the teeth are coming in straight and that there are no congenital problems.

Shortly after the deciduous teeth have erupted, the permanent teeth begin to grow beneath them. Permanent teeth erupt sooner in larger breeds of dog. Permanent incisors erupt by two to five

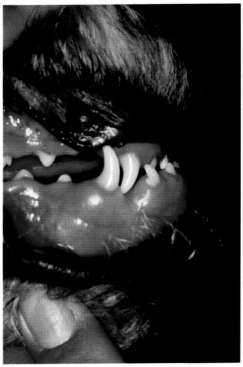

Puppy teeth.

months of age. By six to seven months of age, all permanent teeth should be in place; there are a total of 42 permanent teeth in the dog. At six months of age, a dental evaluation should be performed to make sure that the permanent teeth have erupted properly and that there are no dental abnormalities, especially retained puppy teeth.

A problem that sometimes occurs in young dogs is retained deciduous teeth. This means that the puppy teeth remain when they should have been lost and can cause crowding in the mouth. As a general rule, no two teeth of the same type should be occupying the same place at the same time. If not corrected early, this can cause permanent changes to the dental pattern. These retained teeth can be removed by your veterinarian to allow room for the permanent teeth to erupt. Radiographs are usually taken first to confirm that there are in fact permanent teeth available to erupt and that they are not impacted.

It is also important to realize that the upper and lower jaws grow at different rates and independently from one another. This is a normal occurrence but because the puppy and adult teeth grow in so quickly, they may create a problem of dental "interlock" as the upper and lower jaws grow at different rates. This is another reason why dogs should have dental checkups at eight weeks of age (when the puppy teeth have all erupted) and again at six to seven months of age (when the permanent teeth have all erupted). Corrections of tooth placement are referred to as orthodontics.

TOOTH ANATOMY

The terminology used to describe teeth is similar whether the patient is animal or human. Animals have incisors, canine teeth, premolars and molars. Each tooth has four surfaces and this is important when it comes to understanding the need for comprehensive dental cleaning. The labial surface of a tooth faces the lips; the lingual surface faces the tongue; the occlusal surface is the biting and chewing area; and the contact surface is that area between adjacent teeth. When brushing the teeth, most of the attention is focused on the outer labial aspects of the teeth because these are most accessible, but it is important to remember that plaque can form on all surfaces and all surfaces need cleaning.

The part of the tooth that extends above the gumline, and that we can see, is called the crown. This is the part of the tooth that we can clean at home. The uppermost layer of the crown is the enamel, which forms a hard protective covering for the underlying dentin. This dentin consists of dense material and constitutes the bulk of the tooth. It can be sensitive to both heat and cold and therefore needs to be covered by a healthy layer of enamel.

The tooth root is that portion below the gumline, just as the crown is that portion above the gumline. Cementum covers the tooth root and helps anchor the tooth to the underlying bone. The central core of the tooth root is called the pulp. The pulp is soft and contains nerves and blood vessels. If the pulp becomes exposed, the tooth becomes very painful. In this case the tooth can be repaired by special endodontic procedures or by extracting the tooth.

The tooth itself is anchored in the periodontium, which consists of the gums (gingiva), supporting ligaments, the cementum, and bone. An understanding of this aspect of oral anatomy is critical because it is in this space, between the teeth and the gums, where pockets develop and gingivitis occurs. The gums are the first line of defense against periodontal disease and this is a point worth noting. In time, if dental health care is not maintained, periodontal disease results, there is loss of supporting bone, and the teeth loosen and fall out. Accompanying infection can spread via the bloodstream to the liver, kidneys and heart, causing other medical problems. Proper home care and regular veterinary dental prophylaxis maintain the teeth and gums in a healthy state so that they might last the pet's whole life.

BITE

Most people can appreciate that the teeth should meet in a normal manner and certainly there are many people that have worn braces to straighten their own teeth. In dogs, normal occlusion (the meeting of upper and lower teeth) is often referred to as "scissors bite." With a normal bite the upper incisors should end up just in front of the lower incisors when the mouth is closed. There are many other rules that apply to how the molars and premolars should meet, where the canines should rest and how the jaws should be opposed when the mouth is closed. If the bite is abnormal, there will be abnormal tooth wear, perhaps pain in chewing and sometimes difficulty eating. Of course some breeds have been created with abnormal bites and this must also be appreciated. Breeds such as the Bulldog are supposed to have an undershot jaw, called prognathism. In most breeds, however, this is a genetic fault and the animal should definitely not be used for breeding. The opposite problem is an overshot jaw, or brachygnathism, which is an abnormality in all breeds. These animals should also not be used for breeding. It is important to note that many orthodontic problems are not genetic in origin but result from dental interlock when the upper and lower jaws grow at different rates. When this malocclusion interferes with dental function, correction can be attempted with orthodontics. Of course orthodontics should not be used for cosmetic purposes in purebreds with heritable defects, since they can still pass the problems along to future generations.

THE NEED FOR PROPER DENTAL CARE

We learn from a very young age how important it is to take care of our teeth, the necessity of regular dental checkups, and the danger of tartar and gum disease. It is

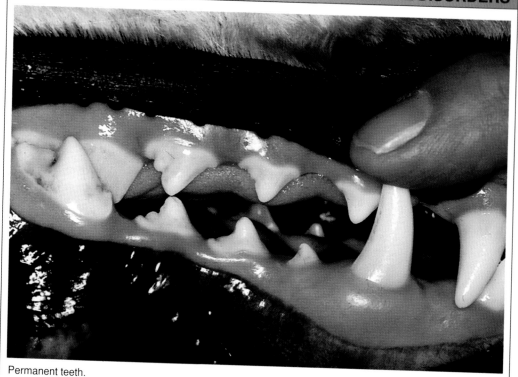

Permanent teeth.

Anatomy of a tooth (Reprinted with permission from M. Tholen. The role of the technician in veterinary dental medicine. 1. Dental anatomy and pathology, *Veterinary Technician* 1984, 5:286-291).

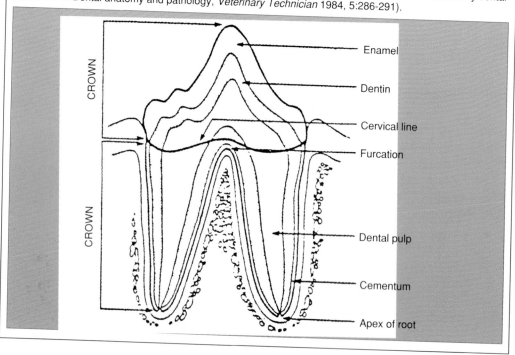

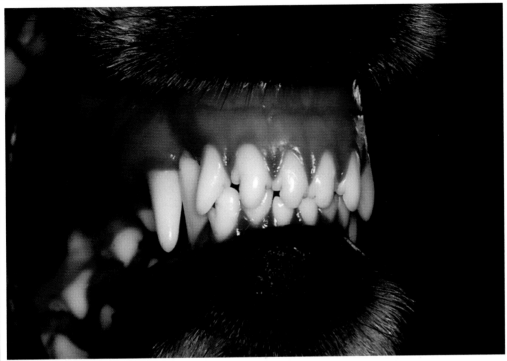

Normal (scissors) bite.

Periodontal disease progression (Courtesy of Petcom, Inc.).

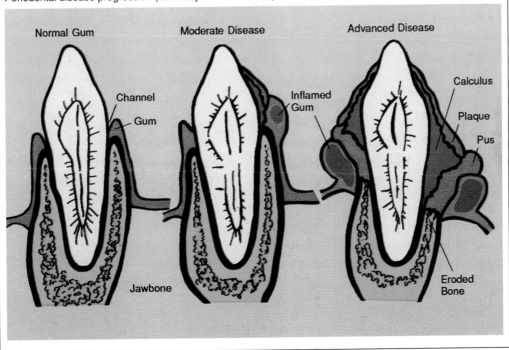

therefore hard to believe that, until a few years ago, veterinary dentistry consisted only of routine cleaning procedures and extracting or "pulling" bad teeth. Veterinary dentistry is now an approved specialty, recognized by the American Veterinary Medical Association, and is enjoying much popularity as both owners and veterinarians realize the benefits of routine dental care for pets.

Our thinking about health care in general has changed greatly in recent years. Rather than be preoccupied with how to treat diseases, we are realizing that the key to good health is prevention. This concept is usually expressed as wellness, meaning that health comes from preventing disease, rather than waiting for it to occur and then be treated. Wellness is more than a fad and it is fortunate that the concepts are being applied to our pets. Unfortunately, although everyone appreciates the need for dental care, most pets do not receive adequate attention for their dental needs and are suffering for it.

It is a sad statistic that more than 85% of dogs older than four years of age have periodontal disease. Periodontal disease is the most common cause of both tooth loss and bad breath and is so prevalent that many people have just come to consider it normal. After all, don't all dogs have "doggy breath"? Obviously, there is a great need for dental care in these animals, but for some reason they are not receiving this care and are

suffering from an entirely preventable disease. The process doesn't end there. If periodontal disease continues and the gums start bleeding, bacteria growing in the pockets created around the teeth get released into the bloodstream, where they can travel to the heart, liver and kidneys. As if that is not bad enough, chronic periodontal disease results in loss of anchoring bone and the teeth eventually fall out.

As we care for our pets better, and they live longer lives, dental care becomes a more critical issue. Just as vaccinations help prevent our pets from getting a number of different diseases, periodic veterinary dental checkups and regular home care help prevent periodontal infection, loss of teeth, bad breath, tartar buildup, and associated infections. Actually, when you consider that the average person is very aware of the need for dental visits, tooth brushing, dental flossing, tartar control and fluoride treatments, it is amazing that pet dental health has been such a neglected issue. If there was a virus affecting 85% of dogs over four years of age, there would be panic in the pet-owning public. And yet dental care is sometimes neglected even though most problems are entirely preventable. Even if you take your pet to the veterinarian every six months for a dental cleaning, it is not enough. Who would think of allowing their children not to brush between dental visits? Regular home care is as important as veterinary dental care and the reasons are fairly straightforward.

To truly appreciate the need for dental care it is important to understand plaque and calculus and how they fit into the picture of dental health. Plaque is a combination of bacteria, bits of food, and saliva that adheres to the teeth on a daily basis. This plaque, once it forms, cannot be rinsed away with water; that's how tenaciously it hangs on to the teeth. It can only be removed by brushing, veterinary dental instruments, or safe chew products (such as Nylabone® and Gumabone™). Now is the time to remove this plaque (daily) before it causes any serious problems.

Plaque collects below the gumline and starts to lift the gum away from the tooth. The "pocket" that is formed in this region not only collects bacteria and plaque but damages the attachments that hold the tooth in place and the underlying bone to which it is anchored. At this stage, brushing at home will not do any good because you can't get under the gum margin to arrest the damage. Veterinary intervention can halt the process of periodontal disease if caught before permanent damage has occurred.

In time, if plaque is allowed to remain on your pet's teeth, it becomes mineralized and is called tartar (calculus). This hard, rough material is an excellent breeding ground for bacteria, and, unlike plaque, calculus cannot be removed from the teeth by brushing. Tartar buildup doesn't just happen by accident. Dogs that are fed soft food rather than kibble have a higher incidence of tartar and some breeds are more affected than others. Small breeds of dogs appear to have more problems with tartar than do larger dogs, and dogs with a lot of muzzle hair such as Poodles, schnauzers and terriers also have more problems. Toy breeds that tend to open-mouth breathe are more prone to tartar because their mouths become dry. If your pet does have tartar buildup, it will need to be removed by veterinary prophylaxis. Do not try to remove it yourself by scraping as you might do considerable damage to the supporting structures of the teeth as well as to the enamel. There are some things you can do at home, and some things that are best left to your veterinarian.

The first stage of dental disease associated with plaque and calculus is called gingivitis. It occurs when the bacterial population around the teeth is approximately ten to 20 times greater than normal. At this time the margins of the gums may become reddened to reflect the inflammation occurring there. Gingivitis may start to occur in pups as young as nine months of age but can become severe by the time a dog is two years old. Gingivitis is completely reversible with proper veterinary attention and home care. If the process continues, however, there is damage to the anchoring

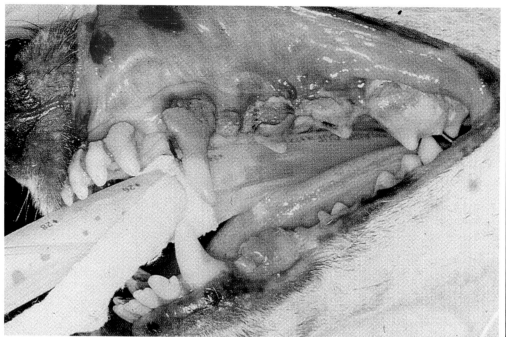

Severe tartar accumulation on a dog's teeth.

Broken tooth.

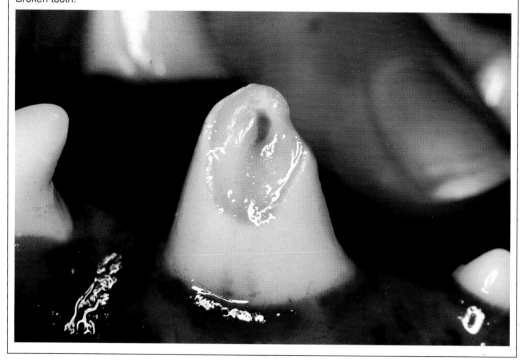

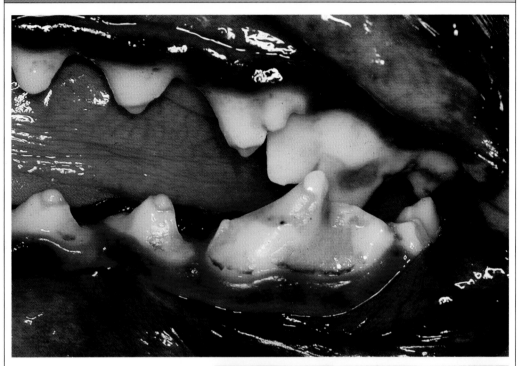

Pitting of the teeth from distemper infection.

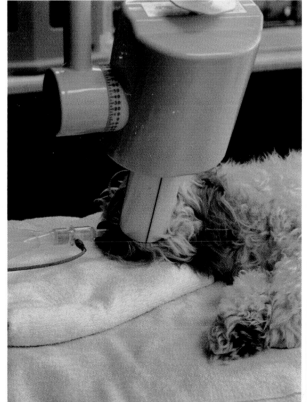

Dental radiographs are taken with the same kind of machine used in a regular dentist's office.

attachments of the teeth; we refer to this as periodontitis. Gingivitis may persist for years without progressing to periodontitis. Even this can often be reversed with appropriate attention, but, as the process continues, the damage caused can be permanent. Don't let this happen to your dog—those teeth are meant to last a lifetime!

What if pets do develop periodontitis and eventually lose their teeth? Is that so bad? Well, part of the problem is that pets with periodontal disease have infected gums as well as infections around the roots of the teeth. This is often first noted as bad breath and most owners consider this an esthetic concern more than a medical issue. The fact is that infection will end up causing the gums to bleed as well as allowing pus to accumulate under the gums. Owners may never see evidence of bleeding gums unless they closely inspect chew toys or bones for flecks of blood. When a dog's gums are infected (gingivitis), every time the dog chews, the impact on the teeth force microbes deeper into the tissues and eventually into the bloodstream. The bacteria may circulate around the body and end up in a variety of organs, especially the heart, liver or kidneys, where they can do serious damage.

The good news is that all of these problems are entirely preventable. Plaque can be removed at home by regular brushing and by using oral rinses. Regular veterinary visits for dental evaluation should be scheduled every six to 12 months. The dental prophylaxis procedure will remove tartar and even plaque below the gumline. Pets encouraged to eat dry foods and given appropriate chew toys (of which Nylabone® and Gumabone™ are the safest and most affordable in the long run) will also have fewer problems with plaque and tartar.

OTHER PROBLEMS

In people, a discussion of dental health would of course include the topic of cavities. In dogs, we talk about caries, the bacterial destruction of the tooth surface. Caries are more often apparent in the enamel but might also be seen in the cementum if the tooth root has been exposed by ongoing periodontal disease. Caries are not as common in dogs as they are in people for several reasons. First, the pH of dog saliva is different than in people and not as conducive to the bacteria that initiate caries. Second, most dogs eat a diet low in fermentable carbohydrates (sugars) which promotes the growth of caries-causing bacteria in people. In dogs, caries are most often found in the upper molars, which tend to have more "pits" than the other teeth. In general, caries are seen in teeth secondary to gingivitis and periodontitis where the inflammation in the gums exposes the tooth root to bacterial damage.

Dogs can suffer from broken teeth, most often from chewing on objects that are too hard for them, such as stones. If only the enamel is fractured, the tooth will probably self-heal. If the fracture extends into the dentin, the ensuing inflammation usually is sufficient to insulate the sensitive inner pulp. If, however, the pulp is breached, endodontic treatment (root canal therapy) is needed or the tooth must be extracted.

The enamel is prone to other insults than just fracture. While the enamel is forming, it is susceptible to damage, especially from viruses and drugs. The distemper virus, in particular, can cause irreversible pitting and discoloration of the teeth. Tetracyclines, when administered to pregnant females or to pups less than six months of age, can also discolor the teeth.

BASIC VETERINARY DENTAL CARE— DENTAL PROPHYLAXIS

As you are no doubt now aware, proper dental care is critical for our pets. Unfortunately, even daily home care is not completely sufficient for your dog's dental health. Just as you need to schedule regular visits with your own dentist, your dog needs periodic visits with your veterinarian. A thorough dental evaluation should be performed once or twice a year, and there are many steps to this process. Some of the most important steps are a complete dental examination, the removal of calculus from the teeth, cleaning below the gumline and polishing the teeth. Sound familiar?—these are some of the same steps your dentist does in

evaluating your teeth.

The dental evaluation and prophylaxis (or "prophy" for short) procedure should be done as often as necessary to keep the teeth as healthy as possible. This varies from animal to animal depending on the age, breed, conformation of the teeth, individual tendencies, and the willingness of owners to clean their pet's teeth regularly at home. If you have been doing a good job at home, the prophylaxis will be a relatively easy procedure of cleaning those aspects of the teeth that can't be accessed at home.

A thorough examination of the mouth is done at the time of the dental checkup to evaluate problems and to identify areas that might need more attention at home. This often involves using a periodontal probe (just like at your dentist's office) to explore the depth of pockets around each tooth. Deep pockets mean that bacteria have access to the sensitive regions under the gumline. The deeper aspects of the teeth are evaluated by dental radiographs, which can show the attachments of the teeth to the underlying bone.

Many veterinarians keep a written history of your pet's dental health on a special chart using graphic symbols to indicate any evidence of dental problems. Like the rest of the medical record, it serves to identify problem areas and record them for future consideration. It allows veterinarians to see at a glance how your dog's dental picture has

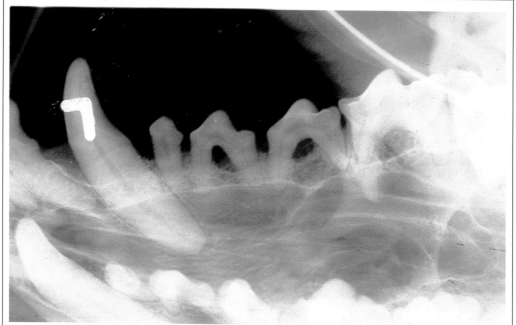

Dental radiographs help identify disorders that may not be evident on visual inspection.

Polishing of the teeth to remove rough areas on the tooth surface.

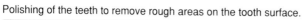

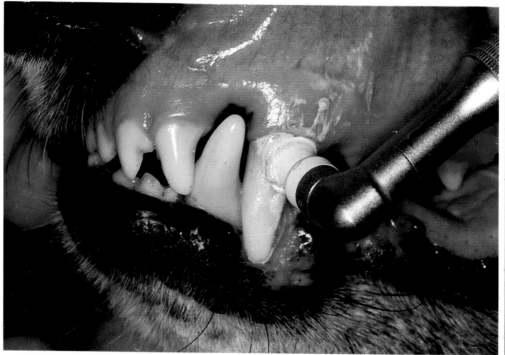

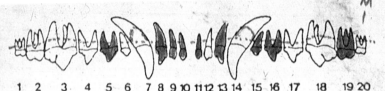

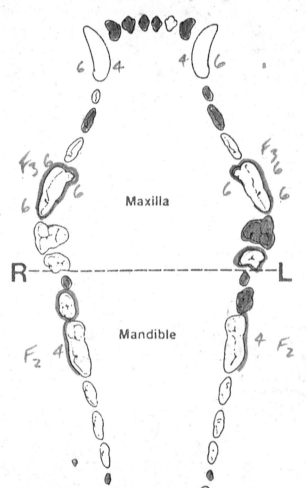

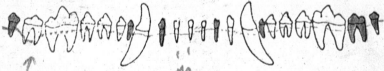

A dental chart is used to keep a record of a pet's dental health.

changed over the years and where problems may be expected in the future.

The procedure known as the dental prophylaxis involves several steps to clean the teeth, above and below the gumline, and to polish them so plaque has a harder time adhering to the tooth surface. The goal is to slow or prevent the development of periodontal disease by treating those areas that cannot be effectively cleaned by home dental care.

Because the cleaning extends beneath the sensitive gumline, dogs must be anesthetized to do a comprehensive cleaning. While people can appreciate what a dentist is trying to do for them and will allow injections of local anesthetic and sometimes painful procedures, it is unreasonable to expect this of our pets. When under general anesthesia, the dog can have its teeth effectively and efficiently evaluated and cleaned, and it can wake up without fear or apprehension. The newer anesthetics, particularly isoflurane, make anesthesia, even in older pets, quite safe as long as they are in good general health. If there are any questions about a pet's health, veterinarians will often perform blood tests, and sometimes an electrocardiogram (ECG) before attempting any anesthetic procedure.

Once the dog is anesthetized, most of the plaque and calculus is removed from the teeth by scaling. This can be done manually, but in most cases the preliminary work is done with ultrasonic scalers that disrupt and remove calculus by their high frequency vibrations. Although many people do not realize this, the ultrasonic scalers don't actually touch the tooth surface to disrupt the calculus. In fact, if they are used improperly, they can act like a miniature jackhammer and produce pitting of the enamel surface. Once again, scaling is a valuable procedure because it removes plaque and calculus from all portions of the teeth (both above and below the gumline), removes inflammatory tissue where it occurs, and creates a smooth tooth surface to decrease plaque buildup on the teeth.

After most of the plaque and calculus is removed by mechanical scaling methods, hand scalers are used to complete the prophylaxis procedure by removing any remaining plaque and calculus from under the gumline. A variety of dental tools are used for this, including scalers, hoes, files and curettes. It must be remembered that the most important phase of the dental "prophy" is cleaning under the gumline. Root planing is used to remove dental calculus, plaque, and cementum on the root surface, which creates an extremely smooth, glasslike surface and helps to reduce the potential for future plaque adherence.

After all of this intense cleaning is finished, we're still not done. We've managed to clean the teeth of plaque and calculus, but we need to polish the teeth to remove any rough areas on the tooth surface that might have resulted from plaque and calculus accumulation or even by the scaling procedure itself. The polishing is performed by applying pumice "prophy" pastes to the tooth and using a polisher to rotate the pumice against the tooth. This polishes the tooth surface and helps to remove stains.

After polishing, we're still not done. It's time for a fluoride treatment. The fluoride gel applied helps to desensitize the teeth, helps kill bacteria that contribute to plaque formation, and helps with enamel repair.

For anyone who has witnessed a "prophy" procedure, he can appreciate how tedious it is to clean and polish all aspects of the teeth, but the benefits can be appreciated by all. The teeth are cleaner (and therefore the breath smells better) and are more resistant to plaque buildup, making home care easier and more effective. And, most importantly, with healthy teeth, our pets are healthier themselves.

DENTAL HOME CARE

Just as you wouldn't think of neglecting your own teeth between dental visits, your pet needs dental attention more often than once every six to 12 months. In order to prevent gum disease and tooth loss, it becomes important to keep a pet's teeth clean on a day-to-day basis.

Don't underestimate the value of cleaning your pet's teeth at home. Since plaque develops daily you should begin routine cleaning

procedures by the time your pet is about six months of age. At this age your pet will quickly learn to accept teeth cleaning as part of a routine home care ritual. If you're starting with an older pet, don't worry—it may take a little more time and patience but the benefits are worth it. There are several things you can do at home to keep your pet's teeth healthy between veterinary dental checkups.

CHEWING FOR DENTAL WELL BEING

It may sound obvious, but the more dogs chew, the cleaner the teeth become. Some pets are better chewers than others, and it is the actual chewing itself that gets the job done. The longer a dog spends chewing at something the longer the abrasive action of chewing will scrub the teeth clean. On the other hand, if a dog just gulps a biscuit as a treat rather than chewing it, there is very little benefit.

It has been shown that hard foods, such as kibble, clean the teeth more than soft foods. Remember, it is the action of chewing that cleans the teeth. If your dog is a "gulper," the kibble will probably not remain in the mouth long enough to get the job done. The same is often true of biscuits. If they are accepted as a treat and eaten quickly, they will not work as well as if they are chewed thoroughly and completely. Because many of the biscuits available have more than 100 calories apiece, use them only as directed by the manufacturer; consider also the low-calorie varieties. The advantage of

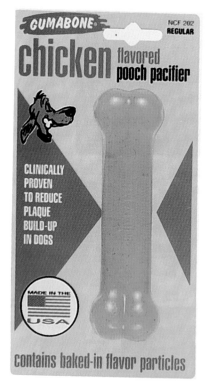

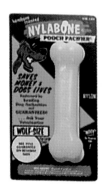

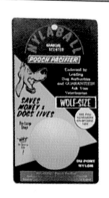

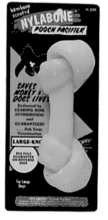

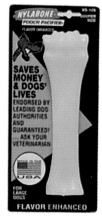

Nylabone dental devices, available from fine pet shops everywhere, come in a variety of sizes, shapes and colors! Responsible owners, to ensure the good health of their dogs' mouths, provide one or more of these chew toys on a regular basis. Photographs courtesy of Nylabone.

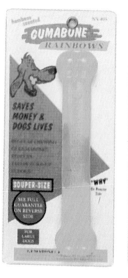

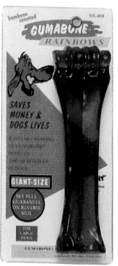

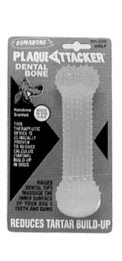

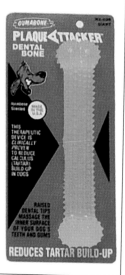

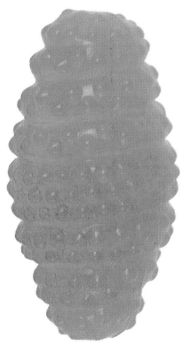

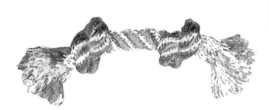

Dental floss exercisers and polyurethane dog bones with raised dental tips are among the dental device breakthroughs introduced to the dog world by Nylabone. These wonderfully effective chew toys are loved both by dogs and veterinarians the world over. All Nylabone products are available in pet shops. Photographs courtesy of Nylabone.

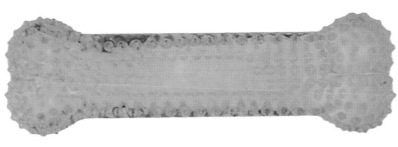

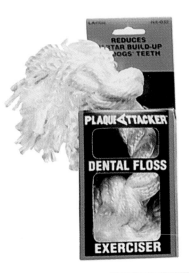

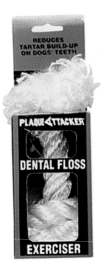

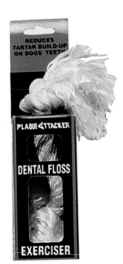

biscuits is that the vast majority of dogs will gladly accept them; some are more particular when it comes to chew toys and treats. One product (i.e., CHOOZ™), made of cheese protein (without the fat), poultry meal and gelatin (without sugar, salt or preservatives) is microwaveable and therefore its texture can be varied to suit the individual taste of each dog.

Rawhide chew sticks, strips and toys are usually helpful because they are well accepted by many dogs and the time spent chewing them is much longer (on average) than for biscuits. The longer dogs chew, the more the rawhide comes in contact with the teeth and the cleaner the teeth become. Rawhide appears to be fairly safe for dogs and a very useful daily tool to help keep their teeth clean, but dogs do occasionally choke on softened rawhide strips.

Nylon chew toys from Nylabone® are excellent chewing abrasives for dogs. Some dogs love their chew toys and spend hours a day with them; others seem disinterested. They come in a variety of sizes and shapes, from bones to balls to flying discs, to provide dogs with chewing exercise and fun. One product (Plaque Attacker™) has raised "dental tips" to combat plaque and tartar and is shaped to reach inner and outer aspects of the teeth. There is even a chew toy with nylon strands that functions like dental floss to remove destructive plaque from between the teeth and beneath the gumline; it is called Nylafloss™.

Give your pets a variety of chewing options and you will quickly learn which ones they spend the most time chewing. Whichever safe products encourage your pet to chew will do their part to help remove plaque and calculus.

An important consideration in the choice of chewing supplements is safety. Do not give your dog real bones under any circumstances. Although they will have some desirable cleaning effects on the teeth, they are potentially very dangerous. Not only can they cause vomiting and diarrhea, but there is a very real danger that they will cause an obstruction or cause a puncture in the digestive tract. When there are so many safe chewing supplements available, it doesn't make sense to risk your dog's health with real bones.

Chewing is great for the teeth, but some teeth benefit more than others from the exercise. Since dogs chew with their molars and premolars, these teeth benefit most. The large canine teeth are really designed for ripping rather than chewing and so do not benefit as much from chewing. It is important to stress that the act of chewing helps remove dental calculus. The pet that eats soft food and refuses chew toys needs to have more dental care by a veterinarian and more home care by the pet owner.

BRUSHING THE TEETH

You should be brushing your pet's teeth at least twice weekly, daily if you can manage it. It's not as difficult as you might imagine and, after the initial fuss, it shouldn't be traumatic for either your pet or yourself.

Step one is to pick an appropriate pet toothbrush. Save yourself time and money by not buying a child's toothbrush for the job—it won't work for you. Not only are the bristles of a child's toothbrush too hard for pets but even the shape of the brush never seems to fit the pet's mouth and teeth correctly. The ideal pet toothbrush will have a long handle to give you good access to the teeth, an angled head to better fit a pet's mouth and extra soft bristles to add to your pet's comfort. If you select this or a similar type of brush, your pet will accept the process better and you'll be able to do a better job. Another option is the brush and gum massage tools that fit over your finger. Some people find it easier to "finger brush" their pets' teeth while others prefer a standard pet toothbrush; the choice is yours.

Step two is to select an appropriate dentifrice. The ideal pet dentifrice is an enzymatic toothpaste that is specially formulated for dogs. These pet toothpastes contain no detergents, baking soda or salt which are often found in human products and may be harmful to pets. Fluorides may be incorporated into the toothpaste to help control the bacteria that contribute to plaque. Ask your veterinarian for advice and don't use human products—they won't

do the job for you. Once you select your pet dentifrice, take the time to apply it properly to the brush to get the most benefit. Rather than leaving a strip of paste on top of the bristles, squirt the paste between the bristles. This allows the dentifrice to spend the most time in contact with the teeth and, after all, that is the entire purpose of brushing.

Step three is to get the brush with dentifrice into your pet's mouth and get those teeth, all of them, brushed. Most pets accept brushing if they are approached in a gentle manner. If you can start them young enough, it's quite easy, but even older pets will accept the process if you're gentle and patient. If your dog is not used to having its teeth brushed, start slowly. You can use a washcloth or a piece of gauze to wipe the teeth, front and back, in the same manner you will eventually be using a toothbrush. Do this twice daily for about two weeks and your pet should be familiar with the approach. Then, take your special pet toothbrush and soak it in warm water and start brushing daily for several days. When your pet accepts this brushing, start with your pet toothpaste and you're on your way.

When your pet has learned to allow you to brush the teeth, make sure your technique takes full advantage of the situation. The bristles should be placed at the gum margin (where the teeth and gums meet) at an angle of 45 degrees (to the long axis of the tooth), and moved in a gentle oval

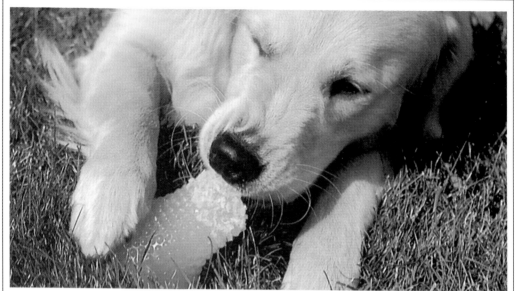

Golden Retriever enjoying good dental health and great fun with his Gumabone Plaque Attacker. Photograph by Karen Taylor.

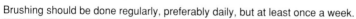

Brushing should be done regularly, preferably daily, but at least once a week.

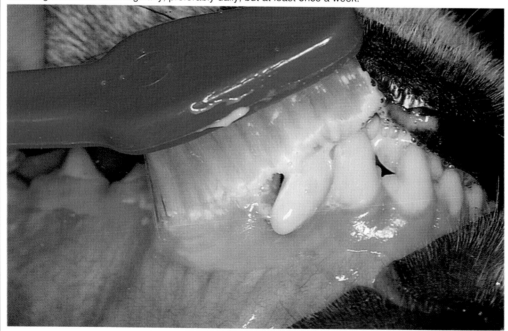

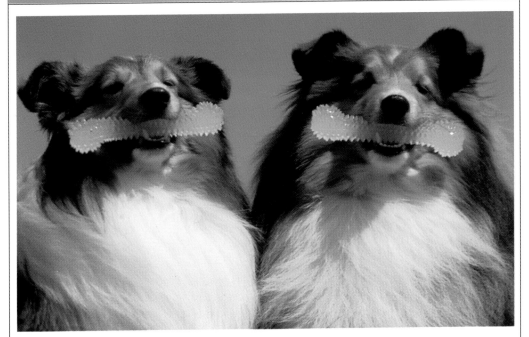

Above: Gumabone® Plaque Attacker™. Raised "dental tips" attack plaque and tartar buildup. Spiral design ensures that the inside surface of teeth and gums will be massaged while chewing.

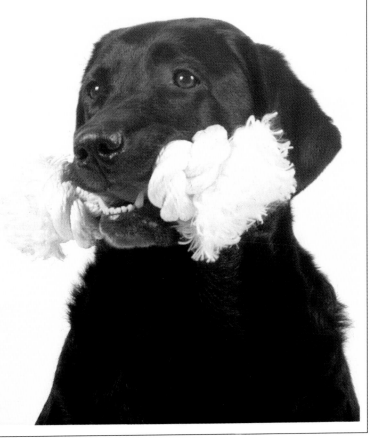

Right: Nylafloss™ dental device, with hambone-flavored nylon strands, helps remove destructive plaque between the teeth and beneath the gum line.

pattern. Be sure to gently force the bristle ends into the area around the base of the tooth as well as into the space between the teeth. Ten short back-and-forth motions should be completed in the same position and then the brush should be lifted and moved to a new position and the process repeated. This cleans the teeth and avoids aggressive "scrubbing" actions. The process should be continued, section by section, covering three or four teeth at a time until all teeth are done. For hard-to-reach teeth, the brush is inserted vertically and the "heel" of the brush used to generate ten short up-and-down strokes in each location.

Brushing the teeth will be very effective if you take time to make sure the dentifrice makes adequate contact with the teeth and that you do all of the teeth. Remember to get the bristles well into the gum margins and the space between the teeth because these are the areas where tartar is most likely to form.

An excellent followup to brushing is to use dental rinses and sprays that aid in reducing plaque and inflammation. As an extra bonus, they also help dogs with bad breath. The antiseptic action of these products help disinfect the mouth and help discourage plaque formation. The best results are reported with the use of fluorides, chlorhexidine, alexidine, antibiotics, enzymes such as dextranase, and acetate compounds of zinc and manganese. Studies on a chlorhexidine-based product suggested that two daily rinses almost completely inhibited the development of plaque, calculus and gingivitis. These chemical plaque-controlling agents are not a substitute for proper dental prophylaxis. Calculus must be removed from the teeth and the teeth polished before using these agents.

Zinc ascorbate cysteine (ZAC) compounds have also shown promising results both with and without brushing. For those persons who feel they just cannot brush their pet's teeth, this provides a valuable option. The gel cleans and freshens the mouth and is usually well accepted by pets. The product also appears to hasten healing of gum tissue and removes plaque from the surface of the teeth. Clearly, if you don't feel comfortable brushing your pet's teeth, this is an easy option you really should consider.

To be truly effective, you must have regular veterinary dental checkups and periodic prophylaxis to help remove calculus (tartar) from the teeth and polish them so that plaque has a harder time adhering to the teeth. Neither brushing nor rinsing will remove tartar but, combined with routine veterinary dental care, will help your pet's teeth remain healthy for a lifetime.

HEREDITARY DENTAL PROBLEMS

It should be little surprise that some dental problems are more common in some breeds than others. Although some problems are clearly genetic, others are more developmental in nature. Since over 300 different breeds have been created, with different stature, conformation and breed standards, diversity is to be expected. For example, some breeds have been created that have a shorter upper jaw than a lower jaw and are described as being brachycephalic. The brachycephalic breeds include the Bulldog, Boxer, Pekingese and Boston Terrier, among others. Because of the way these dogs have been bred, all are expected to have an undershot jaw, termed prognathism. This abnormality has become "normal" in these breeds. On the other hand, an overshot jaw is abnormal in all breeds.

Malocclusion

Malocclusion refers to any abnormality in how the upper and lower teeth meet. There are five types of malocclusion recognized in dogs: undershot, overshot, level, reverse scissors and open. Remember that the normal "bite" is the scissors bite in which the teeth of the upper jaw are positioned just in front of those of the lower jaw.

Malocclusion is the most common genetic dental problem and is often a major concern to breeders and those involved in conformation. A good example is prognathism or undershot jaw seen in Bulldogs, Boxers, Pekingese and Boston Terriers. This bite is considered abnormal in breeds that are supposed to have a normal "scissors" bite.

The opposite condition is known as brachygnathism or overshot jaw. This condition, in which the upper jaw protrudes above the lower jaw, is considered abnormal in all breeds. It has been most reported in the Cocker Spaniel, in which it may be referred to as "pig jaw."

Level bite is another malocclusive disorder in which the front teeth meet end to end rather than the top incisors being just slightly in front of the bottom incisors. It is considered a minor form of prognathism. Level bite is acceptable in several breeds and owners should consult the breed standard for their own particular breed.

The reverse scissors bite occurs when the upper incisors fall just behind the lower incisors. If an actual gap is evident, the condition would be more correctly described as overshot jaw. The reverse scissors bite is called for in some breeds, including the Afghan Hound, Boxer, Bullmastiff, English Toy Spaniel, Pekingese, Shih Tzu, Boston Terrier, Bulldog, and French Bulldog.

Open bite occurs when there is a gap between the top and bottom incisors (of at least 5 mm) when the mouth is closed. It can occur on its own or in conjunction with any of the other malocclusions. Open bite can be concentrated in a line by inbreeding. It is suspected to be a recessive trait but this has yet to be proven.

It is important to note that malocclusion can and often does result from a genetic condition known as achondroplasia, a defect in cartilage growth and development. This is transmitted as

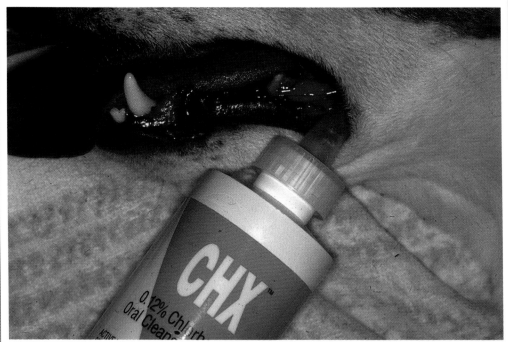

Antiseptic rinses are an important adjunct to home dental care.

Undershot bite.

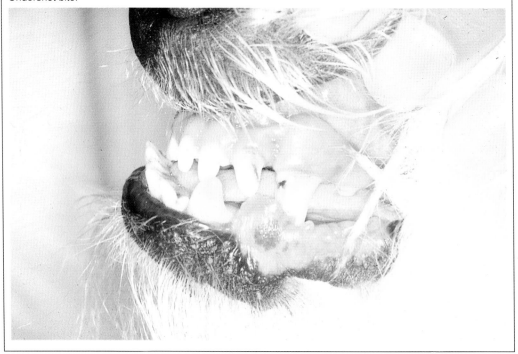

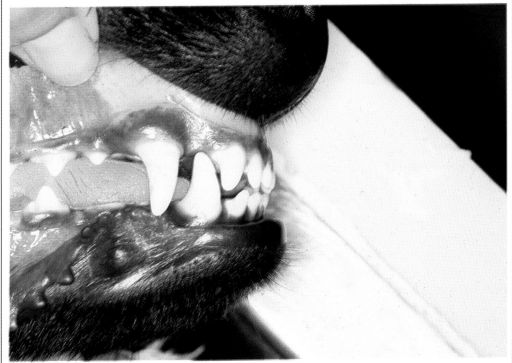

Level bite.

Reverse scissors bite.

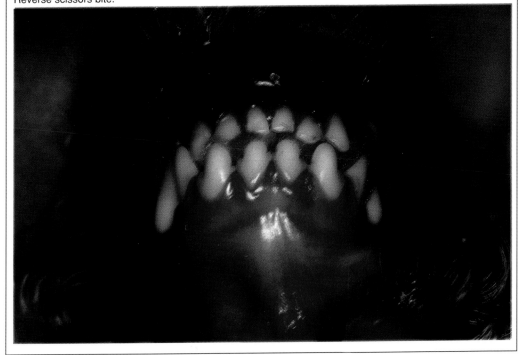

an autosomal dominant trait with variable expressivity. For those unfamiliar with the parlance of genetics, this means that pups can be affected if either parent carries the gene, but that some pups will be more affected than others. Although the gene pattern responsible for this condition is carried by many small breeds, including the Basset Hound, Miniature Poodle and Scottish Terrier, the Dachshund seems to be particularly at risk. It should be realized that malocclusion is almost never seen in dogs that have not been bred by man. We have manipulated the genes of domesticated dogs by breeding them intensively and concentrated these bad genes in many breeds of dog.

Wry mouth is another dental abnormality in which an overshot or undershot condition only affects one side of the head, the left or right. Genetically it is a form of brachygnathism or prognathism and is obviously abnormal in all breeds.

Retention of Deciduous Teeth

The deciduous or puppy teeth are normally completely erupted by eight weeks of age and then fall out and are replaced by the permanent teeth. The permanent teeth are usually completely in place by six to seven months of age. If the puppy teeth do not fall out on schedule, they can cause many problems by their effective "crowding" of the other teeth. When the puppy teeth don't fall out, we refer to the condition as retention of deciduous teeth.

There is little doubt that there is a strong genetic basis for the retention of deciduous teeth, but the actual genetic pattern has not yet been characterized. If the lower canine teeth are displaced centrally, toward the tongue, the condition is often referred to as "base narrow." This can cause severe problems as the lower canines impact on the upper gums rather than the upper canines and cause gum damage, periodontal pockets, and even tracts into the nasal cavity, better known as oronasal fistulas. In the Collie, the tendency to create an elongated head has also resulted in a potential base narrow configuration.

All pups should have dental checkups at eight weeks of age and six to seven months of age to check for proper occlusion and possible retention of deciduous teeth. If caught early enough, the puppy teeth can be removed to make room for the permanent teeth before any real damage is done. If not caught early enough, the displacement of the permanent teeth will need to be corrected with orthodontic procedures. This orthodontic movement should be started at six to ten months of age and may take as little as five to ten days to move the lower canines back into proper position. In older dogs, it may take three to six weeks or even longer. Until the genetics of retained deciduous teeth have been fully characterized, it is suggested that animals with this condition not be used for breeding.

Missing and Extra Teeth

Missing teeth, or anodontia, is common in dogs and may be inherited. The premolar teeth are the most likely to be missing in the dog. It is important not to confuse anodontia with tooth loss that occurs because of periodontal disease of other causes. Anodontia refers to those teeth missing since birth or in early puppyhood. Radiography will confirm that there is no tooth root in the area and that the problem is not due to impaction of the tooth beneath the gumline.

Extra teeth, known as supernumerary teeth, may also occur in the dog and are particularly prevalent in spaniels, hounds, and Greyhounds. Just as the premolars are most likely to be missing in anodontia, these teeth are also the most likely to produce extra (supernumerary) teeth. These extra teeth need to be extracted if they are causing crowding of the other teeth.

ORAL GROWTHS

There are a variety of oral growths that occur in the dog. Some are malignant and definitely not good news, while others are troublesome, but benign.

Benign tumors of the mouth are fairly common in dogs. Of all the tumors that dogs may get, benign oral tumors account for just under 5% of them. The most common benign tumors are called epulis,

ameloblastoma, and gingival hyperplasia.

The epulis family (epulides) includes many oral growths, some of which are invasive and some aren't. The ones that aren't invasive may be removed surgically but the others are more bothersome, even though they are not malignant. Radiation therapy is sometimes used to help treat these invasive forms.

Gingival hyperplasia refers to an overgrowth of gum tissue and since it occurs not uncommonly in Collies and a number of other large breeds, an inherited cause has been suggested. In many dogs, gingival hyperplasia does not need to be treated because it is not doing any harm, even though it is unsightly. If it causes periodontal disease because of its location, treatment with electrosurgery, in which the tissue is cauterized with an electric current, is often helpful.

The incidence of malignant oral cancers is not high and recent studies seem to indicate that less than one dog in a thousand will be affected by these tumors. The most common oral malignancies include melanomas, squamous cell carcinomas, and fibrosarcomas. It has been reported that German Shorthaired Pointers, Weimaraners, Golden Retrievers, and Boxers are at greater risk that other breeds for developing malignant oral cancers. Oral melanomas tend to affect breeds with dark gums such as Scottish Terriers, black Cocker Spaniels, and Boston Terriers. For reasons

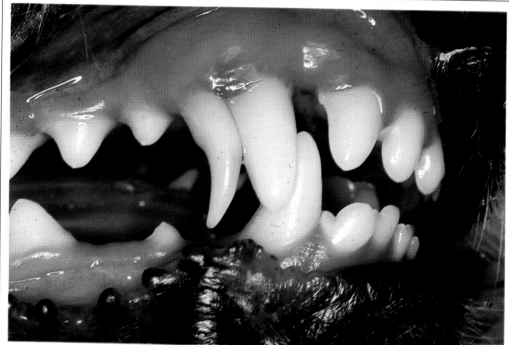

Example of retained deciduous teeth.

Gingival hyperplasia.

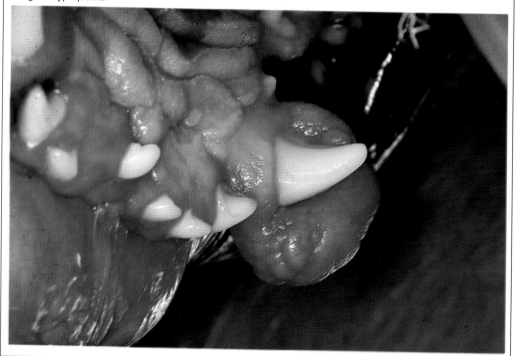

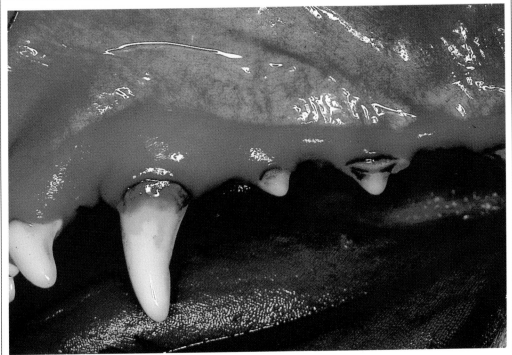

Gingivitis, the beginning of dental disease.

Orthodontic headgear used to help reposition teeth.

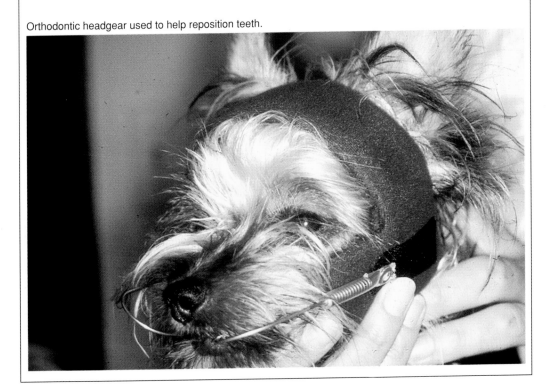

that are not yet known, oral cancers tend to occur more often in male dogs than in females.

SPECIAL PROCEDURES

It is comforting to know that a high level of sophistication in the field of veterinary dentistry is available for our pets. Routine dental prophylaxis keeps the teeth clean and polished and even removes calculus from under the gums. Regular brushing of the teeth at home, mouth rinses and chewing exercises help prevent plaque buildup and the development of gingivitis. But what if our pets have special dental needs? What can be done then?

If there is a problem out of the ordinary that can't be dealt with by a regular veterinarian, there is another option—the veterinary dentist. The American Veterinary Dental College (AVDC) was established by the American Veterinary Medical Association in 1988. Board-certified diplomates of the American Veterinary Dental College are specialists who are trained to evaluate and treat a variety of dental problems in our pets. They are recognized by certain initials following their names (Dipl. AVDC) that denote their discipline and are allowed by the AVMA to use the word "specialist" in their titles.

Because of the major strides made in the field of veterinary dentistry lately, many of the same procedures used in human dentistry are available for our pets. Some of the major accomplishments in veterinary dentistry are expertise in periodontics, endodontics, orthodontics, and restorations. Veterinary dentists may also be involved in a number of different surgical and medical aspects of oral diseases.

Periodontics

Periodontics is the branch of dentistry concerned with the gum tissue (gingiva) and the supporting tissues for the teeth. Most people are familiar with the term gingivitis, which is an inflammation of the gums. The most common cause for this, of course, is poor oral hygiene. When bacteria accumulates on the teeth throughout the day and combines with saliva and food, plaque develops. If the plaque is not removed from the teeth it will build up and then undergo a process of mineralization. Once this occurs, the plaque becomes calculus (tartar).

The good news is that gingivitis is preventable with proper dental care. Even after gingivitis has developed, the condition can be reversed by removing the plaque and calculus from the teeth, above and below the gumline. Over time, however, inflammation of the gums leads to "pockets" of infection that start to erode the bone that ultimately supports the teeth. When bone starts to be lost, gingivitis becomes periodontitis. Once bone loss has started, professional help is critical, and the destruction may be only partially reversible. Specialized gum and bone surgeries are sometimes necessary to slow the progression of gum disease and prevent the loss of teeth.

Since gingivitis is completely reversible, it makes sense to prevent the problem rather than trying to treat it with less than complete success. The routine dental cleaning or "prophy" should be performed every six months or as recommended by a veterinarian. Prevention is the only way to decrease this periodontal disease and allow our pets to keep all of their teeth for as long as possible, hopefully their whole lives.

Endodontics

Endodontics deals with the internal portions of the tooth, especially the sensitive tooth pulp, which consists of nerves, blood vessels, and loose connective tissue. When the tooth pulp is damaged there are two options: pull the tooth or perform endodontic treatment. The latter option consists of root canal therapy. The damaged pulp is capped (pulpotomy) or removed (pulpectomy) and then the crown can be restored. The emphasis in veterinary dentistry is to save teeth and not extract teeth. Even part of the tooth can be saved by endodontic procedures so that the crown can be restored.

Orthodontics

Orthodontic procedures are used to straighten teeth. Yes, some dogs do wear braces. The principle of orthodontics is that if pressure is applied to a tooth, over time the tooth will move as the bone around the tooth remodels. Since bone doesn't form overnight, tooth movement is a gradual process. Not every dog with crooked teeth needs orthodontics. In fact, it is unethical to use orthodontics on a purebred so that it does better in the show ring. Some things are best left up to nature. And yet, there is a very real need for orthodontics in dogs that have poorly positioned and painful teeth, can't close their mouths properly, or can't eat properly. Orthodontics does not alter the genetics of a bad bite and therefore can not be used by breeders as a method of improving their breeding stock. Orthodontic cases in veterinary medicine require the specialist to have considerable experience to be able to predict the eventual position of the corrected teeth.

Restorations

When a tooth is damaged but we still want to save it, the tooth can be repaired with a synthetic device such as a crown. A crown replaces the function and structure of a damaged tooth and protects the portion of the tooth that remains. It can be made to closely match the function and appearance of the original tooth.

This specialized branch of veterinary dentistry is known as prosthodontics, the construction of artificial appliances used in the restorative process. These procedures can be accomplished by placing implants in the bones of

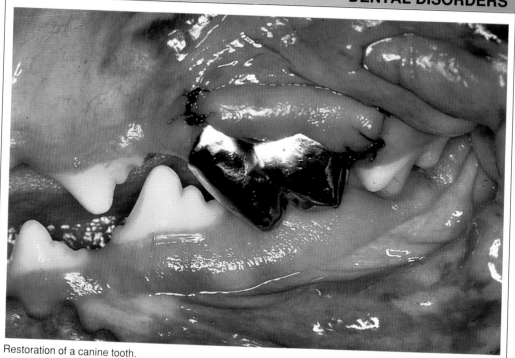

Restoration of a canine tooth.

the jaw and attaching "teeth" to them. There's nothing simple about making a crown for a dog. Crowns are generally used in working dogs (such as police dogs) but can be fabricated for any pet that fractures a tooth.

Damaged or discolored teeth can also be restored by direct bonding procedures. In these restorations a bonding material, an acrylic ceramic, is bonded to the tooth structure by using a light-cured material. This lighting helps fuse the restorative to the tooth.

Oral Surgery

Veterinary dentists perform a variety of surgical procedures, not all of which may involve teeth. A surgical approach is needed for endodontic and restorative procedures but also may be necessary for disorders of the tongue, lips, cheeks and palate. The veterinary dentist is concerned with all aspects of oral health, not just the teeth.

One of the most common oral surgeries is to correct palate defects, such as cleft palate. Sometimes defects can be repaired but occasionally complete reconstructive procedures are warranted. The veterinary oral surgeon is trained to perform extensive surgical techniques of the oral tissues and skull.

DISEASES OF THE MOUTH AND THROAT

There are a number of diseases that affect the oral cavity and many of these are referred to veterinary dental specialists. For instance, stomatitis, which is an inflammation in the mouth, may result from a variety of different potential causes and therefore most cases require careful scrutiny. The reason for careful evaluation is that the ultimate cause can be very difficult to diagnose, and an incomplete evaluation may mean incomplete control. For this reason many veterinarians count on a veterinary dentist for help in making as accurate a diagnosis as possible so a comprehensive treatment plan can be initiated.

Diseases of the throat, including the tonsils, pharynx, larynx, and salivary glands, can also be evaluated by the dental specialist. Veterinary dentists may also be involved in the management of dental cancers.

As in most areas of veterinary medicine, there may be crossover between areas of expertise in specific aspects of oral health. For instance, problems with the lips may be dealt with by dermatologists or dentists. Also, some oral diseases are related to diseases of the skin and may be managed by dermatologists. Veterinary surgeons may be involved in reconstructive surgeries of the head and face, including the mouth. Veterinary oncologists, specialists in cancer in animals, may be involved in the treatment of tumors in the mouth. Specialists in internal medicine may deal with problems in the throat area or internal diseases that may involve the mouth.

Because of the complexity of oral medicine, and veterinary medicine in general, it is imperative that excellent communication be maintained by veterinarians and the specialists to whom they refer cases. The key to overall success in pet health is the primary care veterinarian who knows the most about the pet and owner. For pets with oral problems, they have never had as many excellent health care options as they do today.

ADDITIONAL READING

Lyon, KF: Dental prophylaxis. *Pet Focus*, 1990; 2(1): 27-29.

Lyon, KF: Dental home care. *Pet Focus*, 1990; 2(3): 40-43.

Lyon, KF: Veterinary dentistry. *Pet Focus*, 1990; 2(6): 102-103.

Publisher's note: *The foregoing chapter was adapted from* Dog Owner's Guide to Proper Dental Care *by Kenneth Lyon, DVM, and Lowell Ackerman, DVM (TFH Publications, Inc.).*

Index

Page numbers in **boldface** refer to illustrations.